1001
Questions, Answers
& Case Studies
In Endovascular Procedures

First Edition

Abdullah Jibawi
MBBS MS FRCS AVS MD
Consultant Vascular and Endovascular Surgeon

British Library cataloguing in publication data are available

The photographs used from 3rd parties are exclusively used from pictures released under Creative Commons into the public domain.

ISBN 978-1-9997500-3-9
web: vssmasterclass.co.uk
email: admin@vssmasterclass.co.uk

DISCLAIMERS

The material included in this book was prepared by the author(s) in their personal capacity. The opinions expressed in this book are the authors' own and do not reflect the view of any health institution that the author(s) employed by or affiliated to.

The author makes no representation, express or implied, that the drug dosages or other therapeutic recommendations in this book are correct. Readers must therefore always check the product information and clinical procedures with the most up-to-date published product information and data sheets provided by the manufacturers, and the most recent codes of conduct and safety regulations. The author(s) and the publisher do not accept responsibility or legal liability for any errors in the text, or for the misuse or misapplication of material in this work. Except where otherwise stated, drug dosages and recommendations are for the non-pregnant adult who is not breastfeeding.

Contents

CHAPTER 2   **81**
Iliac Endovascular Therapies Q&A   **81**

CHAPTER 3   **167**
SFA Endovascular Therapies Q&A   **167**

CHAPTER 4   **213**
POPLITEAL (+/- SFA and/or Tibials) Endovascular Therapies Q&A   **213**

CHAPTER 9   **303**
Endovascular Visual Quiz   **303**

CHAPTER 10   **343**
Endovascular Decision-Making Quiz   **343**

Forward

"An expert is a person who has made all the mistakes that can be made in a very narrow field."

NIELS BOHR, the Father of Quantum Theory and Nobel Prize winner

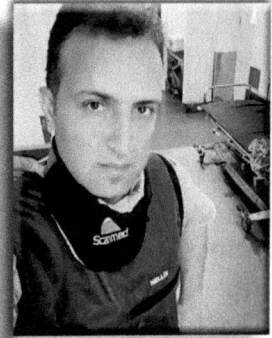

The Origins of Passion: A Glimpse into the Past
From the very inception of this book, "1001 Endovascular Questions, Answers, and Case Studies", the journey has been nothing short of a rollercoaster ride — laden with remarkable insights, enriching challenges, and moments of epiphany. A little over 15 years ago, as I navigated the intricate corridors of general surgery in Wales, I crossed paths with an exceptionally talented vascular surgeons. This fortuitous encounter not only exposed me to the nuances of the vascular world but also led to my maiden introduction to the marvel of endovascular surgery. I was amazed by the radical shift from the traditional, larger incisions of laparotomies to the precise, minimalistic access points needed for inserting stents in aortic aneurysms. This evolution in approach was truly a medical renaissance.

The Leicester Chapter: Gaining Ground in a Pioneering Environment
The winds of destiny soon ushered me into the renowned Leicester Royal Infirmary, a beacon in the UK's vascular arena. The institution was pulsating with innovation and knowledge, thanks to the presence of stalwarts like Dr. Amman Bolia. Working closely with him, I witnessed firsthand the genius behind his groundbreaking subintimal angioplasty and ingenious tools like the Bolia catheter, all of which have left indelible footprints in the sands of endovascular surgery. But Dr. Bolia wasn't the only titan there. Professor Sir Peter Bell's unparalleled educational abilities bridged theory with practicality, while Prof Ross Naylor's meticulous research and unwavering standards set new benchmarks, especially concerning carotid artery diseases.

Academic Forays: Bridging Theories with Real-World Practices
Two significant academic collaborations further refined my perspective on vascular surgery. Firstly, working in tandem with the University of Oxford, I co-authored the seminal "Oxford Current Surgical Guidelines" reference book. This pioneering venture sought to transform evidence-based surgical guidelines into a surgeon's daily practice, bringing textbook knowledge directly to the operating table. Following this, my joint Doctorate Degree with the University of Oxford and Sussex delved deep into innovative strategies aimed at enhancing outcomes in vascular surgery. These academic pursuits were not just about amassing knowledge; they were about embracing the art of seamlessly integrating theoretical constructs into palpable, real-world surgical interventions.

A Stint with Prof Waquar Yusuf: Mastering the Intricacies of EVAR
Along side my academic collaborations, before diving deep into the dynamic environment of the Royal Free Hospital, I had the immense fortune of being mentored by a luminary in endovascular surgery – Prof Waquar Yusuf. Prof Yusuf's astute mind and profound wisdom dramatically shaped my understanding of the intricacies of endovascular aortic aneurysm stent repair (EVAR). His unparalleled skills in planning, designing, and executing complex endovascular procedures left a lasting impression on me.

It's hardly surprising to learn that Prof Yusuf has the distinction of reporting the very first case of treating a ruptured aneurysm utilizing the EVAR technique. Training under such an innovative and groundbreaking expert was truly a masterclass in understanding the nitty-gritty details of our field. The art of biomechanics in endovascular surgery, the precision required in our interventions, and the beauty of nuanced understanding - these lessons were instilled in me during this phase.

Under his able guidance, I undertook and completed the prestigious Royal College AVS course, earning the esteemed accolade of an accredited vascular scientist, with special focus on haemodynamics and biomechanics. This feat was further accentuated when I was awarded the full certificate by the Society for Vascular Scientists in the UK. Prof Yusuf didn't just teach me procedures; he taught me to appreciate the art and science of endovascular practice in its fullest depth and breadth.

A New Chapter: The Royal Free Hospital and Beyond
My professional narrative took yet another vibrant turn with my tenure at the Royal Free Hospital. Immersed in an environment of excellence, I was fortunate to train under and work alongside global giants like Prof Krassi Ivancev and Prof George Hamilton. Their exhaustive knowledge, meticulous planning, and relentless pursuit of perfection significantly influenced my surgical approach, decision-making processes, and overall perspective on endovascular techniques.

St. George's University Hospital: Merging History with Modernity
Lastly, my association with St George's University Hospital, an institution steeped in historical significance since 1733, brought my journey full circle. At St George's, I encountered a unique blend of age-old medical wisdom and cutting-edge endovascular practices. The legacy of pioneers like the anatomist John Hunter merged beautifully with contemporary endovascular surgeons and interventionalists, offering a comprehensive learning experience like no other.

The Tapestry of Experience: From Ideas to Paper
Drawing from these diverse yet interconnected experiences, this book emerged as a tapestry of knowledge, insights, and practical wisdom. My innate inclination to sketch ideas and elucidate complex concepts through diagrams found its rightful place in this volume. As I present this work to the next generation, my aspiration is to ignite a paradigm shift in their endovascular understanding and practice.

In Gratitude: Synergy and Interdependence
As I reflect on the culmination of experiences and knowledge enshrined within this book, I realize it is genuinely a synergistic product of the many brilliant minds I've been fortunate to engage with. While the journey of endovascular surgery is narrated through my lens, it is, in essence, a collective tapestry woven by the profound interactions, debates, and collaborations with numerous esteemed peers, mentors, and students.

There's a core belief I've come to uphold firmly over the years: interdependence holds a higher value than mere independence. Every chapter, every case study, every piece of advice in this book resonates with the shared wisdom, the collective effort, and the mutual respect I've shared with my peers. To all the students who questioned and challenged, the colleagues who brainstormed and debated, and the mentors who guided and critiqued – your invaluable contributions have indelibly shaped this work.

In a field as dynamic and intricate as ours, the journey of learning is ceaseless. It is my profound hope that "1001 Endovascular Questions, Answers, and Case Studies" stands testament to the essence of collaborative learning, and more importantly, inspires the next generation to embrace the spirit of synergy in their own unique journeys.

In the end, while this tome reflects my journey, learnings, and insights, it's crucial to highlight that these perspectives are deeply personal. They are born out of my experiences and do not necessarily mirror the official viewpoints of the esteemed institutions with which I've been privileged to be associated.

Mr. Abdullah Jibawi
Consultant Vascular and Endovascular Surgeon

Preface

"1001 Questions, Answers and Case Studies in Endovascular Procedures" stands out as an irreplaceable ally on this invigorating path. Whether a seasoned expert or a novice entering the world of endovascular procedures, this volume unfolds a comprehensive, enlightening, and pioneering landscape covering the vast terrain of peripheral vascular diseases.

Our journey begins with an A to Z power review chapter, designed to elevate your grasp of endovascular techniques, enriched with biomechanical and hemodynamic principles. Delving deep into pivotal concepts such as pushability, stress, strain, and blood flow analysis, we painstakingly unpack the multifaceted world of vascular interventions, all portrayed through stunning illustrations, priming you for an enriched level of proficiency.

Chapters two to eight steer you through a curated collection of case studies, each echoing real-world scenarios. Each step, potential complication, eventual outcome, and nuanced biomechanical consideration is intricately laid out, supplemented by vivid visuals that bring the narrative to life.

Venturing further, chapters six to eight introduce you to more complex domains, like ruptured aneurysm endovascular repair and innovative methods for bypass and in-stent complications. Every challenge faced in these intricate cases is highlighted, emphasizing complications and their resolution strategies.

The "Endovascular Decision-Making Quiz" in Chapter 10 sharpens your clinical judgment. Concurrently, the "Endovascular Evidence Review" in Chapter 11 integrates the latest research findings and insights into your daily practice.

A unique and invaluable feature of this edition is the linkage of every chapter with live cases, diligently curated from the InCathLab portal, each resonating with the core concept of the corresponding chapter. Moreover, an exciting integration is the addition of simulation cases from our SIMPOD masterclass. These simulation cases serve as a tangible tool, providing readers and candidates an unparalleled opportunity for hands-on practice and training, enriching the learning experience wherever simulations are available.

Chapters 12 and 13, the "Endovascular Charts Quiz" and the "Endovascular Mind Mapping Quiz," respectively, challenge your cognitive abilities, ensuring a holistic understanding of the field's diagnostic and procedural facets.

Drawing from vast expertise housed in leading UK centers, "1001 Questions, Answers and Case Studies in Endovascular Procedures" fills a significant void in endovascular literature. More than a repository of knowledge, this work challenges, enlightens, and inspires, weaving theory and practice seamlessly and provoking reflection, broadening understanding, and refining the vital skills the realm demands.

I cordially invite you to embark on this illuminating voyage with us, exploring, discerning, and mastering the vast and intricate expanse of endovascular procedures.

Acknowledgements

In the mosaic of interactions that have enriched my journey, a special acknowledgment is owed to my esteemed colleagues at St Peters Hospital. I extend my heartfelt gratitude to Mr. Tahir Ali, Dr Shirish Prabhudesai, and Dr. Alex Chapman. All have been instrumental in honing my professional perspective. Their contributions to my understanding of the field, our mutual efforts in standardizing complex procedures, and their innovative solutions to challenging cases have been invaluable. But above all, it's our shared commitment to the well-being and care of our patients that truly binds us. Their mentorship and partnership, combined with our shared dedication, have left an indelible mark on my practice.

CHAPTER 1
A TO Z
ENDOVASCULAR
POWER REVIEW

ANATOMY

In the following diagram, name the labeled arteries as appropriate.

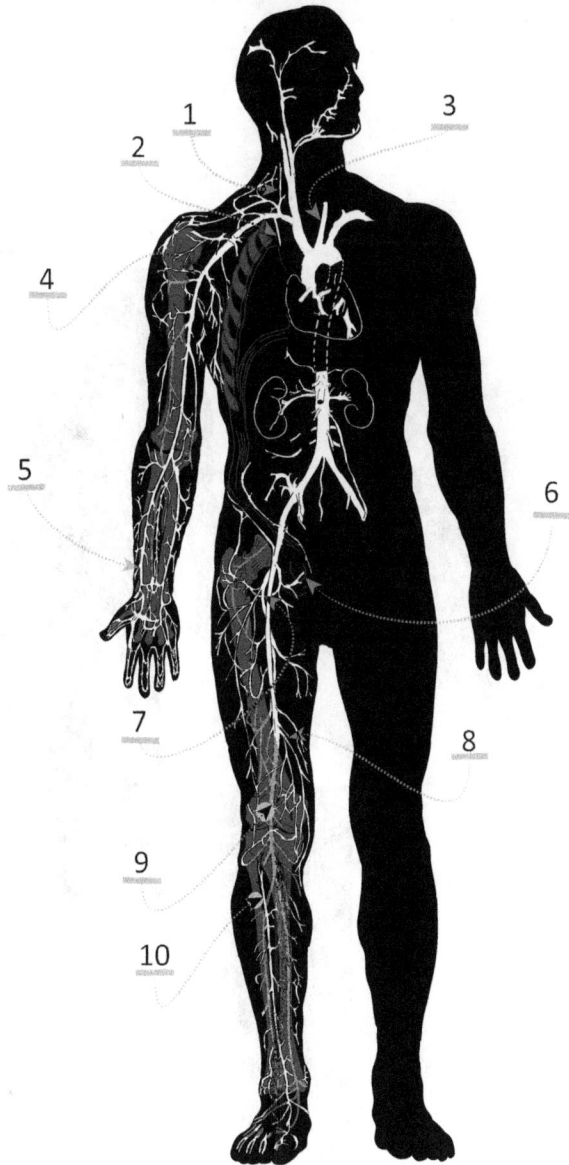

1. Right common carotid artery   2. Internal thoracic artery, aka the internal mammary artery.   3. Left common carotid artery
4. Brachial artery   5. Radial artery   6. Internal pudendal artery   7. Femoral profunda artery   8. Superior genicular artery
9.Popliteal artery   10. Anterior tibial artery

In the following diagram, name the labeled arteries as appropriate:

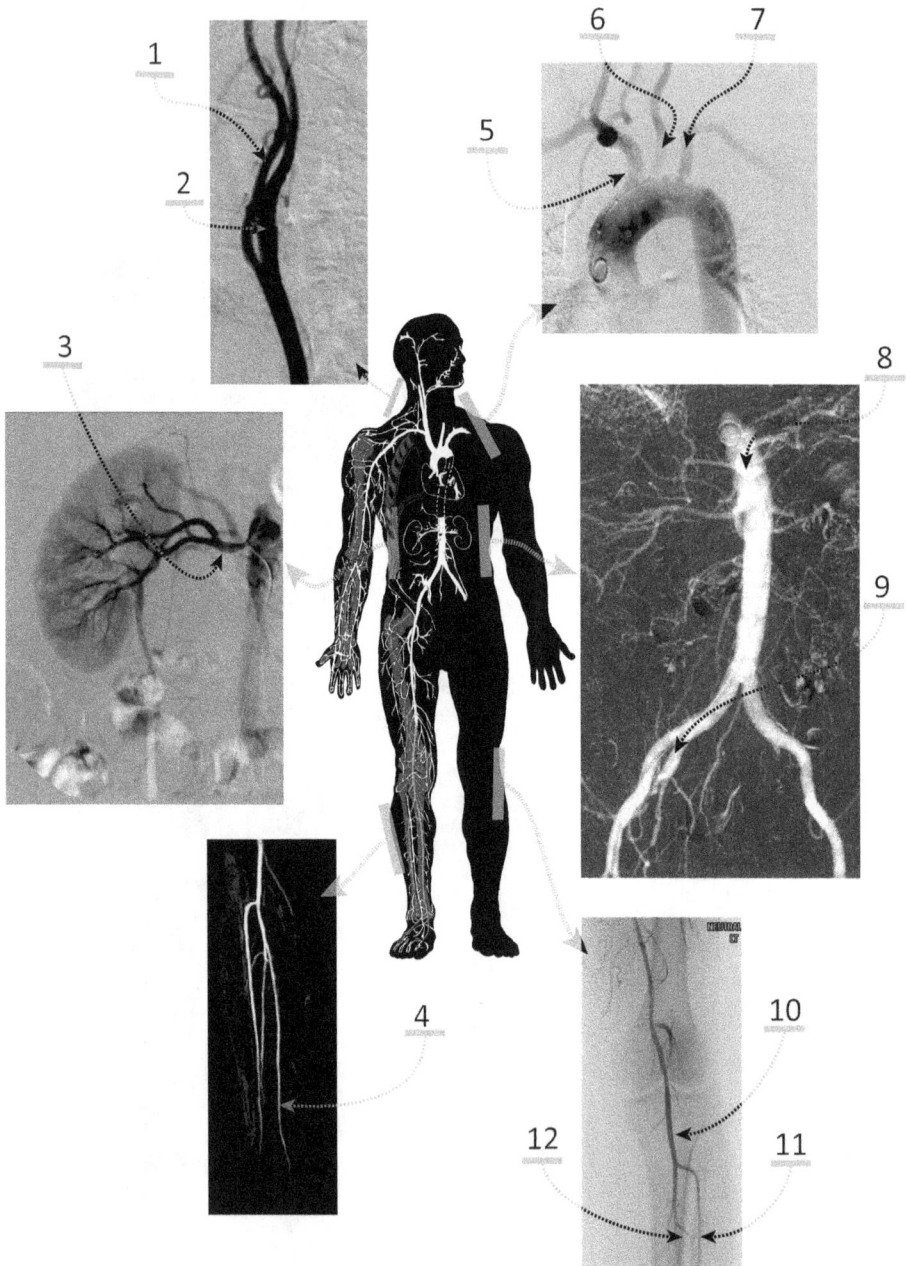

1

2

3

6   7

5

8

9

4

10

12   11

1. External carotid artery   2. Internal carotid artery.   3. Right renal artery   4. Posterior tibial artery   5. Brachiocephalic artery   6. Left common carotid artery   7. Left subclavian artery 8. Abdominal aorta   9.Internal iliac artery   10. Popliteal artery 11.Anterior tibial artery   12. Peroneal artery

In the following diagram, name the labeled arteries as appropriate

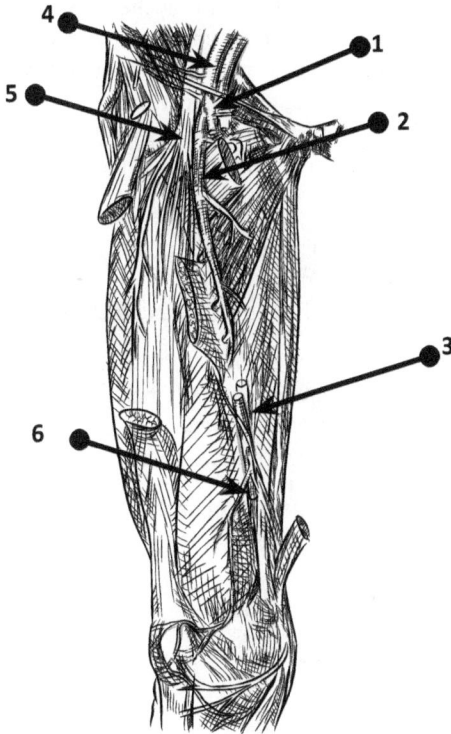

1. Common Femoral Artery (CFA)
2. Profunda Artery (PFA)
3. Superficial Femoral Artery (SFA)
4. External Iliac Artery
5. Femoral Nerve
6. Adductor Hiatus

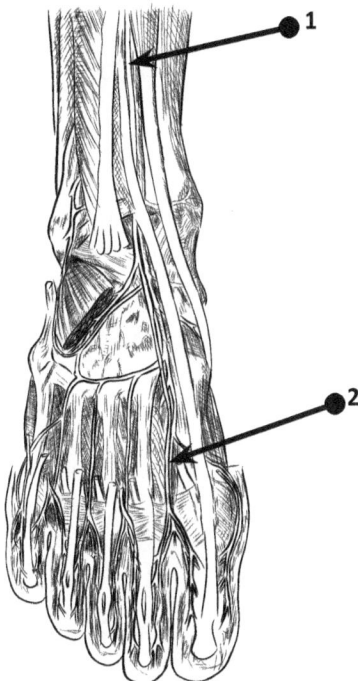

1. Anterior Tibial Artery
2. Dorsalis Pedis

What is the Hunter's Canal, and what structures pass through it?

Hunter's Canal, also known as the adductor canal, is an intermuscular passage in the middle third of the thigh. It contains the femoral artery and vein, and the saphenous nerve.

What are the branches of the celiac trunk, and which organs do they primarily supply?

The celiac trunk has three major branches: the left gastric artery (supplies the lesser curvature of the stomach), the splenic artery (supplies the spleen, pancreatic branches, and short gastric arteries), and the common hepatic artery (gives off proper hepatic artery for the liver and the gastroduodenal artery for the stomach and first part of the duodenum).

What structures do the anterior and posterior spinal arteries supply?

The anterior spinal artery supplies the anterior two-thirds of the spinal cord, including the anterior and lateral corticospinal tracts. The posterior spinal arteries supply the posterior one-third of the spinal cord, including the dorsal columns.

Which artery is the primary blood supply to the midgut, and what structures does this include?

The superior mesenteric artery is the primary blood supply to the midgut, which includes the distal half of the duodenum, the jejunum, ileum, cecum, appendix, ascending colon, and the proximal two-thirds of the transverse colon.

What vascular structure is commonly used as a graft in coronary artery bypass surgery, and why?

The internal thoracic (mammary) artery is commonly used as a graft in coronary artery bypass surgery due to its size.

Which artery runs alongside the sciatic nerve in the posterior thigh?

The profunda femoris artery.

Which artery can be palpated against the ischial tuberosity when the hip is flexed?

The internal pudendal artery.

Which artery gives off branches that anastomose around the head of the femur in the acetabular notch?

The obturator artery.

Which vessel runs with the deep peroneal nerve along the anterior compartment of the leg?

The anterior tibial artery.

Which artery travels through the transverse foramina?

The vertebral artery.

In a CT angiogram of the chest, which artery is seen branching from the aortic arch between the brachio-cephalic trunk and the left subclavian artery?

The left common carotid artery

In a CT angiogram of the head, what are the first two branches of the internal carotid artery within the brain?

The ophthalmic artery and the posterior communicating artery.

In a CT angiogram of the abdomen, what is the first major branch of the abdominal aorta?

The celiac trunk.

In a CT angiogram of the neck, what is the name of the artery that branches from the external carotid artery just above the level of the hyoid bone?

The lingual artery.

In a CT angiogram of the abdomen, what vessels are seen branching off the celiac trunk?

The left gastric artery, the common hepatic artery, and the splenic artery.

On a CT angiogram of the pelvis, which artery typically gives off the obturator artery?

The internal iliac artery.

Name the following anatomical numbers and regions in the popliteal artery area:

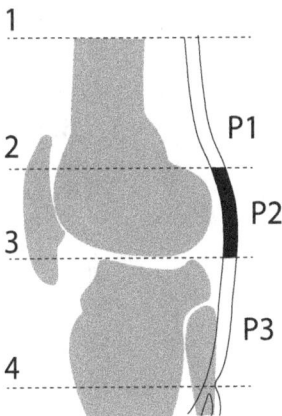

1. Hunter Canal Level
2. Proximal edge of patella
3. Centre of knee joint space
4- Origin of anterior tibial artery
P1. First popliteal artery region
P2. Second popliteal artery region
P3. Third popliteal artery region

ACCESS

At what point should you consider utilizing a brachial approach right from the start of the situation?

CONSIDER BRACHIAL APPROACH IN THE FOLLOWING:
Aorta:
Aortic occlusion
Iliac Arteries:
Bilateral critical/diffuse iliac occlusive disease
Common Femoral Artery:
Bilateral common femoral artery occlusion (where endovascular procedure is the only indicated method)
Renal Arteries:
Acute downward angle at origin of renal arteries
Mesenteric Arteries:
Selective catheterization of or endovascular intervention in mesenteric arteries
Subclavian Arteries:
Retrograde approach to endovascular therapy for subclavian lesions
Axillary Arteries:
Axillary lesions
Other Considerations:
Severe infrarenal occlusive disease
When femoral puncture is contraindicated due to recent surgery
Pseudoaneurysm
More favorable angle of approach

What is the primary entry point for the following vascular regions:

Region	Entry
Brachiocephalic/Carotid	Femorals or left brachial
Subclavian	Femorals or ipsilateral brachial
Visceral Celiac/SMA	Femorals or left brachial
Renal	Femorals or left brachial
Aortoiliac Infrarenal	Femorals or left brachial
Common iliac	Contralateral femoral / or ipsilateral
Internal iliac	Contralateral femoral / or left brachial
External iliac	Contralateral femoral / or ipsilateral
Infrainguinal Femoral	Ipsilateral femoral / or contralateral
Popliteal	Ipsilateral femoral
Tibial Pedal	Ipsilateral femoral

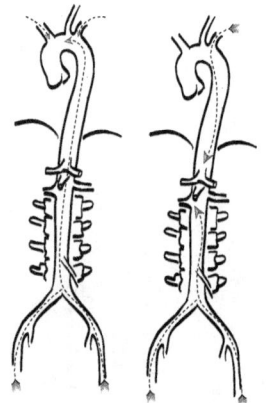

Which regions should be avoided during femoral puncture, and why?

AVOID THE FOLLOWING PUNCTURE POINTS:
Proximal SFA: can cause puncture site thrombosis.
Proximal PFA: difficulty in compression afterwards and risk of dissection.
CFA bifurcation: risk of disrupting plaque (common area for plaque formation)
Distal EIA: higher risk for a retroperitoneal bleeding

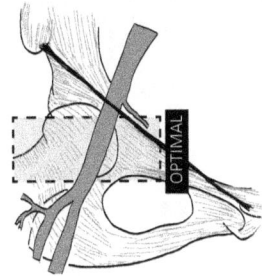

If the guidewire is unable to pass through the needle despite the presence of a pulastile backflow, what should the operator expect/do?

IF GUIDEWIRE IS NOT PASSING THROUGH:
Most likely the wire is hitting the arterial back wall. Withdrawing the needle slightly back, and possibly changing the angle slightly, should allow the wire to pass through

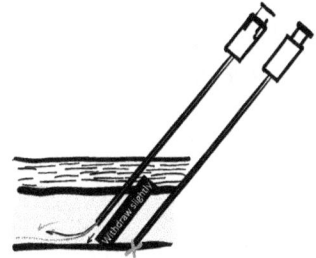

In an obese patient, the femoral areas can be better exposed by?

In Obese Patients:
use tape to secure the abdominal pannus.

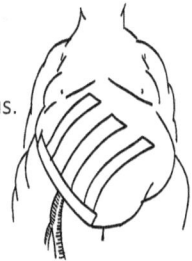

Which side is typically preferred for axillary or brachial access and what is the reason for this?

Access Via Left Brachial:
The left side is often chosen to prevent crossing the carotid arteries while handling catheters and wires, as this can potentially lead to embolisation and stroke.

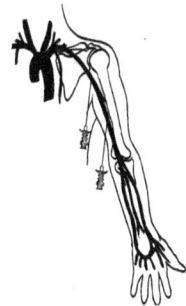

The access sheath size for brachial artery is ?

6Fr sheath, with prediltation usually using 4fr sheath and catheter first.

Where should the operator stand to perform a retrograde iliac angioplasty?

Operator position:
Should always work forehand; therefore, for right handed operators, they should stand on patient's right (and C-Arm on left) for iliacs and femoral retrograde access.

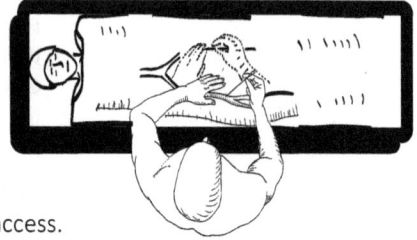

What access is available for difficult iliac cases?

Contralateral femoral access.
Brachial (7Fr usually needed- higher complication rate than femoral and longer tools needed).
Axillary (higher complication rate)

What alternatives are available when there is insufficient working room to perform the procedure via femoral access?

Transbrachial approach across an aortic aneurysm.
Securing a partially inserted femoral sheath.
Placing the sheath in the proximal SFA via percutaneous insertion or cutdown procedure.

Puncture-related retroperitoneal bleeding. How does it happen usually and what makes it worse?

Puncture-related Retroperitoneal bleeding.
A groin puncture that is too far proximal may enter the distal EIA and cause hemorrhage into retroperitoneal space. If this is unrecognized, pressure at the skin puncture site in the groin, which is somewhat distal to the arterial puncture site, may exacerbate the bleeding hemorrhage by creating additional outflow resistance.

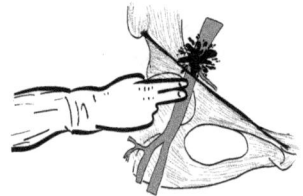

What are the components needed in a puncture set?

PUNCTURE SET COMPONENTS:
Sterile towel
Scalpel
Haemostat
Puncture needle
Syringe
Wire

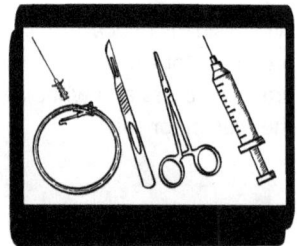

What is the typical behavior of the guidewire when crossing an aneurysm?

GUIDEWIRE WITHIN THE ANEURYSM:
The guidewire has a tendency to accumulate or bunch up within the aorta. To overcome this, a multi-purpose catheter (such as Cobra C2) with a simple curve, can be employed to guide the guidewire through convoluted iliac and aortic segments.

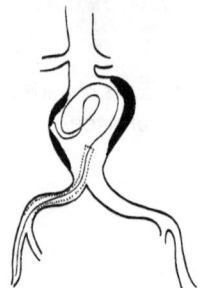

The axillary artery punctures is usually located at?

Just lateral to the axilla and is in reality is a high brachial artery puncture

What should you do to puncture a pulseless femoral artery?

Detect the artery by palpation.
Examine previous arteriograms, and the location of the artery in relation to the femoral head.
Use Fluoroscopy to identify vascular calcification and assist in guiding the puncture.
Consider alternative entry sites if this was not possible.

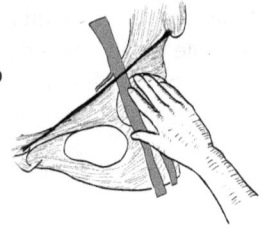

List common complications from femoral artery catheterization?

Minor bleeding or hematoma: Reported frequency ranges from 6.0% to 10.0%.
Major bleeding or hematoma: Occurs in approximately 1.0% to 2.4% of cases and may require transfusion, surgery, or delayed discharge. The threshold for complication according to SCVIR (Society of Interventional Radiology) is 3.0%.
Pseudoaneurysm: Occurs in about 0.5% to 5.0% of cases.
Rare:
Occlusion (thrombosis or dissection): Occurs in approximately 0.3% to 1.0%.
Distal embolization: Reported frequency is less than 0.5%.

What 2nd accesses to consider for difficult SFA case?

Retrograde popliteal.
Limitation in treating proximal lesions .: best to treat them first.

Before arterial access, what should the operator palpate?

Arterial pulse.
Calcified artery (if no pulse).
Anatomical landmarks including pubic tubercle, inguinal ligament path, and anterior superior iliac spine (ASIS).

A double-wall puncture is:

DOUBLE-WALL PUNCTURE:
In this femoral puncture technique, the needle is inserted across front and back arterial walls. The needle is then withdrawn gradually till a pulsatile back bleeding is evident.

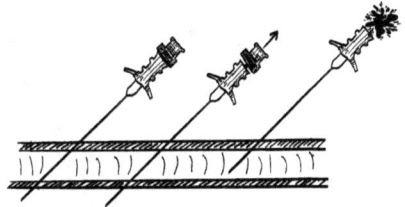

How should the patient be positioned for a retrograde popliteal approach?

Prone

AORTA

What treatment option is available for an isolated but significant focal lesion in the infrarenal abdominal aorta?

ISOLATED AORTIC LESIONS
These can treated by performing balloon angioplasty.

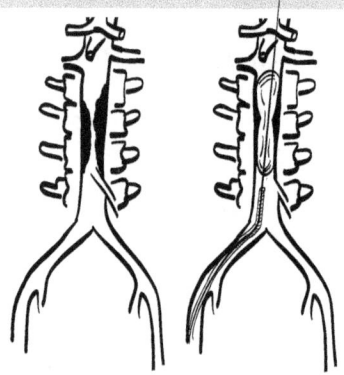

How can a more extensive lesion involving the infrarenal aorta and its bifurcation be treated?

The complex lesion is treated by retrogradely placing guidewires through each femoral artery, followed by aortic balloon angioplasty and the use of kissing balloons to dilate the bifurcation. A CERAB procedure (see below) can also be considered.

How to perform CERAB?

A lesion in the infrarenal aorta and iliac arteries can be addressed via multi-stent reconstruction, involving insertion of guidewires, aortic stent delivery, guidewire retraction and re advancement to insert a bilateral iliac kissing stents (see diagram).

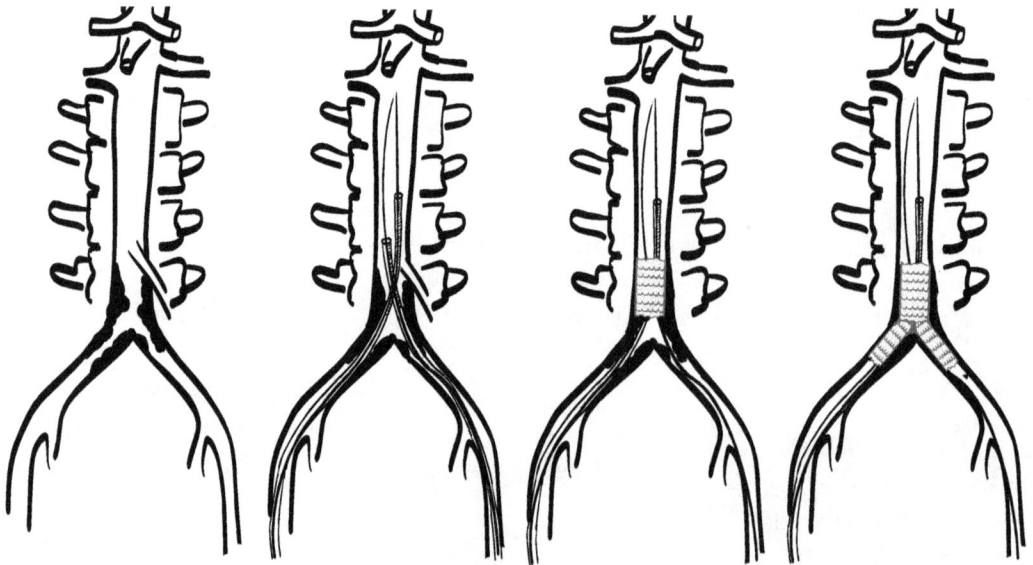

BALLOON ANGIOPLASTY

What does the process of dilating the atherosclerotic waist during angioplasty involve?

During angioplasty, the atherosclerotic waist is dilated by placing the balloon catheter within the lesion, shaping the balloon at low pressure, increasing pressure to reveal the waist, observing a residual stenosis at low pressure, and achieving complete dilation at high (nominal) pressure.

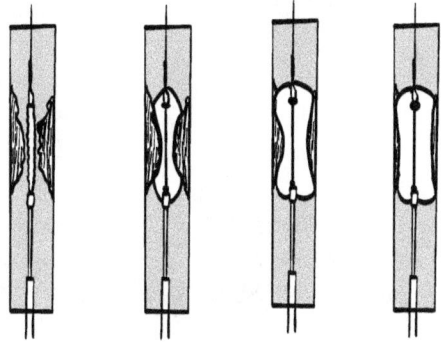

What are the methods used to evaluate the outcomes of a balloon angioplasty procedure?

Results of balloon angioplasty are evaluated through completion arteriogram, magnified view, oblique projection, pressure measurement, intravascular ultrasound, clinical evaluation, and assessment of hemodynamic stability, extremity pulse/color, and flank pain.

What elements constitute the balloon in an angioplasty catheter?

Shaft: The long, flexible part of the catheter that allows navigation through blood vessels. Its size, often measured in French, impacts manoeuvrability and device compatibility.

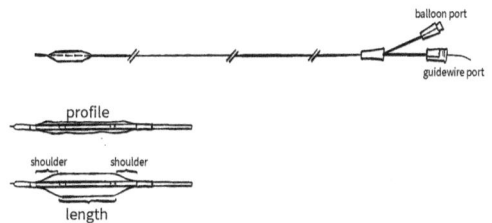

Profile: The catheter's diameter, including the deflated balloon. Lower profiles are more effective in smaller or complex vessels.

Balloon Length: Corresponds to the length of the vessel section that can be dilated at once. It should match the length of the lesion being treated.

Balloon Diameter: The width of the balloon should align with the vessel size to ensure effective dilation without damaging the vessel.

Shoulder: The transition part between the inflated balloon and the catheter shaft. A smooth shoulder prevents plaque or thrombus trapping during operation.

What is the mechanical impact resulting from balloon angioplasty?

MECHANICAL EFFECT OF BALLOON ANGIOPLASTY:
Balloon dilatation involves using a catheter to apply radial force to atherosclerotic lesions, causing plaque fracture and possible dissection, often noted in final angiographic studies.

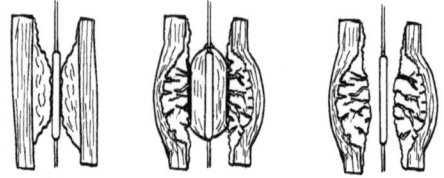

How is the angioplasty of the Superficial Femoral Artery (SFA) performed?

ANGIOPLASTY FOR SFA STENOSIS:
a guidewire is placed across the stenosis via an ipsilateral or contralateral femoral artery puncture. A sheath is inserted for lesion evaluation and balloon passage. The lesion is dilated with the balloon and its position is verified post-dilation through completion arteriography.

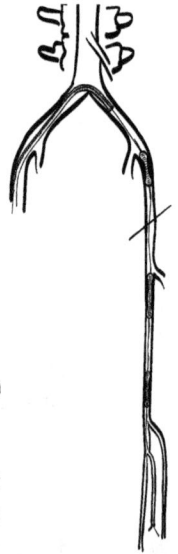

What is the optimal approach for performing angioplasty on multiple lesions?

In angioplasty of multiple lesions, the approach is from proximal to distal, treating all lesions within the same artery, dilating the proximal lesion first in sequential lesions across different arteries, and selectively dilating critical areas in a diffusely diseased artery.

BIOMECHANICS

Describe the relationship and distinctions between force, pressure, stress, and strain, in the context of arterial biomechanics?

Force is a vector quantity that results in the movement, deformation, or change in the state of motion of an object.
Pressure, in the context of arteries, is the force exerted by the blood per unit area on the artery walls.
Stress is similar to pressure but more specific in the sense that it refers to the internal resistance a material (arterial wall in this case) exerts against deformation.
Strain is the deformation that results from stress, specifically, the relative change in shape or size of an object due to applied stress.

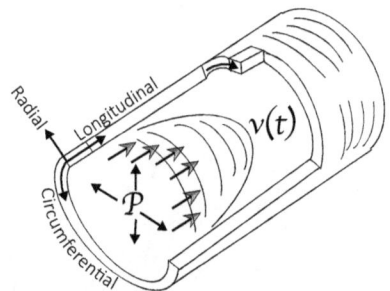

How can those be applied in the context of arterial tree

In arteries, for example, the force of the blood flow (due to blood pressure) applies stress to the artery walls, resulting in a strain or deformation of these walls. The interplay between these concepts allows arteries to accommodate changes in blood pressure and volume while maintaining their integrity and function.

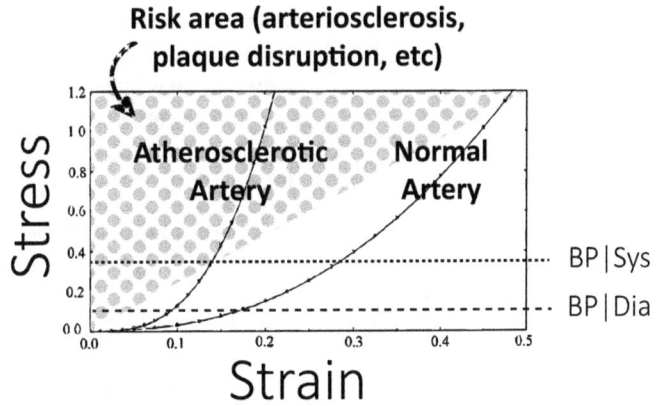

Risk area (arteriosclerosis, plaque disruption, etc)

Explain the relationship between stress and the forces of bending, twisting, and elongation in the arterial wall?

The forces of bending, twisting, and elongation can lead to increased stress within the arterial wall. Stress is the artery's internal response to resist these external forces. When an artery bends, twists, or elongates, its walls are subjected to changes in mechanical load which in turn results in stress. The level of stress depends on the magnitude of these forces and the material properties of the arterial wall. Excessive or repetitive stress may lead to structural changes or damage in the artery over time, impacting its ability to function properly.

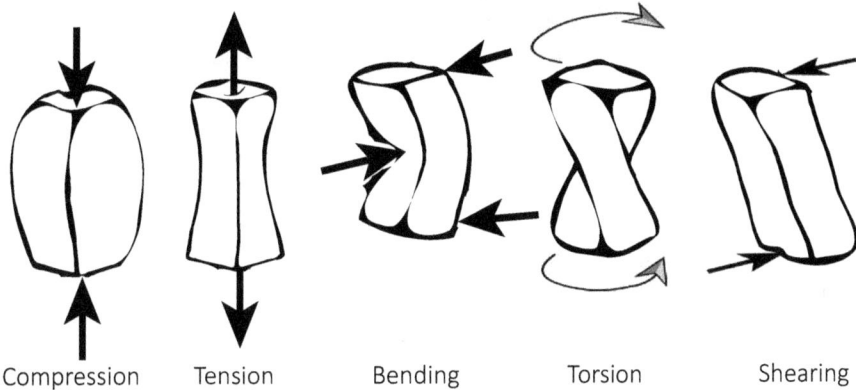

Compression   Tension   Bending   Torsion   Shearing

What methods are used to quantify the stress within the arterial wall?

The stress in the arterial wall is typically estimated using computational models, which incorporate parameters like blood pressure, blood flow velocity, and arterial wall properties. It's challenging to measure stress directly in vivo due to the complex and dynamic nature of arteries.

Techniques like intravascular ultrasound (IVUS) or optical coherence tomography (OCT) can provide images of the arterial wall from which measurements like wall thickness or diameter can be derived, and these measurements are then used in combination with blood pressure to estimate wall stress. Additionally, techniques like strain elastography or magnetic resonance elastography can provide information about tissue deformation, which can also help estimate stress.

What is the mathematical formula used to calculate the stress experienced by the arterial wall?

The stress (σ) experienced in the arterial wall can be calculated using the formula derived from Laplace's law:

$$\sigma = Pr/t$$

where P is the blood pressure inside the artery, r is the radius of the artery, and t is the thickness of the arterial wall. This formula applies primarily to cylindrical vessels under the assumption of thin-wall and steady-state conditions.

Why is stress a more useful measure in arterial biomechanics than forces?

Stress, which is force per unit area, is more insightful than force alone in arterial biomechanics because it takes into account the area over which the force is distributed. This is crucial because the same force can have different effects on the arterial wall depending on the area it's acting upon. Furthermore, stress can be directly related to strain, providing a measure of deformation in the artery. This helps in understanding the impact on the arterial structure and function, as well as the risk of mechanical failure or damage such as dissection or aneurysm formation. Therefore, stress provides a more detailed and comprehensive understanding of the biomechanical behavior of arteries.

What is the mathematical relationship between stress and strain?

The relationship between stress (σ) and strain (ε) is given by Hooke's law in the elastic deformation region:

$$\sigma = E * \varepsilon$$

where σ represents stress, ε represents strain and E represents Young's modulus of elasticity.

This formula indicates that stress is directly proportional to strain, with the proportionality constant being the material's modulus of elasticity. However, it's important to note that this law only holds true within the elastic limit of the material. In the case of biological tissues such as arteries, which often display nonlinear behavior, the relationship between stress and strain can be more complex

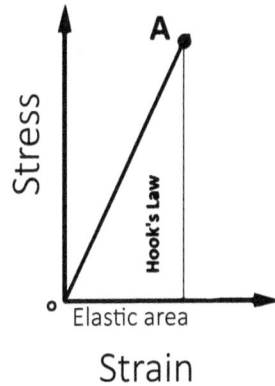

Describe how alterations in stress and strain can facilitate smoother insertion and positioning of guidewires, catheters, and sheaths?

Alterations in stress and strain can influence the ease of entry and setup of guidewires, catheters, and sheaths. Specifically, manipulating these parameters, by appropriate skilful tools selection and handling, can decrease the friction and resistance encountered during insertion. A device designed to minimize the stress it exerts on the vessel wall (lower strain) will reduce the risk of vessel injury and improve navigability. Furthermore, the flexibility and elasticity of these devices can also be adjusted to better conform to the vascular pathway, reducing the applied stress and strain on both the device and the vessel wall. This can be particularly important in tortuous or stenotic vessels. Thus, understanding and controlling stress and strain in the design and application of these devices can greatly enhance their performance and safety in vascular procedures.

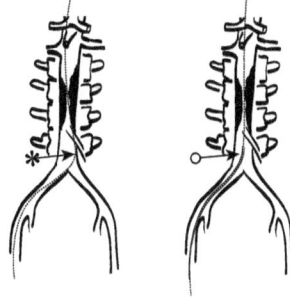

Describe how torque techniques, safari wire techniques, and the use of low-profile catheters and sheaths can minimize strain and facilitate the smoother insertion and setup of wires, catheters, and sheaths?

Torque techniques, safari wire techniques, and low-profile catheters and sheaths are all examples of methods used to minimize strain on the vessel wall during insertion.

Torque techniques, for example, allow for better control and manipulation of the wire or catheter, thus reducing the stress and strain applied on the vessel wall during navigation. This then allows the pushing force to move the wire forward.

The safari wire technique uses a long guidewire (inserted and fixed from two insertion points) that provides extra support and stability, reducing the forces applied to the arterial wall and lowering the risk of injury.

Lastly, **low-profile catheters** and sheaths have a smaller diameter and are more flexible. Their design reduces the stress and strain on the vessel during insertion, facilitating smoother entry and reducing the risk of damaging the vessel.

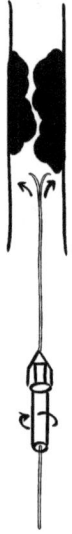

Can you provide an example demonstrating the use of torque techniques, safari wire technique, and low-profile catheters and sheaths in arterial procedures?

An example could be an angioplasty procedure to treat an arterial blockage in the contralateral SFA. In this case, torque techniques would be used to carefully navigate the guidewire through the vascular system to the blockage site. The safari wire technique could be employed to give added support and stability to the guidewire, reducing the forces exerted on the artery wall and focusing the forces onto the wire line. Lastly, a low-profile balloon catheter, which has a smaller diameter and flexibility, would be threaded over the guidewire to the blockage. This design minimizes the stress and strain on the vessel walls during insertion, allowing for smoother entry and minimizing the risk of vessel damage. Once the catheter is in place at the blockage site, the balloon can be inflated to open up the blocked artery, and then deflated and withdrawn.

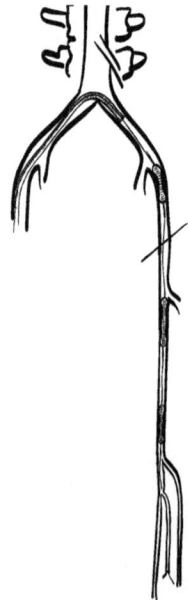

Can you explain how the stress and strain alter in both the stented and un-stented sections of an artery?

Insertion of a stent to treat stenosis modifies the stress and strain distributions in the arterial wall. In the stented area, stress and strain are generally reduced due to the load-bearing role of the stent. It provides structural support, reducing the vessel's deformation under the forces exerted by the blood flow.

However, the presence of a stent can create regions of increased stress (stress concentrations) at the edges of the stent, where the stent ends and the un-stented artery

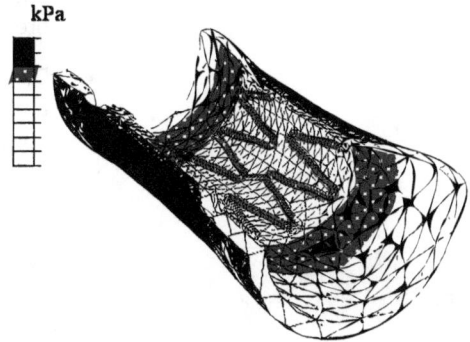

begins. This can increase strain in these regions. Over time, this might lead to restenosis or even vessel injury in the un-stented sections. Such effects underline the importance of the design and placement of stents in preventing complications.

What occurs when a stent is placed at the juncture of the femoral and popliteal arteries?

When a stent is deployed at the intersection of the femoral and popliteal arteries, despite its therapeutic benefits, it's sub-jected to considerable deformations owing to routine patient activities. The legs, during regular body movement, experience multiaxial deformations with up to 60% rotation and 20% contraction when transitioning from an extended position. Therefore, the stent in this region undergoes substantial multi-axial displacements, as well as bending, torsion, tension, and compression during the walking cycle.

Provide a framework that can be applied to analyze the biomechanics of a specific vessel segment and its interaction with a proposed stent or bypass?

When analyzing the biomechanical properties of a system like a vessel (artery or vein), the following model can be helpful:

- **Structure Identification:** Understand the structural com-ponents of the system. For blood vessels, consider the three main layers: tunica intima, tunica media, and tunica adventitia. Each has distinct properties and functions.

- **Material Properties:** Identify the biomechanical prop-erties of each structural component. This could include elasticity, viscosity, anisotropy (the condition where a ma-terial's properties differ based on the direction of meas-urement), incompressibility, and residual stresses.

- **Functionality**: Evaluate how these properties contribute to the function of the system. For blood vessels, this involves understanding the regulation of blood flow and pressure.

- **Load Analysis**: Consider the various forces applied to the system under normal physiological conditions, as well as under stress. For a blood vessel, this would include blood pressure and shear stress from blood flow.

- **Behavior Under Stress - the stress/strain relation**: Study the system's response to stress and deformation. How does it react to cyclical stresses (hysteresis) or sustained deformation (stress relaxation).

BYPASS

How is balloon angioplasty performed on an aorto-bifem bypass graft ?

ANGIOPLASTY FOR AORTO-BIFEMORAL BYPASS: A femoral sheath and guidewire are placed, a balloon is positioned in the relevant stenotic areas, inflated appropriately, and finally completion arteriography is conducted through a proximally placed flush catheter.

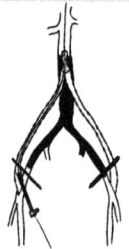

How is balloon angioplasty performed on an infrainguinal bypass graft using an antegrade approach?

ANTEGRADE ANGIOPLASTY FOR FEMPOP BYPASS: Interventions on infrainguinal bypass grafts involve placing an antegrade femoral sheath, performing arteriography, guiding a wire across the graft lesion, removing the catheter, performing balloon angioplasty, and completing with a final arteriography, maintaining wire access throughout.

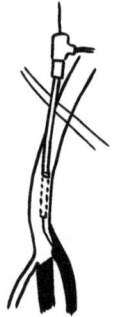

How is balloon angioplasty performed on an infrainguinal bypass graft using an up-and-over approach?

A proximal graft lesion in an infrainguinal bypass from the common femoral artery is addressed through arteriography, guidewire passage, balloon angioplasty, and completion arteriography using an up-and-over sheath.

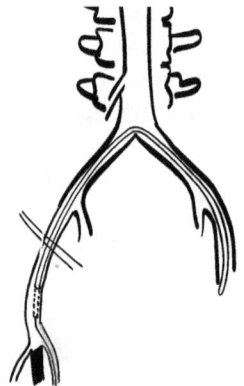

How is balloon angioplasty performed on an iliac anastomosis ?

A selective catheter is used to direct the guidewire across the anastomosis.

CANNULATION

What are the steps involved in setting up a carotid artery access?

Carotid sheath placement involves the following steps: A standard femoral access sheath is inserted, followed by a catheter into the left common carotid artery. After adjusting the C-Arm for optimal viewing, a guidewire is advanced into the external carotid artery. The selective catheter is moved over this guidewire, which is then replaced by an exchange guidewire. Finally, the catheter is removed and the sheath is advanced over the exchange guidewire.

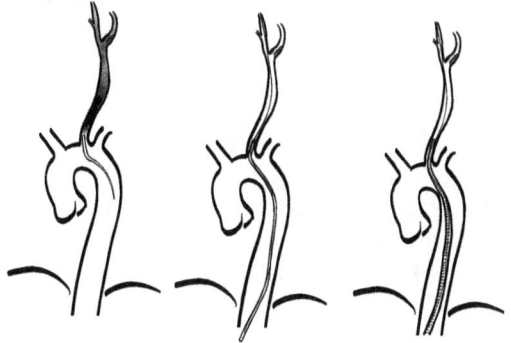

How is the 'up and over' method implemented for positioning a destination sheath?

UP AND OVER SHEATH INSERTION:
Sheath placement involves directing a stiff guidewire towards a safer branch artery, such as the internal iliac artery, advancing the sheath to the common iliac artery, and then replacing the exchange guidewire and dilator with a guidewire that crosses the arterial lesion.

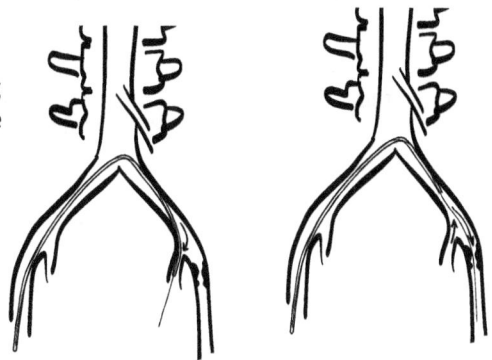

How can the <u>right</u> subclavian artery be catheterized from a femoral access point?

RIGHT SUBCLAVIAN ARTERY CATHETARIZATION:
The technique involves introducing a guidewire into the ascending aorta and advancing a selective cerebral catheter over it. After removing the guidewire, the catheter adjusts to its shape and is slowly rotated clockwise while being withdrawn. As the catheter tip enters the arch branch, the guidewire is then advanced to ensure secure access.

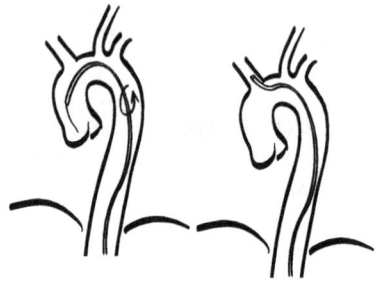

How can the <u>left</u> subclavian artery be catheterized from a femoral access point?

LEFT SUBCLAVIAN ARTERY CATHETARIZATION:
First, a guidewire is inserted into the ascending aorta. Then, a flush catheter is positioned to perform an arch aortogram, typically in the left anterior oblique (LAO) position. Once the origin of the artery and the lesion are identified, the flush catheter is replaced with a simple-curve catheter, which is slightly withdrawn and rotated to guide the catheter tip into the artery's origin. Finally, a selective guidewire is advanced into the artery, followed by potential advancement of the catheter as well.

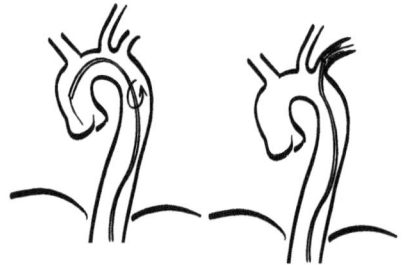

Explain the procedure to cannulate the tibial arteries antegradely

ANTERIOR TIBIAL ARTERY CANNULATION:
Guidewire passage beyond the below-knee popliteal artery typically follows the route of the peroneal artery. To access the anterior tibial artery or posterior tibial artery, a steerable hydrophilic-coated guidewire can be utilized. The steerable guidewire, guided by a bent-tip catheter for example, is directed into the anterior tibial artery despite its challenging angle of origin.

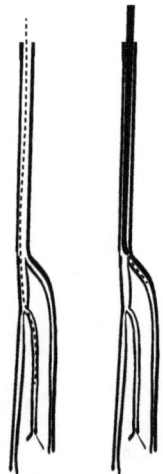

Explain the procedure to cannulate the SFA using the profunda as an aid.

SFA CANNULATION USING PFA:

The initial guidewire is directed towards the deep femoral artery. A steerable guidewire is then used to navigate into the superficial femoral artery. A selective catheter is passed over the guidewire in the deep femoral artery, allowing access to the SFA. The catheter is gradually withdrawn while injecting contrast to locate the femoral bifurcation. Finally, the guidewire is advanced through the selective catheter and into the SFA.

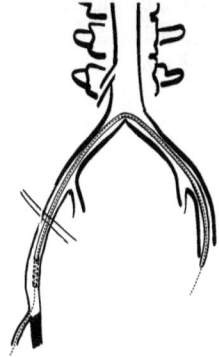

What are the steps involved in setting up an "up and over" iliac access?

UP AND OVER ILIAC ACCESS:

The up-and-over sheath placement involves advancing a suitable catheter and a guidewire over the aortic bifurcation, withdrawing the catheter to enter the contralateral iliac orifice, replacing them with an exchange guidewire, and moving the sheath over this guidewire. The sheath's placement is adjusted, the dilator is removed, and the sheath is prepared for use.

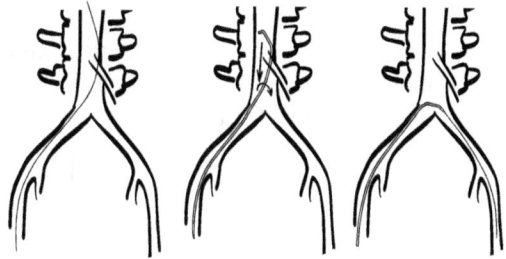

What measures can be taken to prevent the catheter tip from popping out of the iliac artery and inadvertently pulling the guidewire during the process of up and over iliac cannulation?

UP AND OVER ILIAC UNSTABLE CATHETER:

Advance the guidewire into the contralateral iliac system as far as possible before inserting the catheter. During the catheter insertion, pay close attention to the movement of the catheter tip, particularly if the artery is diseased. If the catheter tip encounters resistance, refrain from applying further forward pressure.

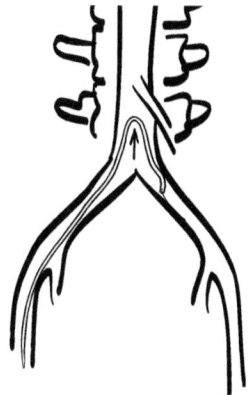

Explain the procedure to avoid cannulating the internal iliac artery instead of the EIA.

CANNULATING EIA:

When advancing the guidewire into the contralateral iliac artery, it often enters the internal iliac artery, particularly if the iliac system is tortuous. To address this, the catheter is retracted towards the common iliac artery, and the guidewire is pulled back to the catheter tip. To navigate the guidewire in an anterolateral direction, a torque maneuver is employed. Subsequently, the guidewire is further advanced into the external iliac artery, followed by the catheter.

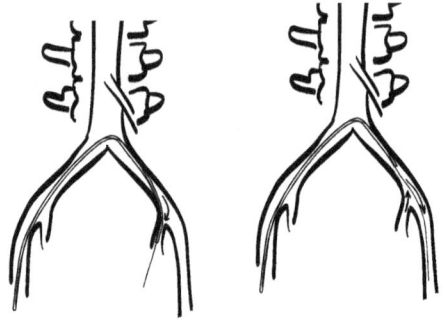

What is the catheter type and position for performing cerebral arteriography?

CANNULATING AORTIC ARCH BRANCHES:

The arch branches are each accessed using a simple-curve selective cerebral catheter that is carefully navigated into them. To prevent the catheter from retracting back into the arch from the artery, it's essential to position the catheter's tip at a depth of several centimeters within the artery. During the administration of the contrast medium, it is normal to observe some backlash or bouncing back of the catheter.

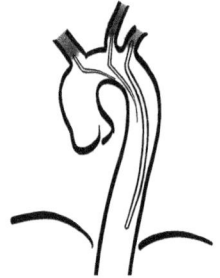

How can a stent be crossed safely?

CANNULATING STENTS:

After deploying a stent, avoid potential false passages, typically by using a J-tip guidewire to avoid passing through the stent's struts.

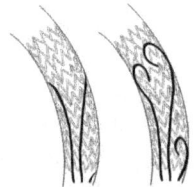

Explain the procedure for crossing the aortic bifurcation.

CROSSING THE AORTIC BIFURCATION:

A Hook-shaped catheter is guided over the guidewire, and both are retracted until the catheter's head is just proximal to the aortic bifurcation, and the guidewire is removed. The catheter's head takes its shape, and it is rotated towards the opposite side while being slowly withdrawn, while the guidewire is advanced into the catheter head.

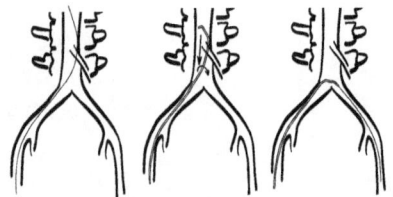

How retrograde or trans-brachial catheterization of the subclavian artery is done?

RETROGRADE CANNULATION OF SUBCLAVIAN:

First, a brachial puncture is performed using a micropuncture set, and a guidewire is inserted in a retrograde manner into the proximal subclavian artery. A selective catheter is then placed over the guidewire. Next, to avoid the guidewire advancing into the ascending aorta, a simple-curve or hook-shaped selective catheter is guided into the distal arch. The guidewire is then removed, and the catheter is directed posterolaterally. Finally, the guidewire is redirected into the descending aorta.

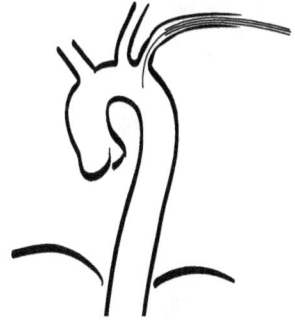

Explain the procedure for cathetarization of the renal artery.

CANNULATION OF RENAL ARTERY:

First, a guidewire is inserted into the aorta. Then, an arteriographic catheter is placed to capture images of the aorta and renal arteries. Following that, the arteriographic catheter is swapped with a cobra catheter, which is carefully withdrawn along the posterolateral aortic wall until its tip reaches the renal artery. Finally, the guidewire is threaded through the renal artery lesion.

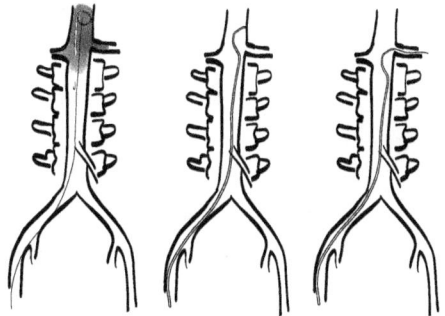

CATHETERS

What is meant by "Walk along" the guidewire to remove catheter.?

"Walk along" the guidewire refers to the technique of gradually and carefully sliding the catheter along the length of the guidewire in order to remove it.

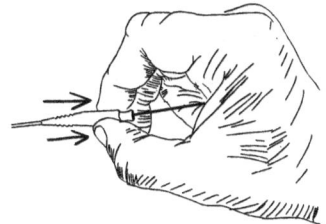

What distinguishes single curve catheters from complex curve catheters?

Single curve catheters rely on a primary curve to define their functionality, while complex curve catheters incorporate both a primary curve and, in some cases, additional secondary curves to gain more suitable shapes for the intended purpose

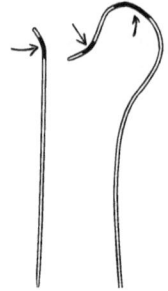

As the guidewire is positioned, the shape of the catheter head undergoes changes. Describe?

CATHETER-WIRE INTERACTIONS:
The position of the guidewire can significantly alter the shape of catheter heads, particularly for flush catheters and complex-curve selective catheters, whereby the presence of a guidewire within the shaft of a hook-shaped visceral catheter causes the catheter head's hook to splay out, and as the floppy part of the guidewire tip exits the catheter, the head of the catheter splays further, eventually straightening out completely when the firm portion of the guidewire shaft occupies the curved portion of the catheter head and exits it.

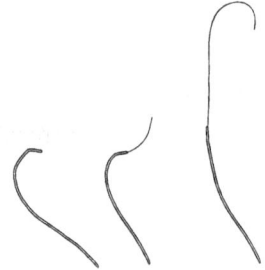

In what way can a guidewire be altered or affected when a catheter is passed over it?

CATHETER-WIRE INTERACTIONS:
To enhance guidewire rigidity, a catheter is used. If a guidewire can't cross a lesion, it's partially retracted, and a straight catheter is inserted over it. The guidewire's tip then probes the lesion before advancing through it.

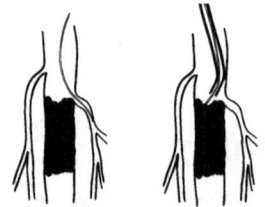

What is the catheter type and position for performing visceral arteriography?

VISCERAL ANGIOGRAPHY
A C2 cobra catheter is employed for the purpose of gaining access to the renal artery. For a detailed arteriography to be conducted, it's essential that the catheter's tip be within the artery. In the case of the celiac and superior mesenteric arteries' selective arteriography, a hook-shaped catheter is utilized.

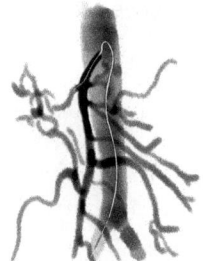

In the event that the catheter fails to progress through the entry site using the firm portion of the guidewire, what course of action should be taken?

Exchange for a stiffer guidewire

NAME THE FOLLOWING CATHETERS:

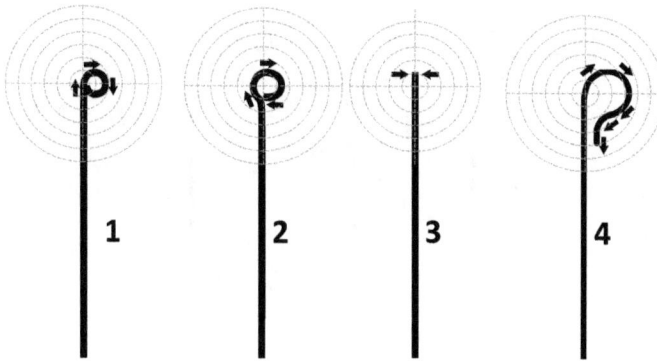

FLUSH CATHETERS
1- Pigtail
2- TR Flush
3- Straight
4- Universal (UF)

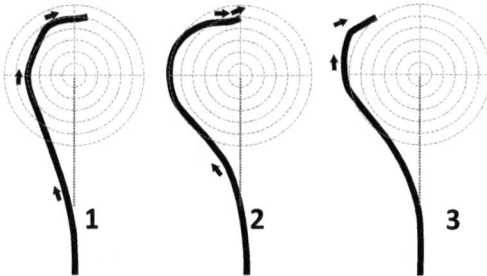

Headhunter CATHETERS
1- H1
2- H2
3- H1H

1g

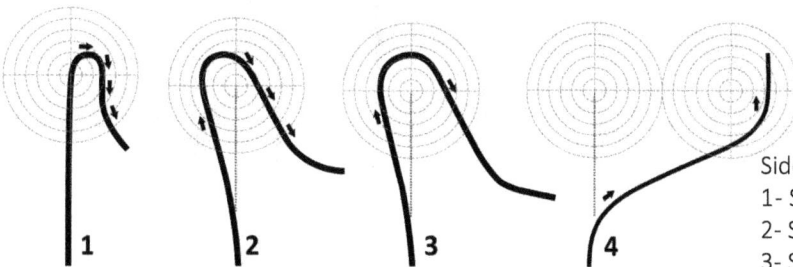

Sidewinder CATHETERS
1- Sim 1
2- Sim 2
3- Sim 3
4- Sim 4

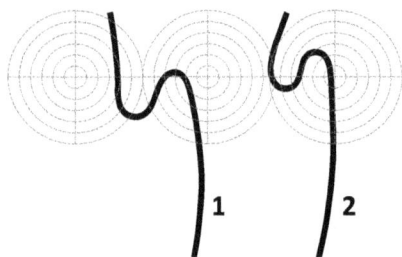

Newton CATHETERS
1- HN3
2- HN4

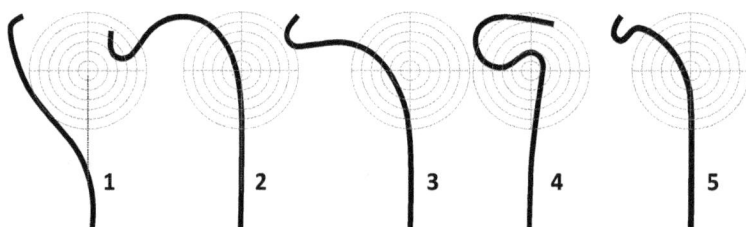

Bentson CATHETERS
1- JB1
2- JB2
3- JB3
4- MAN
5- CK1

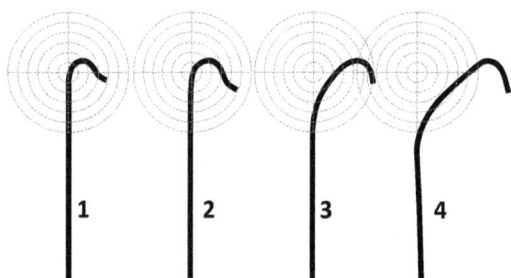

Shephard Hook
CATHETERS
1- SHK 0.8
2- SHK 1.0
3- RDC 1
4- RDC

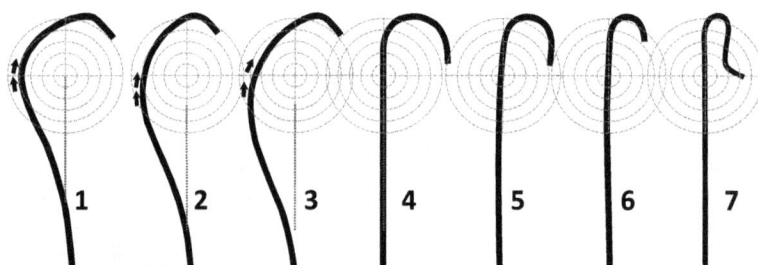

Cobra CATHETERS
1- C1
2- C2
3- C3
4- RC1
5- RC2
6- RC3
7- USL2(VS)

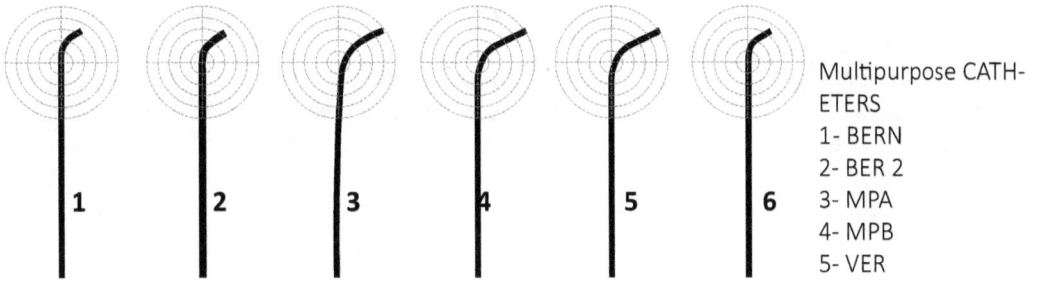

Multipurpose CATHETERS
1- BERN
2- BER 2
3- MPA
4- MPB
5- VER

What's the maximum flow rate in the following catheters:

Flush multi sidehole catheter- 4Fr- 65cm length?	19 mL/sec
Flush multi sidehole catheter- 4Fr- 100cm length?	15 mL/sec
Flush multi sidehole catheter- 5Fr- 65cm length?	32 mL/sec
Flush multi sidehole catheter- 5Fr- 100cm length?	27 mL/sec
Selective end hole catheter -- 5Fr- 65cm length?	15 mL/sec
Selective end hole catheter -- 5Fr- 100cm length?	11 mL/sec

COMPLICATIONS

In the event of balloon rupture on a calcified plaque, what steps should be taken in the management approach?

BALLOON RUPTURE:
If rupture occurs and bloody fluid is returned, replace the balloon with a more puncture-resistant one, possibly needing a larger sheath for accommodation. Gradually dilate the lesion with the balloon's shoulder to avoid the sharpest parts. If needed, place a stent for further support, noting that sharp lesions might occasionally perforate the balloon during the stent's placement.

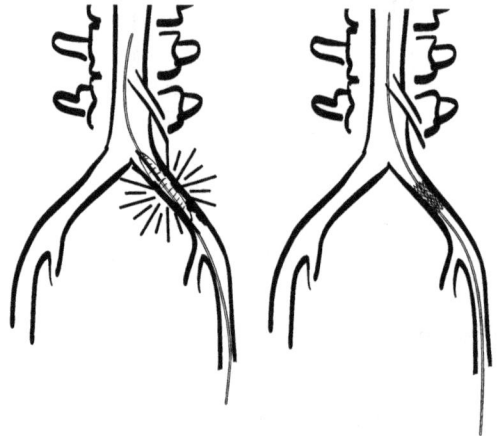

How should a tilted balloon-expandable stent be addressed or managed?

TILTED BALLOON-EXPANDABLE STENT
To overcome challenges posed by artery curvature and lesion location during stent placement, a guidewire is passed through the stenosis, a stent is positioned with incomplete wall opposition, balloon angioplasty is performed on the protruding stent end, and an additional stent may be placed if needed to enhance contact with the arterial wall.

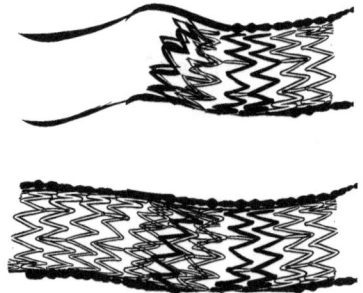

What causes the formation of a kinked sheath and how does it obstruct the passage of a stent?

KINKED SHEATH
In a tortuous artery, the kinking of the sheath after removing the dilator prevents the passage of the stent-mounted balloon through the tortuous iliac artery.

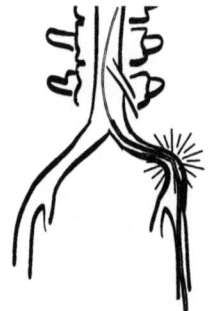

What should be done when the balloon does not deflate or deflates slowly?

Use a large, empty syringe to produce more negative pressure and aspirate the balloon, creating minimal emptying, then ensure continuous aspiration by pulling the plunger back to the syringe's rubber seal, and locking it in position.

What are the strategies for managing an acute near occlusive dissection at the angioplasty site?

ACUTE NEAR OCCLUSIVE DISSECTION
To treat post-angioplasty near occlusive dissection, conduct arteriography, introduce and remove a dilator, pass a stent-loaded balloon through a sheath to the dissection site, inflate it to deploy the stent, and secure the dissection flap.

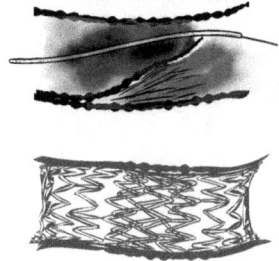

How should one address the collapse of a self-expanding stent in its midsection?

COLLAPSED STENT
The procedure includes guidewire placement, balloon angioplasty, and, if necessary, placement of a balloon-expandable stent to address stenosis-related complications.

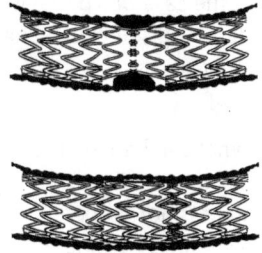

What should be done if the balloon herniates past the lesion during inflation?

HERNIATED BALLOON
Keep the guidewire through the stenosis, allow the balloon to migrate out of the lesion as it forms, deflate and advance the balloon catheter so one radiopaque marker is beyond the lesion before reinflating it, apply traction to hold it in place if it tries to pop out, and consider substituting the catheter for one with a longer balloon if necessary.

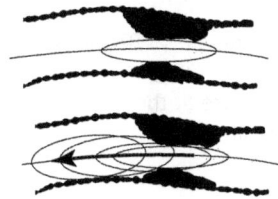

What to do for a dissection found at the end of a stent?

DISSECTION
To repair a dissection during stent placement, a guidewire is placed across the lesion, followed by the placement of an additional stent with slight overlap, effectively repairing the dissection.

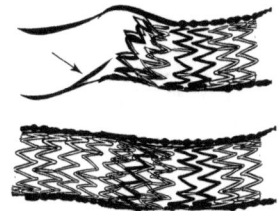

What should be done if the end of the self-expanding device fails to expand?

To correct incomplete expansion of a self-expanding stent, angioplasty is performed along the stent's entire length using a balloon catheter, with priority given to dilating the stent body before the ends to prevent balloon rupture.

What measures can be taken to ensure the accuracy of Self-expanding stent deployment?

PRECISE DEPLOYMENT

For precise deployment in iliac artery lesions, choose between antegrade or retrograde approaches for Wallstent placement, ensuring accurate positioning of the proximal end through retrograde approach and addressing limited working space by placing the distal end first via antegrade approach, considering the excess length of the upper end extending into the proximal external iliac artery and the unpredictable final stent length as it extends into the undiseased common femoral artery.

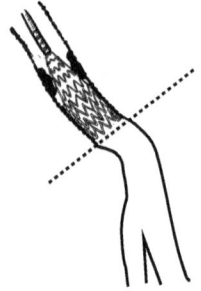

What should be done in the case of a partially deployed self-expanding stent?

In cases where limited working room between the stent deployment site and arterial entry site causes impingement of the stent by the access sheath, stent deployment can be facilitated by partially withdrawing the hemostatic access sheath or using a sheath with a radiopaque tip.

What can happen if a balloon-expandable stent is not properly mounted on the guidewire, causing it to dislodge and shoot forward off the balloon during inflation?

STENT DISLODGED WRONGLY

The stent is deployed in a neutral position after manipulating the guidewire, exchanging to a smaller balloon, and flaring one end of the stent before using the correct-sized balloon.

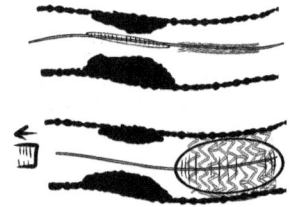

What is the procedure for handling an arterial rupture at the angioplasty site?

Reinsert and reinflate the angioplasty balloon to halt bleeding.

CONTRAST

What are the common rate of injection in doing:

Arch aortogram	30 mL over 2 sec (15 for 30)
Carotid arteriography?	12 mL over 2 sec (4 for 8)
Descending thoracic?	30 mL over 2 sec (15 for 30)
Renal	8 mL over 2 sec (4 for 8)

Aortoiliac	18-24 mL over 3 sec (8 for 24)
Femoral	10 mL over 2 sec (5 for 10)
Tibio-paedal	4-12 mL over 2-3 sec (3 for 9)

| What does the term "rate of contrast" refer to when using an injection device for angiography? | The term "rate of contrast" refers to the speed at which the contrast agent is delivered into the patient's bloodstream through the injection device during an angiographic procedure. This rate is usually measured in millilitres per second (ml/s). It influences the quality of imaging and needs to be adjusted based on the type of procedure and the patient's condition. |

DILATORS

| How is the dilator's diameter is measured? | By quoting the outside diameter (in French) |

DISSECTION

How should a stent be placed following a dissection?

STENTING FOR DISSECTION
Identify any dissection caused by balloon angioplasty through contrast retained in the arterial wall and flow streaming effects, keep the guidewire access stable, and then use a stent at the original angioplasty site (overlapping where needed) to close the false channels.

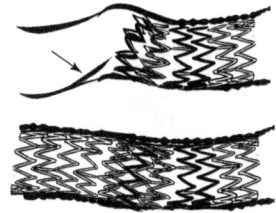

What are the different degrees of dissection that can occur after angioplasty?

DISSECTION DEGREE
A dissection flaps can restrict or obstruct flow, or can be non-flow limiting.

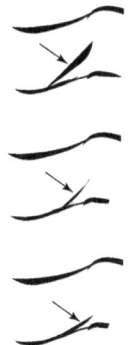

How is residual stenosis managed following angioplasty?

Arterial pressure measurement helps determine the significance of the lesion, repeat dilatation can be performed with higher pressure and longer expansion times, and a stent can be placed to treat any remaining significant lesion.

GUIDEWIRES

How to stiffen the floppy tip of the guidewire?

STIFFEN A FLOPPY GUIDEWIRE
By applying one-handed traction through a specific gripping technique involving the thumb, forefinger, and other fingers.

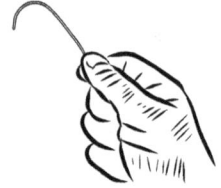

What are the key properties of any guidewire? What characterize each property?

Penetrability, pushability, trackability, torquability, steerability, bending, and lubricity.

Penetrability refers to the ability to puncture different types of lesions, with stiffer lesions requiring greater penetrability. Pushability is the force needed to advance the wire through a lesion, while trackability relates to the wire's ability to navigate bends. Torquability involves the wire's transmission of torque for controlled drilling strategies.
Steerability depends on the wire tip's responsiveness and the transmission of torque from the proximal to distal ends. Bending allows the wire to navigate stiff tissues like calcium. Lubricity relates to the ease of wire movement and depends on factors such as the encountered tissue, bends, and length of the lesion.

How to allow the elbow of buckled guidewire to become the leading edge?

The eccentric lesion is probed by the tip of the guidewire, where the leading edge avoids entering the lesion's lumen but the flexible tip starts to buckle, forming a gentle bend; the guidewire is advanced as long as the bend progresses smoothly until it emerges from the other end of the lesion, allowing for removal of the buckle; however, this buckling technique is suitable only for moderately diseased arterial segments, as in cases of critical or severely preocclusive lesions, the buckle may penetrate below the innermost layer of the artery (subintimal).

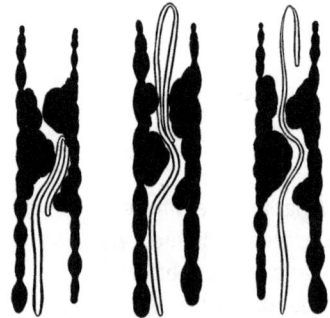

What factors affect wire steerability?

Steerability depends on factors such as the absence of a terminal coil on a single core wire, the lateral support provided by the wire, and the utilization of specially designed wires capable of transmitting torque (e.g., wires with dual or composite core).

What to do to enhance the manoeuvrability of a guidewire tip?

ENHANCING MANOEUVRABILITY
The curvature at the tip of the guidewire can be modified by trapping it between the thumb and the edge of a haemostat, and pulling it along the metal edge of the clamp to achieve a tighter curvature, which is particularly beneficial when employing 0.014 guidewires.

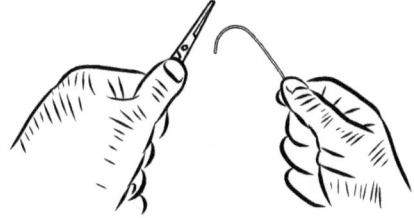

What is the optimal wire length required for the following procedures:

Catheterization of dialysis access | 50-80

General arteriography | 145cm

Arteriography for the arch and carotid | 180-210

Carotid interventions | 200-300

What are the Factors influencing penetrability

Tip load, tapered tip, wire support, and lateral support.

In the following diagram, describe the different interactions between the guidewire and a lesion:

(1) leading edge of the guidewire getting caught on the proximal end of the stenosis, causing the floppy tip to buckle and allowing another part of the guidewire to traverse the lesion.
(2) guidewire tip encountering plaque and being unable to locate the eccentric lumen.
(3) guidewire successfully passing through the lesion on its first attempt.
(4) floppy tip starting to buckle but getting caught on a plaque ledge, preventing it from crossing the lesion.

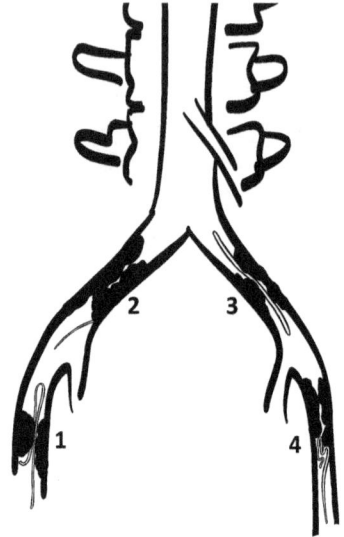

What is the tip length and weight for each of the following:

Asahi Gladiu Guidewire

ASAHI GLADIU
3cm soft tip
1g to cause 2mm bend in the distal 10mm of the wire

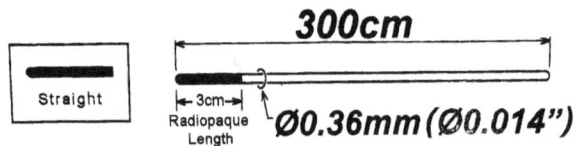

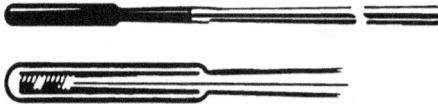

Straight

300cm

3cm
Radiopaque
Length

Ø0.36mm (Ø0.014")

Command 18ST

COMMAND 18ST
3cm soft tip
4g to cause 2mm bend in the distal 10mm of the wire

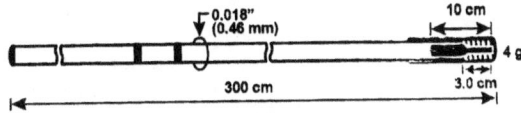

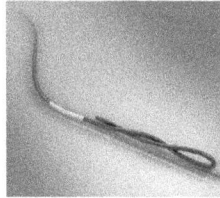

V18

8 cm soft tip

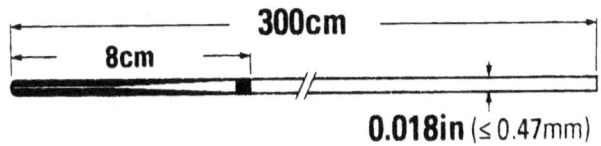

HAEMODYNAMICS

Explain what a fluid is and contrast it with solid and gas states of matter?

A fluid is a substance that undergoes constant deformation or flow. Unlike gases, fluids create a free surface and unlike solids, they do not significantly resist deformation, allowing them to conform to the shape of their containers. Fluids are subject to pressure stress, which can influence their flow, and they can also withstand minimal shear stress.

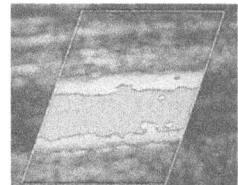

How can we describe the behaviour of fluid (and therefore the physics of blood flow)?

Similar to describing the motion of any physical object, i.e. using Newton's laws of physics.
Newton's laws of motion are three physical laws that form the basis for classical mechanics. They describe the relationship between the forces acting on a body and its motion due to those forces.
1.   First law: The velocity of a body remains constant unless the body is acted upon by an external force.
2.   Second law: The acceleration a of a body is parallel and directly proportional to the net force F and inversely proportional to the mass m, i.e., F = ma.
3.   Third law: The mutual forces of action and reaction between two bodies are equal, opposite and collinear.

Is blood a Newtonian fluid or not?

Blood behaves as a non-Newtonian fluid, meaning its viscosity changes under different flow conditions. In large vessels, blood acts as a Newtonian fluid with constant viscosity, while in smaller vessels, due to interaction between red blood cells and vessel walls, its behavior changes.

What are the specific equations that are applicable to fluid dynamics?

Principles such as Bernoulli's equation and Poiseuille's law also come into play, dictating how changes in pressure, vessel diameter, and blood viscosity impact flow rate.

What are the two main factors that affect blood flow?

The two main factors affecting blood flow are blood pressure and resistance. Blood pressure is the force exerted by blood against the walls of blood vessels, driving the blood flow. Resistance is influenced by factors like vessel diameter, blood viscosity, and the length of the blood vessels, which can hinder the flow.

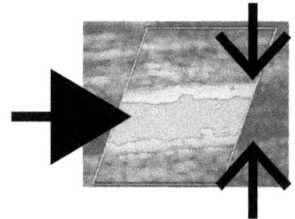

The flow (Q) can be calculated using Ohm's equation:

$$Q = \frac{\Delta P}{R}$$

$$Q\,(mL/s) = \frac{\Delta P\,(dyne/cm^2)}{R\,(poise)}$$

What are the energy forces driving the blood flow?

The energy propelling blood flow primarily comes from three sources: 1) Pressure energy, which is produced by the pumping action of the heart, 2) Kinetic energy, originating from the mass of moving blood and reliant on both the density and speed of the fluid, and 3) Gravitational (or potential) energy, generated due to the influence of gravity on the column of blood.

Specify the formula utilized for determining the kinetic energy of blood?

The kinetic energy of blood, or any moving object, can be calculated using the equation $KE = 1/2\ m\ v^2$, where 'm' is the mass of the object (blood in this case) and 'v' is its velocity.

List the elements that influence resistance to fluid flow?

Flow resistance is primarily affected by three factors: the viscosity of the fluid, the length of the path the fluid is traveling, and the diameter of the path. Specifically, an increase in fluid viscosity or path length will increase resistance, while an increase in path diameter will decrease it. This relationship is outlined by Poiseuille's law in fluid dynamics.

$$Q = (\pi P\ \Delta r^4) / (8\eta L)$$

where:

Q is the flow rate
P is the pressure difference between the two ends
Δr is the radius of the pipe
η is the viscosity of the fluid
L is the length of the pipe

What are the different forms of blood circulation observed within blood vessels?

There are three types of blood flow:

1) Laminar flow consists of blood cells moving in layered paths, sliding over one another at increasing velocities. Initially, this forms a parabolic flow, which, at higher flow rates, changes to a plug flow where most blood cells move at high velocities within a confined range.

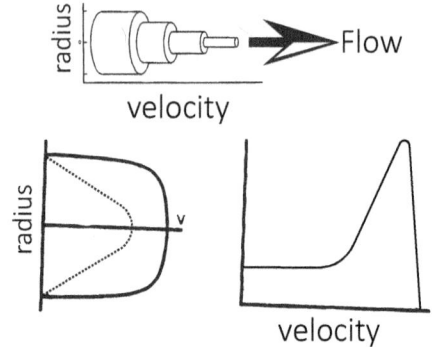

2) Disturbed flow happens at high velocities where fluid particles gain enough momentum to disrupt adjacent layers, causing small eddies and eventually leading to a complete turbulent flow.

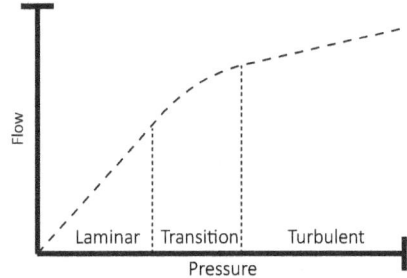

3) Turbulent flow arises when the Reynolds number (Re), a factor involving tube diameter, fluid density, viscosity, and flow velocity, exceeds 2000. The velocity required for turbulence is inversely related to vessel diameter. For instance, a 1 mm diameter vessel requires a velocity of 7.5 m/s, while a 10 mm diameter vessel needs a velocity of just 0.75 m/s to produce turbulence.

How does the pulsating flow pattern in the arteries influence its flow profile?

The pulsatile nature of flow in the arteries, due to rhythmic heart contractions, creates a changing flow profile. During systole (heart contraction), the flow is high and the profile tends to be more parabolic. But during diastole (heart relaxation), the flow is lower and can become flat or 'plug-like'. Thus, this pulsatile nature leads to variable flow profiles in the arterial system.

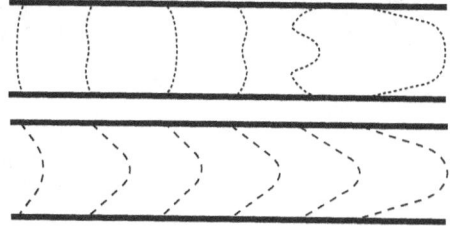

How does the flow pattern alter when blood reaches a bifurcation or a branching point in the vessel?

During laminar flow, a boundary layer, with a specific thickness, develops next to the vessel wall within the fluid. As the vessel branches or bifurcates, the fluid flow becomes detached, creating a free boundary between two regions of flow. This is referred to as boundary layer separation, which appears on both edges of the bifurcating artery. The inner wall, relative to the flow divider line, experiences the highest velocity, while the outer wall sees the lowest. In areas of low shear stress, the flow may even reverse direction. This concept also applies to bifurcations at 90-degree angles.

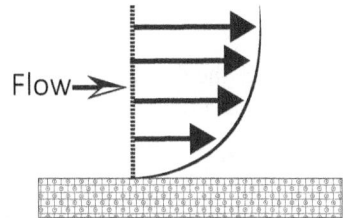

Flow→

How does the flow pattern change when the artery follows a curved path?

The blood flow undergoes centrifugal forces within a curved vessel. This force shifts the peak velocity from the vessel's center towards the outer edge, as illustrated in the diagram.

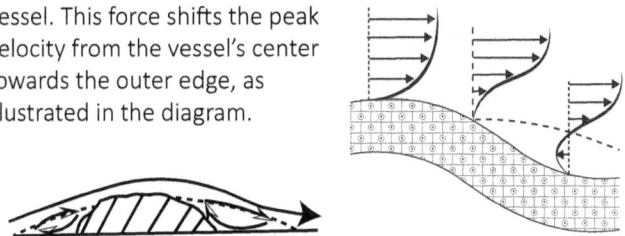

Describe the relation between blood flow, pressure, and level of arterial stenosis.

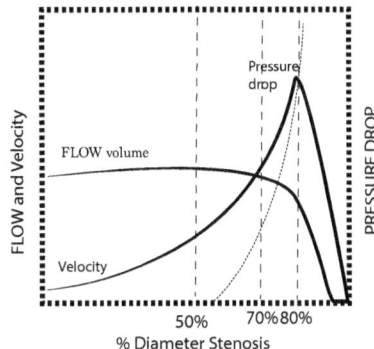

Pressure drop

FLOW and Velocity

FLOW volume

PRESSURE DROP

Velocity

50%   70% 80%

% Diameter Stenosis

How does a stenosis or narrowing of the vessel affect the pattern of blood flow?

As the vessel diameter narrows, causing changes in flow speed and pressure, separation lines form within the fluid. The central stream, with its high velocity, continues to move forward. However, the lower velocity flow along the boundaries tends to reverse direction.

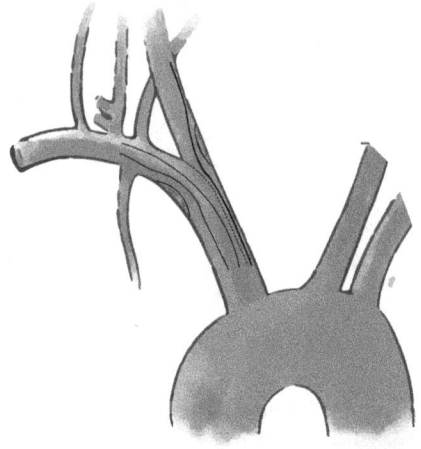

How does the flow of blood impact the vessel wall?

The flow of blood exerts shear stress on the vessel walls, which can influence vessel health and function. Constant laminar flow is generally beneficial, promoting a healthy endothelium and suppressing inflammation. However, areas of disturbed flow, such as at bifurcations or curved segments, can lead to endothelial dysfunction, inflammation, and are often sites of atherosclerotic plaque development.

HEPARIN

List the appropriate amount of heparin needed for each procedure:

A) Procedure: Renal

Heparin Amount: 50-75

B) Procedure: Aortoiliac (Simple)

Heparin Amount: 25-50

C) Procedure: Femoro-popliteal (Simple)

Heparin Amount: 25-75

D) Procedure: Tibial

Heparin Amount: 75-100

E) Procedure: Brachioce-phalic

Heparin Amount: 100

F) Procedure: Aortoiliac (Complex)

Heparin Amount: 50-75

G) Procedure: Femoro-popliteal (Complex)

Heparin Amount: 50-100

IMAGING

What strategies can be employed to enhance spatial orientation during endovascular procedures?

Various tools and techniques, such as the use of contrast media to visualize vessels (puff contrast), creating a roadmap within the vasculature. Internal landmarks, such as vascular calcifications and surgical clips, external landmarks, rulers, clamps, and stent markers.
Other methods include studying anatomy, mental mapping of the case, training on simulators, and utilizing imaging technologies.

How can you confirm that the guidewire is truly positioned within the lumen?

Large perigenicular collaterals can potentially mislead a guidewire trying to cross lesions in the superficial femoral or popliteal artery. Under fluoroscopy, the guidewire might seem to have passed the stenosis, but it might be actually in a parallel collateral. Only through contrast administration can the actual guidewire path be revealed, indicating that the lesion remains un-crossed.

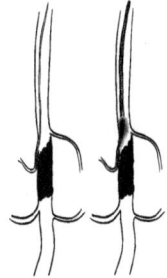

What impact can oblique projections of the iliac and femoral bifurcations have?

Standard anteroposterior projection for aortoiliac arteriography may not clearly show occlusive disease at the common iliac artery bifurcation. Contralateral anterior oblique projection helps visualize this. Occlusive disease at the femoral bifurcation can be difficult to see due to overlapping of arteries. An ipsilateral anterior oblique projection can resolve this overlap, improving visualization.

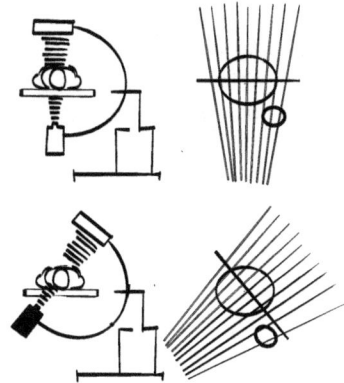

How does placing the image intensifier closer to the patient provide a benefit?

Reduces radiation scatter and expands the visual coverage.

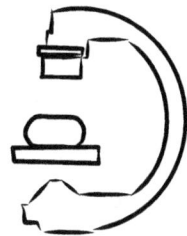

In what way can a magnified oblique view assist in the process of recanalization?

When encountering a complex lesion, the probing guidewire is used. By magnifying the field and utilizing an oblique projection, the entrance to the lesion can be effectively opened up.

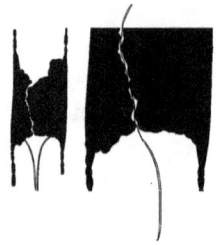

What are the advantages of delayed filming in situations of extended occlusions?

Delayed filming, especially with Digital Subtraction Angiography (DSA), improves the accuracy of occlusion length measurement in arteriography. It reduces overestimation issues found with traditional cut film techniques, aiding in the decision-making for potential recanalization.

Which imaging technique allows for improved visibility of the origin of the renal artery?

Ipsilateral anterior oblique projection

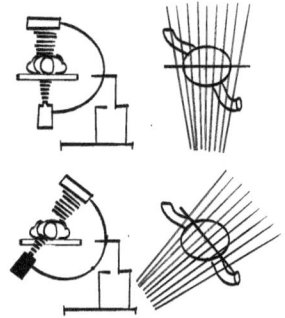

What distinguishes ionic contrast medium from non-ionic contrast medium?

The difference lies in their chemical composition and properties. Ionic contrast media contain positively or negatively charged particles, while non-ionic contrast media do not have charged particles. Ionic contrast media are more likely to cause adverse reactions and have a higher osmolality, which can lead to discomfort. Non-ionic contrast media have a lower risk of adverse reactions and are generally better tolerated by patients.

When is it inappropriate to utilize power injection?

Where there is a risk of arterial injury: fragmented thrombus within an aneurysm, significant recoil from high-pressure injection, constraint of the catheter head within an occlusive lesion leading to potential fragmentation, or when the catheter tip is in direct contact with the aortic wall instead of being freely within its lumen.

What sets AP and LAO projections apart in Arch aortogram imaging?

A 30-45 degree LAO projection is necessary for Arch aortogram imaging to visualize the posterior movement of the aortic arch and to provide better separation of the arch branch origins.

KISSING STENTS

What are the methods for managing a lesion in the aortic bifurcation?

Using the "kissing balloons" technique, two balloon catheters are inserted through each femoral artery, overlapped at the aortic bifurcation stenosis, and inflated simultaneously to dilate the lesion.

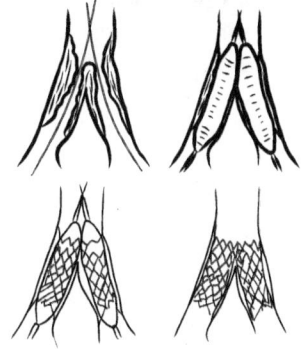

MONORAIL SYSTEM

What distinguishes coaxial systems from monorail systems?

The coaxial balloon angioplasty catheter has a continuous guidewire lumen throughout its entire length, while the monorail balloon angioplasty catheter has a guidewire lumen that extends only partially along the catheter, starting at the tip and exiting along the shaft.

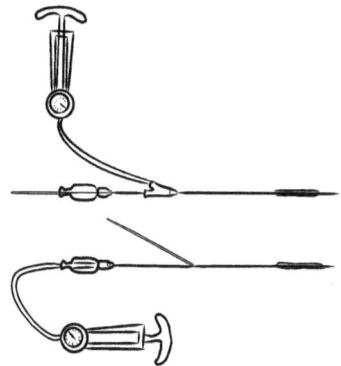

The monorail catheter allows for one-handed insertion, with the operator being able to secure the guidewire with the other hand, and it can be removed by either holding the guidewire steady with one hand while withdrawing the catheter with the other, or by using a two-handed technique when the guidewire and catheter are joined together.

PRESSURE MEASUREMENT

What are the potential pitfalls linked to pressure measurements across occlusive lesions?

Blood pressure fluctuations during pressure measurement both before and after a lesion can impact the results. Measuring pressure in end organ arteries like the renal artery can potentially lower the distal pressure due to the catheter occupying the residual lumen. Poor outflow can lead to pressure equalization across a lesion. While pressure measurements offer quantitative data, they fail to provide a precise measure of flow across a lesion, which is crucial. The significance of occlusive lesions often only appears with exercise, and vasodilators may not accurately mimic these conditions.

PROSTHETIC GRAFT

What's the best access to cannulate a prosthetic grafts in the following locations: Carotid–subclavian, axillo-femoral, femoral–femoral, ilio-femoral, and Infrainguinal graft?

Carotid–subclavian: femoral or brachial
Axillo-femoral: brachial or femoral
Femoral–femoral: femorals
Aorto-femoral: femorals
Ilio-femoral: C/L femoral
Infrainguinal graft: C/L femoral

RADIATION

What are the potential occupational hazards associated with endovascular work, and what safety measures should be taken?

Occupational Hazards for Interventionists Due to Radiation:
- Increased risk of health conditions like cataracts and cancer.
- Strain from heavy protective gear leading to musculoskeletal issues.
- Elevated cancer risk from prolonged radiation exposure.
- Potential skin injuries from radiation.
- Reproductive health concerns.

Safety Measures:
- Stay updated on radiation safety guidelines.
- Use proper shielding like lead aprons.
- Limit radiation doses and fluoroscopy time.
- Monitor exposure using dosimeters.
- Wear ergonomic protective gear.

RECANALIZATION

What is the method of utilizing a puff of contrast into the lesion to aid in recanalization?

After a challenging guidewire insertion, an exchange catheter with multiple side-holes can be used to hold the position through the lesion. This allows contrast delivery through the catheter and fills the lesion. The guidewire can be removed for direct contrast delivery, or a smaller guidewire with an adapter can be utilized.

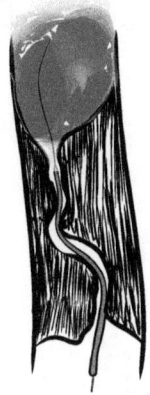

What does buckling of the guidewire and catheter into the distal aorta mean?

This refers to the phenomenon where the guidewire and catheter bend or curve inward as they enter the lower part of the aorta.

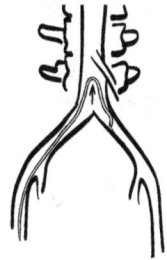

How to deal with this?

A stiffer guidewire can be substituted for the standard guidewire. Additionally, using a long, curved sheath over the aortic bifurcation can minimize tortuosity and friction, allowing for antegrade catheter delivery into the iliac artery, eliminating the need for contralateral access.

What are some helpful methods and techniques that can be utilized to navigate through occlusions?

Navigating occlusions can involve using hydrophilic guidewires and catheters, entry and re-entry catheters from various manufacturers, intravascular ultrasound for lumen identification, lasers, or reverse-direction lesion approach.

What role does the tip of the guidewire play when navigating through severely diseased arterial segments?

To navigate through a lengthy critical lesion, a flexible guidewire can be manoeuvred to make multiple turns, and its tip can be employed to probe the lesion.

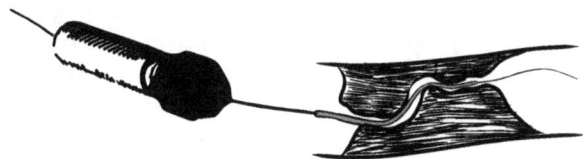

How can the catheter be utilized to navigate or guide the guidewire?

Using a Berenstein catheter (5 Fr) over a guidewire, either steerable or standard, assists in guiding the wire to the desired location. This involves the guidewire entering a collateral near the target lesion, passing a bent-tip Berenstein catheter over it, rotating the catheter to direct the guidewire, and then advancing the wire into the lesion.

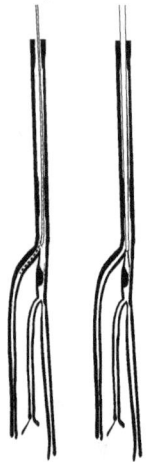

What other advantages of using a wire that can't pass through during sub-clavian recanalization?

In subclavian recanalization, a partially successful guidewire can be left in place as a marker, assisting in an alternate approach to the occlusion. Using fluoroscopy, the distance between the original and new guidewire tips can be estimated more accurately.

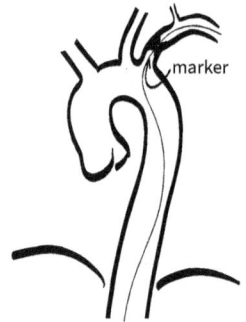

Why might it be unsafe to pass a guidewire retrograde through a common iliac artery occlusion?

The retrograde approach typically guides the guidewire through the lesion and into the subintimal plane, but re-entering the true lumen can be difficult, particularly when dealing with extensive atherosclerotic disease of the aortic bifurcation or severe calcification of the infrarenal aorta.

How to perform recanlisation for iliac more safely then?

Placing a sheath as a platform, using a braided, angled tip catheter to guide a guidewire into the lesion, pushing the guidewire into a promising location with catheter support, progressing the guidewire through the subintimal space into the true lumen, and finally advancing the catheter over the guidewire to access the true lumen.

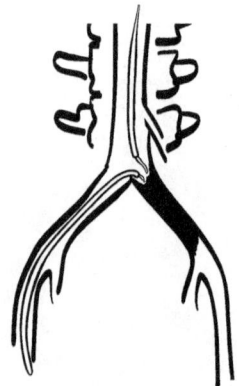

RENAL PROCEDURES

How is balloon angio-
plasty to renal artery is
performed?

This involves cannulation with a cobra catheter, angioplasty
with a balloon
over the guide-
wire, and
completion
arteriography
either via the
balloon catheter
or an alternate
site, with
potential angio-
plasty through a
guiding catheter.

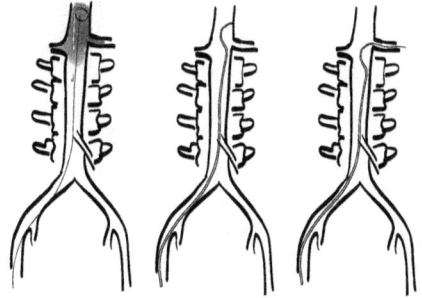

How is balloon stenting
to renal artery is per-
formed?

A guidewire and guiding sheath are positioned in the aorta,
then a selective catheter is inserted into the renal artery,
allowing a balloon catheter to be advanced over the guidewire. A pre-mounted, balloon-expandable stent is placed at
the lesion and inflated, followed by post-stent angiography.

SHEATH

What is the minimum
amount of the wire that
should be inside the
artery before advancing
the sheath over it?

The guidewire should be inserted deep into the vasculature to
position the floppy portion securely, and then the catheter is
advanced over the firmer segment of the guidewire.

What's the method for positioning the sheath as near as possible to the lesion without causing any disruption to it?

For infra-geniculate lesions, max-imize sheath advancement, possi-bly using smaller branches. After guidewire and dilator removal, the sheath tip should be near the lesion.

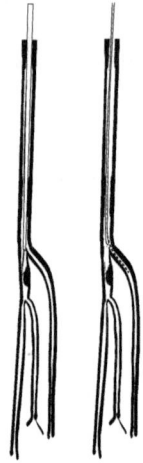

What are the advantages of using a long straight sheath; an up-and-over guiding sheath and the Ansel guiding sheath?

Guiding sheaths offer simpler and more reliable access. They come in several forms, including straight sheaths for balloon angioplasty, long-curved sheaths for crossing the aortic bifurcation, and Ansel sheaths for renal artery procedures.

Is it readily easy to locate the needle tip using ultrasound while puncturing the artery?

If the ultrasound probe is not held perpendicular to the needle's path, this will not be the case.

How do a standard access sheath, a guiding sheath, and a guiding catheter differ from each other?

Standard access sheaths are 12-15 cm, with a valve and side-arm. Guiding sheaths are similar but longer, with a special-ized tip. Guiding catheters, larger and uniquely tipped, can have an adapter added for hemostasis and contrast delivery.

When should you make the knife incision that follows needle puncture and wire insertion?

Once the guidewire is properly positioned within the artery, the 4 or 5 Fr dilator is inserted over it, and upon slight withdrawal, the dilator elevates the skin, pulling out the surrounding tissue, after which the scalpel is utilized to make a precise incision on the skin directly above the dilator.

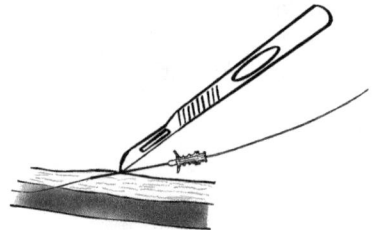

What should be done in case of scarring in the femoral area preventing the entry of the sheath?

The non-dominant hand can be utilized to apply pressure on the tissues surrounding the guidewire and assist in directing the sheath's tip into the artery more forcefully.

What should be done in the case of losing track of the tip of the sheath?

To track the sheath location during balloon angioplasty, methods such as using a radiopaque sheath tip, contrast placement within the sheath, and fluoroscopic observation of the balloon location should be employed.

SIZING

Which combination of location, entry site, and length (cm) is appropriate for balloon angioplasty for:

Carotid
Subclavian
Visceral
Renal
Aorta
Iliac
Femoropopliteal
Infrapopliteal

A) Location: Carotid, Entry site: Femoral, Length (cm): 110-130
H) Location: Subclavian, Entry site: Femoral, Length (cm): 110-120
B) Location: Visceral, Entry site: Femoral, Length (cm): 75-90
I) Location: Renal, Entry site: Femoral, Length (cm): 75-90
C) Location: Aorta, Entry site: Femoral, Length (cm): 65-75
D) Location: Iliac, Entry site: Ipsilateral femoral, Length (cm): 40-75
E) Location: Femoropopliteal, Entry site: Ipsilateral femoral, Length (cm): 75-110
F) Location: Infrapopliteal, Entry site: Ipsilateral femoral, Length (cm): 75-90

SUPERIOR MESENTERIC ARTERY PROCEDURES

How is the catheterization of the celiac and superior mesenteric arteries performed?

Through lateral positioning of an image intensifier, a hook-shaped catheter engages the artery orifice and advances a glidewire, which follows a curved path in the celiac artery or a straighter course in the superior mesenteric artery.

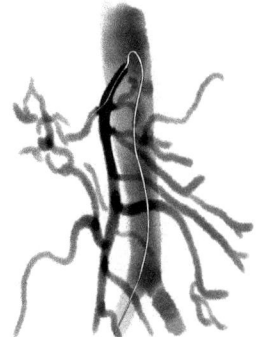

How is the stenting of the superior mesenteric arteries performed?

A guiding sheath is positioned near the SMA and a guidewire is advanced with a supportive catheter, which is then removed; following this, a pre-mounted, low-profile, balloon-expandable stent is advanced into the lesion and placed at the artery's orifice.

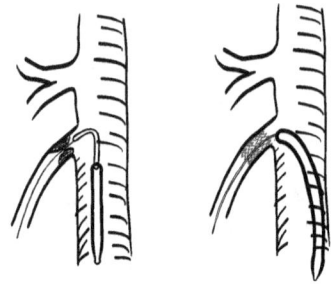

STENTING

How can a self-expandable stent be moved to fit into the diseased area?

Position the guidewire across the lesion, start deploying the stent more proximally, pull back the delivery apparatus to move the stent into the lesion, then continue with the deployment.

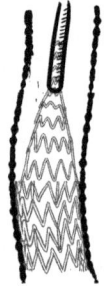

What characteristics define a balloon-expanding stent?

The balloon-expandable stent, made of steel or stainless steel, possesses moderate radiopacity and is characterized by its slotted-tube design, high radial force, and rigidity, and while it tends to shorten with expansion, it performs best at shorter lengths and can be either pre-mounted or fitted onto a balloon of choice.

What is the placement technique for self-expanding stent?

Place the guidewire across the lesion, align the stent delivery catheter over it, while monitoring stent positioning using fluoroscopy, withdraw the valve body to let the stent expand, and after deployment, remove the catheter.

What characteristics define a self-expanding stent?

A self-expanding stent is a flexible, long, wire mesh or slotted tube, usually oversized for the vessel, made from nitinol or light metal alloy, and comes with a delivery catheter and a covering sheath; although it has variable shortening, some do not shorten, and it generally possesses poor radiopacity, though some have markers.

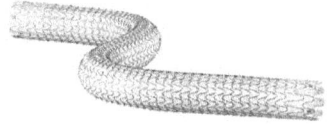

When would it be appropriate to place a balloon-expandable stent without a sheath?

When the guidewire is across a lesion and the artery's tortuosity prevents safe sheath Passage. In that case, guide the pre-mounted stent on an angioplasty balloon beyond the sheath through the lesion, then deploy the stent.

How is an up-and-over angioplasty of the Superficial Femoral Artery (SFA) and Popliteal (Pop) artery performed?

a guidewire is carefully inserted via the contralateral femoral artery, followed by the placement of an up-and-over sheath. After arteriography, the guidewire is advanced across the lesion and balloon angioplasty is performed, concluding with a completion arteriography.

How can a self-expanding stent be tapered?

After guiding the wire through the iliac artery stenosis, deploy the self-expanding stent which tapers naturally with the artery's decreasing diameter, then perform angioplasty from the distal end to the larger proximal end of the stent.

Explain the"Telescope Effect"" observed when using balloon-expandable stent?

For a long iliac artery stenosis, place multiple stents starting with the distal (often smaller) one, then overlap with the proximal (often larger) one inside it to create a telescope effect, preventing metal edge protrusion into the flow stream.

How is a balloon-expandable stent typically placed?

Advance the dilator and sheath through the lesion, then, with the dilator removed, use introducer to set the stent on the balloon, guide it into the sheath, position it via fluoroscopy, expose it by withdrawing the sheath, and deploy it by inflating the balloon.

How can a balloon-expandable stent be tapered?

Guide the guidewire, sheath, and stent-mounted balloon through the iliac artery stenosis, deploy the stent to fit the external iliac artery, then use a larger balloon to expand the stent's top end, forming a slight taper at the iliac bifurcation.

SUBCLAVIAN

How is balloon angioplasty of the subclavian artery performed using a trans-femoral approach?

A guidewire is inserted across the lesion into the subclavian artery, followed by a long sheath with an angioplasty catheter, after which balloon angioplasty is performed on the lesion, and the procedure is concluded with completion arteriography.

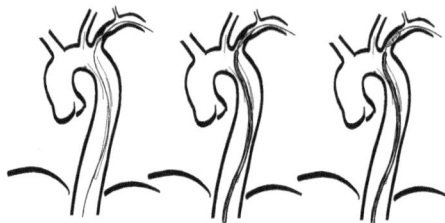

How is stent angioplasty of the subclavian artery performed using a trans-femoral approach?

This involves inserting a long sheath into the proximal subclavian artery, delivering and deploying the stent at the lesion site with caution to prevent sheath-stent engagement and proximity to the vertebral artery origin, followed by completion arteriography.

How is balloon angioplasty of the subclavian artery performed using a trans-brachial approach?

This involves placing a guidewire and sheath through a brachial artery, advancing a balloon catheter into the lesion for angioplasty, and performing completion arteriography post-withdrawal of the balloon.

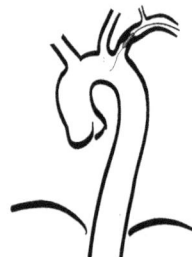

SUBINTIMAL ANGIOPLASTY

How to perform a subintimal angioplasty?

During an angioplasty, a sheath is positioned near the occlusion's origin, an angled-tip braided catheter points away from the largest proximal collateral, the Glidewire probes between the plaque and artery wall, forms a loop which is pushed forward until it re-enters the true lumen, supported and advanced by the catheter.

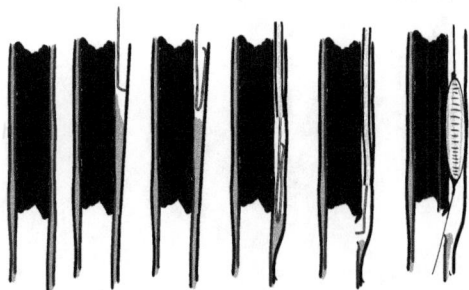

How can one navigate through the subintimal space during subintimal angioplasty?

Manage the guidewire loop effectively by incrementally advancing the catheter to support the guidewire, ensuring its narrowness for easy passage, cautiously advancing it when resistance is encountered, and avoiding excessive advancement that can lead to unpredictable patterns, to maintain its efficacy as a re-entry tool.

How can one perform the re-entry into the true lumen during subintimal angioplasty?

The procedure involves using contrast to visualize the distal segment, manipulating the guidewire and catheter within the true lumen, ensuring guidewire mobility, and confirming catheter placement via additional contrast.

How to use a re-entry catheter during subintimal angioplasty?

The guidewire and catheter, despite initial challenges in re-entry, are manoeuvred through the subintimal space past the arterial lesion and aligned with the true lumen, then a re-entry catheter is utilized, deploying a needle at the tip, which allows successful advancement of the guidewire into the true lumen, after which the needle and re-entry catheter are removed, leaving the guidewire in place.

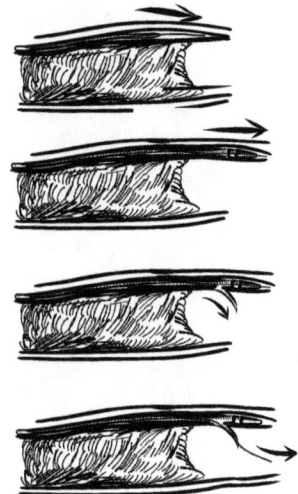

Provide some tips and tricks for performing a subintimal angioplasty?

Entering the subintimal space involves using a braided, stiff angled-tip catheter targeted at the plaque-artery interface, following the stump or the largest end-collateral with an angled Glidewire, while re-entering the true lumen can be achieved by advancing the guidewire into the distal artery stump, and if unsuccessful, balloon angioplasty, a stiff angled-tip catheter, or re-entry catheter can be employed.

TLR

What is meant by the term TLR (Target Lesion Revascularization)

TLR, or Target Lesion Revascularization, is a clinical term used in the context of vascular interventional procedures, such as angioplasty and stenting. It refers to the need for a repeat interventional procedure (such as angioplasty or stent placement) or surgical bypass operation at the specific site of the original treatment, due to the recurrence of significant narrowing or blockage of the blood vessel. This narrowing or blockage is often referred to as restenosis.

Target Lesion Revascularization (TLR) needed

In simpler terms, TLR is a measure of whether the treated section of a blood vessel remains open and functional or whether it narrows again, requiring another procedure to reopen it. It is a common endpoint in clinical studies evaluating the effectiveness of various vascular interventions, as a lower rate of TLR is generally seen as indicative of a more durable and successful initial procedure.

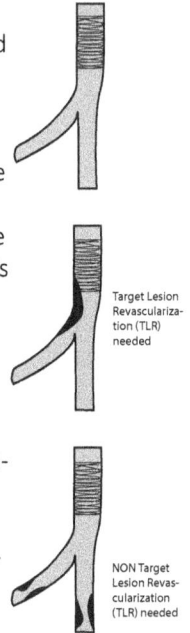

NON Target Lesion Revascularization (TLR) needed

CHAPTER 2
Iliac Endovascular Therapies Q&A

ILIAC CASE: 1

A 65-year-old patient presented with an intermittent claudication in the left leg. He had a previous EVAR done. Duplex scan showed significant narrowing in left iliac EVAR limb and increased flow velocity with possible dissection. A decision was agreed to re-align the left EVAR limb and treat the dissection.

READ CAREFULLY ...

Access	Pre Op checklist, supine, LA, cleaned and draped, Successful left groin puncture (retrograde) under ultrasound guidance
Equipments	Standard (Micro-access. J Wire. Glidewire+Cobra. Amplatz+Proglide. Pigtail. contrast+HepSaline) + Zilver Flex 10x100.
Angiogram Findings	Short dissection in left EIA, kinking of left limb of EVAR
Procedure	Amplatz wire passed through. Zilver Flex stent positioned and deployed
Complications	None observed during the procedure
Closure	Final angiogram demonstrated absence of dissection, closed with femseal

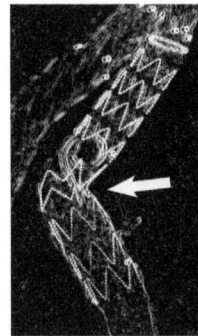

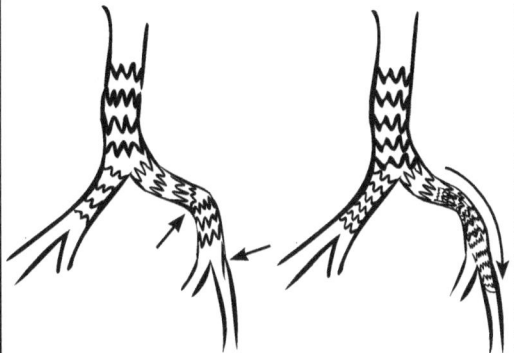

CONCISELY SUMMARIZE THE PROCEDURE USING KEY TERMS (ANSWER BELOW).

CHECK YOUR KNOWLEDGE

ON STRATEGY

When should a stenosis or kinking in the iliac EVAR limb be rectified?

If the severity is high and symptoms manifest in the patient, re-alignment is generally advised.

How pressing is the need for such a re-alignment?

It is of significant urgency, as neglecting it can lead to severe consequences.

While waiting for the re-alignment, what medication should the patient be on?

A mono antiplatelet is the primary recommendation, but there's also a consideration for dual antiplatelet or anticoagulation; however, concrete evidence on this is limited.

Which risk factors should be taken into account for predicting an iliac limb occlusion?

Factors include a small iliac bifurcation diameter, a tortuous and elongated iliac, the necessity for a limb extension, a small EIA diameter, and the absence of antiplatelet treatment.

ON ACCESS

Does contralateral access offer improved control during the procedure?

No. The process of cannulating the opposite limb in a patient who has previously undergone an EVAR can be complex. The extremely sharp division angle may also diminish the instruments' pushability and trackability.

How does a prior procedure affect access to the iliac lesion?

For those with a previous EVAR, there's a risk of dislodging the limb (refer to the Iliac 2 case). For those with a prior Fem-pop, the SFA or brachial route can be considered for smoother access.
In the case of a prior femoral endarterectomy, there's a need to be cautious about dislodging the intimal hyperplasia (as detailed in the following cases).

Is the contrast injected from the access sheath typically sufficient to visualize the CIA and areas above?

No. It's advisable to refrain from doing so as it introduces an unnecessary iodine burden and occasionally leads to dissection.

ON BALLOONING

Is it essential for the balloon to extend past the edge of the limb extension?

For a moulding balloon, it isn't. It's sufficient for the balloon to remain within the limits of the limb since the balloon's shoulder will naturally adjust to form the border.

ON STENTING

Is it suitable to choose a covered stent for iliac limb extension?

When addressing a type Ib endoleak, it is. But if it's to rectify a kink or dissection, it might not be the optimal selection for that situation.

In situations where there's a notable size difference between the EVAR limb and the EIA, what should be the dimension of the uncovered stent?

The size should be appropriate for the EIA, even if it doesn't match the EVAR iliac limb, as in this scenario. One might also think about employing a sandwich technique, as mentioned below.

IN-DEPTH ANALYSIS

SUMMARY OF PROCEDURE PERFORMED: EIA RE-ALIGNMENT OF A PREVIOUS EVAR LIMB. NO COMPLICATIONS.

In this case, the patient underwent an endovascular procedure to address a short dissection in the external iliac and kinking of the left limb of the EVAR. The use of ultrasound guidance for puncture and meticulous stent placement contributed to the success of the intervention, with no complications observed. The final angiogram's confirmation of the absence of dissection showcases the effectiveness of the chosen treatment strategy.

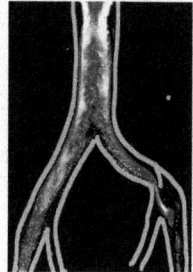

BIOMECHANICAL INSIGHT:

- The presence of the short dissection in the external iliac and the kinking of the left limb of the EVAR indicate the development of abnormal stress patterns, likely due to alterations in blood flow and shear stress within the vasculature. These stress patterns can lead to endothelial dysfunction, neointimal hyperplasia, and potentially graft failure.
- The choice of Zilver Flex stent's radial force, flexibility, and conformability to the vessel wall help alleviate the abnormal stress concentrations and facilitate a more uniform distribution of hemodynamic forces along the treated segment. This, in turn, minimizes the risk of restenosis and promotes long-term patency as compared to the previously dissected area.

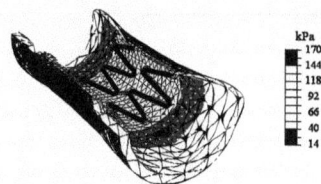

RESEARCH INSIGHT

- A systematic review and meta-analysis (2019) showed that adjunctive stenting is an effective prophylaxis for selected high risk limbs, yet intra-operative identification remains problematic. Most limb occlusions occur in the

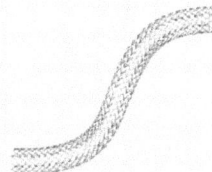

first year after EVAR, emphasising the importance of careful early follow up of high risk patients. In this meta-analysis, 179 at-risk limbs were treated by pre-emptive stenting, which significantly reduced the risk of limb occlusion: not pre-emptively stenting limbs at risk had a negative impact on graft limb patency (odds ratio 4.30).

- In a systematic review, a graft limb kink was present in 42.8% of all cases of graft limb occlusion.
- There are multiple identified risk factors for limb kinking and occlusion. The use of unsupported first-generation endografts was associated with a higher incidence of limb occlusion compared to second-generation supported endografts. Tortuosity of the iliac arteries is a significant cause of kinking and occlusion. Extending the deployment of the endograft into the external iliac artery (EIA) increases the risk of limb thrombosis due to compression or kinking, smaller device size, reduced blood flow, and hypogastric artery occlusion. A narrow distal aorta can complicate endograft deployment, but it is not a frequent cause of limb occlusion. Intra-graft mural thrombus and excessive stent over-sizing also contribute to the risk of limb occlusion.
- REF: PubMed. https://pubmed.ncbi.nlm.nih.gov/31514990/.

MODEL CASE:
Complications of Endovascular Stent Graft Repair

WATCH LIVE:
https://tinyurl.com/
32j9mxt3

NOTES, TIPS AND TRICKS:

ILIAC CASE: 2

A patient of 57 years of age presented with serious periodic claudication in the left lower extremity, having previously had a stent inserted in the left common iliac artery (CIA). He was found to have a blocked superficial femoral artery (SFA). A decision was agreed to perform an angioplasty on the blocked left SFA to re-establish blood circulation and relieve the patient's discomfort.

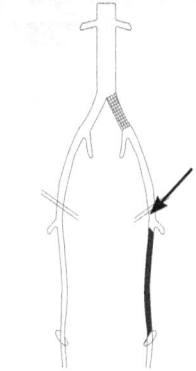

READ CAREFULLY ...

STAGE 1		STAGE 2		STAGE 3	
Access	Pre Op checklist, supine, LA, cleaned and draped, Rt CFA Successfully puncture under ultrasound guidance. 6 Fr sheath, up & over	**Access**	Left CFA cannulation (US-guided retrograde). 7Fr sheath.	**Access**	Via right femoral 7Fr sheath. Angiogram.
		Procedure	Snaring the wire from right groin to left, then tracking destination sheath from right to left over snared wire	**Findings**	Occluded left SFA, flow reconstitutes at adductor hiatus, PT & Peroneal patent, AT occludes distally
Equipments	Standard (Micro-access. J Wire. Glidewire+Cobra. Amplatz+Proglide. Pigtail. contrast+Hep-Saline). Later: 9x59 covered stent			**Procedure**	Attempting to cross SFA occlusion FAILED. Using Outback device, guidewire crossed occlusion FAILED as guidewire stuck in the Outback. POBA to CIA bilaterally and re-aligning left CIA stent.
Complication	Left CIA stent displacement occurred and unable to cannulate C/L iliac.			**Closure**	Femseal

CONCISELY SUMMARIZE THE PROCEDURE USING KEY TERMS (ANSWER BELOW).

CHECK YOUR KNOWLEDGE

ON ACCESS

What are the potential entry sites to treat the SFA occlusion and which one is highly recommended?

Ipsilateral Antegrade femoral: Often not appropriate due to the presence of flush sfa occlusion.
Ipsilateral Retrograde popliteal: It's feasible, but treating iliacs becomes an issue if they're diseased.
Contralateral Retrograde femoral: This might be the most effective and seamless method.

What risks arise from cannulating a stented iliac artery?

The insertion of the sheath might displace the stent

Is it simpler to access a stented iliac through the ipsilateral femoral or the contralateral femoral?

Typically, the ipsilateral approach is more straightforward since the contralateral method demands navigating a curve, which can shift the pressure to the vessel wall instead of maintaining it centralized. However, the ipsilateral approach is not commonly ideal for a direct SFA treatment.

ON RECANALISATION

If the attempt to cannulate the stented iliac from the opposite side is unsuccessful, yet the procedure (recanalization of a flush occlusion of the SFA) remains essential due to a non-healing ulcer, what's the alternative approach?

The next step would be to access through the ipsilateral retrograde femoral (on the left side for this instance), utilize the Safari technique, guide the sheath from the contralateral femoral using the wire, and then move forward with the SFA recanalization, operating from the right groin access such as in this case.

Could the outbreak device itself be the cause of a failed outbreak?

Yes, this could occur if the guidewire becomes trapped, as in this case.

IN-DEPTH ANALYSIS

SUMMARY OF PROCEDURE PERFORMED: Attempted left SFA angioplasty. CIA old stent dislodged. SFA not possible to canalize. bilateral CIA plasty done.

This case highlights the challenges faced where a previous intervention exists. The procedure encountered difficulties such as the displacement of the left CIA stent and unsuccessful attempts to cross the occluded left SFA. The ability to adapt and attempt alternative approaches, such as the use of a Safari wire technique, and the Outback device, demonstrates the importance of persistence and versatility in these procedures.

BIOMECHANICAL INSIGHT:
- The initial displacement of the CIA stent can be attributed to *forces exerted on stent edges during the tracking* of the destination sheath
- The occluded SFA presented a formidable obstacle due to its atheromatous plaque burden, and calcification, which *impeded guidewire advancement* and necessitated multiple attempts at recanalization.
- The use of the Outback device, a specialized re-entry catheter system, aimed to facilitate the successful crossing of the occluded SFA *by leveraging the principles of controlled subintimal dissection* and *targeted re-entry*. However, the wire became entrapped within the device, indicating a possible *issue with the deployment mechanics* or the interaction between the guidewire and the device's lumen.

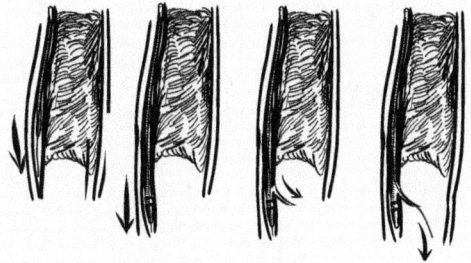

RESEARCH INSIGHT
- A systematic review of 87 studies and 4,665 patients looked at using subintimal angioplasty (SIA) and re-entry devices to cross femoropopliteal (FP) artery chronic total occlusions (CTOs). Re-entry devices (RED) was shown to further assist with true lumen re-entry. The procedural success rate ranged from 64.5%-100% (92.5% for SIA without RED, 88.3% for RED cases). The complication rate ranged from 1.6% - 28% among different studies (cumulative rates: SIA: 9.1%, RED 9.3%). Perforations occurred in 1.6% of the total population.

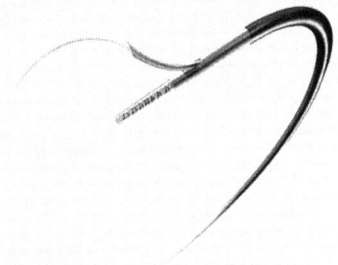

- **REF**: PubMed. https://pubmed.ncbi.nlm.nih.gov/31054801/.

MODEL CASE:
Multi Level Lower Limb Angioplasty
Through Contra-Lateral Access, <u>Outback
Re-Entry Device</u>, Femoral Artery Stenting,
Popliteal Artery Stenting, Btk Angioplasty

WATCH LIVE:
https://tinyurl.
com/4fxb5wwx

NOTES, TIPS AND TRICKS:

ILIAC CASE: 3

A 52-year-old IVDU patient presented with an infected large pseudoaneurysm in the right iliac fossa. CTA demonstrated a large pseudoaneurysm in the right EIA. A decision was agreed to use an EIA covered stent and surgically drain the infected Haematoma.

READ CAREFULLY ...

Access	Pre Op checklist, supine, GA , cleaned and draped, Successful puncture of left CFA (below injection sinus area) under ultrasound guidance. Up and Over approach.
Equipments	Standard (Micro-access. J Wire. Glidewire+Cobra. Amplatz+Proglide. Pigtail. contrast+HepSaline) + Viabhan 8x50 (x2).
Angiogram Findings	Near-occlusion of right EIA with a contrast blush.
Procedure	Amplatz wire passed through. 2x Viabhan covered stent positioned and deployed
Complications	None observed during the procedure
Closure	Final angiogram demonstrated brisk flow, closed with proglide

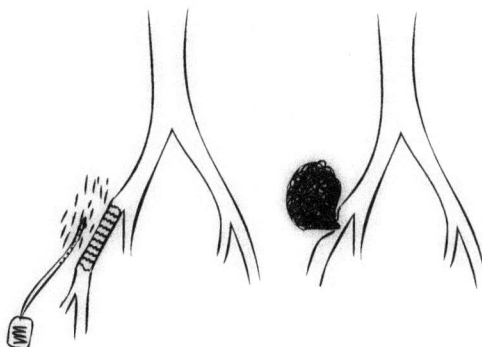

CONCISELY SUMMARIZE THE PROCEDURE USING KEY TERMS (ANSWER BELOW).

CHECK YOUR KNOWLEDGE

Qs ON ACCESS

Is securing USS-guided femoral access challenging in IVDU patients? Are there any other available options?

Yes, securing such access can be difficult because of the presence of scar tissue. In cases where it is difficult or fails, utilizing the SFA for access, and avoiding the groin injection sinus, serves as an alternative approach.

Qs ON RECANALISATION

What challenges do you foresee in achieving cannulation of this patient's EIA from the contralateral approach, extending down to the distal EIA and CFA?

There is a predisposition for the wire to navigate towards the pseudoaneurysm lumen rather than the distal EIA, as experienced in this case. This tendency not only jeopardizes the wire's stability, making it difficult to steer the destination sheath accordingly, but also poses a threat to the aneurysm wall.

In the event that contralateral cannulation is unsuccessful, what alternatives can be considered?

One potential solution could be to initiate access from the ipsilateral side, possibly targeting the SFA, and retrieving the other wire through the aneurysm lumen using a snare.

Qs ON STENTING

What covered stents would be suitable for use in this context?

Viabhan is ideal for emergency procedures involving EIA covered stents.

Is it probable that the stent will end up in the CFA? If so, is there a need for an additional stent?

Yes, it is probable that the stent will land in the CFA. In non-emergency situations involving non-infected IVDU patients, the use of a Supera stent could be considered.

Are Viabhan, Zilver, or Supera approved for use in the CFA?

None of them have received universal approval or licensing for use in the CFA.

Could you elaborate on the flexibility and contractibility of the EIA as it passes beneath the inguinal ligament?

The EIA exhibits a notable degree of mobility as it traces along the pelvic region and transitions into the femoral artery, facilitated by the connective tissue present in the area. This tissue not only anchors the artery but also permits a certain amount of movement, allowing the EIA to adjust to various changes in the positioning of the lower limbs and pelvis occurring during different activities, such as walking and sitting.

A notable filling defect was observed during the final angiography. What could be the cause of this, and how should we proceed?

The filling defect is likely a thrombus, stemming either from wire manipulation or directly from the pseudoaneurysm. Initial recommendation is to perform balloon angioplasty, which has proved successful in this case. Given the urgent nature of the situation, a degree of residual narrowing can be deemed acceptable.

Following the balloon angioplasty, another filling defect was detected. What would be the most prudent course of action, and why?

The appropriate response hinges on the patient's stability. Despite the potential risk to the stent, a conservative approach of not intervening may be reasonable, bearing in mind the probable necessity for stent extraction at a later date. Alternatively, a further balloon angioplasty might be considered. Introducing a supporting Zilver stent remains a contentious option due to the following concerns: a) introducing an additional foreign body to an infected site, and b) the foreseeable requirement to extend the Zilver to the SFA through the profunda, which would consequently influence the future ligation level..

IN-DEPTH ANALYSIS

Procedure : Cover stent to right EIA for a pseudoaneurysm + evacuation of an infected haematoma

Vascular complications and changes associated with IVDU can include:
1. Vessel damage: Repeated injections can lead to scarring, damage, or occlusion of the vessels, making it more challenging to visualize and access the CFA using ultrasound.
2. Infections: IVDU patients have an increased risk of developing local or systemic infections, such as cellulitis, abscess formation, or infective endocarditis, which can complicate the surrounding anatomy and hinder ultrasound-guided access.
3. Vessel wall changes: Chronic inflammation, venous insufficiency, and other vessel wall changes due to IVDU can alter the normal appearance and biomechanics of the CFA, making it more challenging to secure access.
4. Vascular anomalies: IVDU patients may have developed collateral circulation or vascular anomalies as a result of chronic damage to the vasculature, complicating ultrasound-guided access to the CFA.

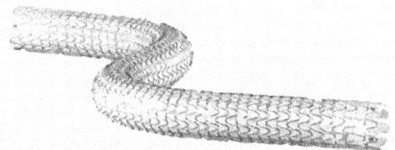

BIOMECHANICAL INSIGHT:
- An essential factor is the **flexibility of the stent**. Given the location in the iliac artery, the stent needs to **accommodate physiological movements** such as hip flexion and extension. The stent's design should allow

for a balance between flexibility and radial strength - a stent that is too flexible might collapse under external pressure, while a stent that is too rigid might not accommodate natural bodily movements.

- The **material properties** of the stent are also crucial. Stents made from nitinol, a nickel-titanium alloy, are commonly used because of their **super-elasticity and shape memory characteristics**. These properties allow the stent to **withstand deformation** and recover its shape **without significant loss of mechanical strength**.

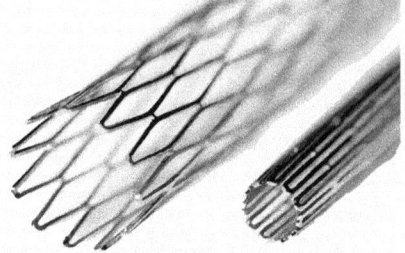

RESEARCH INSIGHT

- A systematic review was conducted on the efficacy and outcome of endovascular treatment of infected iliofemoral arterial pseudoaneurysms with covered stents.
- 35 cases were identified, with 22 pseudoaneurysms located in the femoral area and 13 in the iliac vessels.
- The most common complaints were pulsatile groin mass, sepsis, active bleeding, and groin infection with purulent discharge. S. aureus and Streptococcus species were the most common microbes isolated.
- Factors for the development of infected pseudoaneurysms included intravenous drug use, infection of anastomosis in bypass surgery, cancer, history of multiple hip operations, renal transplantation, and obesity.
- The most commonly used covered stents were Viabhan, Jostent, Fluency, and Wallgraft. In 15 cases, surgical debridement and/or drainage was also performed.
- The mean follow-up was 15.8 months. There were only 2 cases of stent graft thrombosis and 2 patients required an open vascular bypass procedure at a later stage. One death was attributed to procedure-related complications.
- The infection rate of the deployed stent graft in follow-up was 3.4%.
- **REF**: Vasa. 2017 Jan;46(1):5-9.

ILIAC CASE: 4

A 65-year-old patient presented with multiple ulcers and necrosis in the right foot. CTA demonstrated stenotic CFA and occluded right EIA. A decision was agreed to do a right CFA endartrectomy (CFAe) with profundoplasty and iliac recanalisation.

READ CAREFULLY ...

Access	Pre Op checklist, supine, GA, cleaned and draped, Successful CFA Endarteerctomy Performed.
Procedure	Attempt to recanalise the EIA failed. A decision was made to move to a left-to-right fem-fem crossover as patient has a critical ischaemic leg and ulcers

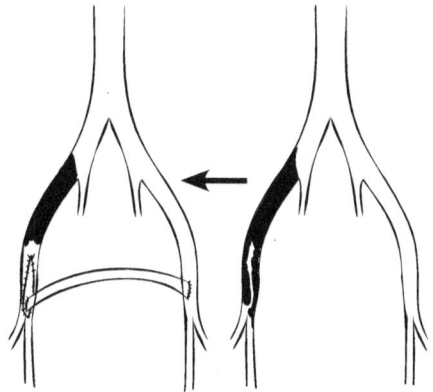

CONCISELY SUMMARIZE THE PROCEDURE USING KEY TERMS (ANSWER BELOW).

CHECK YOUR KNOWLEDGE

Qs ON ACCESS

What is the optimal approach for accessing and managing EIA occlusion during the planning stage of CFA endartrectomy?

An advisable strategy could be to initially puncture the CFA to allow the introduction of a guidewire into the EIA, assuming it is patent. Following this step, undertake CFA endarterectomy, potentially succeeded by balloon angioplasty into the iliac and, if necessary, stenting.

Qs ON RECANALISATION

What are the frequent causes of unsuccessful iliac plasty following CFA endartrectomy?

What are the primary challenges in addressing extensively calcified iliac lesions?

Failures in iliac plasty post-CFA endarterectomy can occur due to issues such as the inability to pass the wire, difficulties in re-entering the lumen, or the onset of significant dissection.

- Assessing calcification extent is challenging, may need advanced imaging like IVUS.
- Severe calcification hinders endovascular navigation and limits conventional treatments.
- Resistant lesions might need alternative strategies like atherectomy or lithoplasty.
- Treating calcification can cause complications, requiring further interventions or surgical procedures.
- If endovascular treatments are nonviable, bypass surgery or endarterectomy may be considered.
- Treatment needs risk-benefit analysis, considering patient's health factors.
- Severe femoropopliteal calcification management requires a multidisciplinary team for optimal outcomes.

IN-DEPTH ANALYSIS

Procedure : ATTEMPTED ILIAC PLASTY FOLLOWING CFA ENDARTERECTOMY 03/2017 - UNABLE TO BREAK BACK. A DECISION WAS MADE TO PROCEED TO A LEFT-TO-RIGHT FEM-FEM CROSSOVER AS PATIENT HAS A CRITICAL ISCHAEMIC LEG AND ULCERS.

This case reflects a complex vascular procedure involving attempted recanalisation of the External Iliac Artery (EIA) following a Right Common Femoral Artery (CFA) endarterectomy and profundo-plasty. The re-entry was not possible, suggesting a significant occlusion or other structural issue. The decision to transition to a left to right femoral-femoral crossover bypass, which is a more complex procedure, underscores the criticality of the situation, particularly given the patient was under general anaesthesia and had critical limb ischemia (CLI). This highlights the importance of flexibility and adaptability in vascular surgery when faced with unexpected intraoperative findings.

HAEMODYNAMIC INSIGHT:

The iliac artery stent and femoro-femoral (fem-fem) crossover grafting are two different approaches to restoring blood flow in the presence of peripheral artery disease, specifically iliac artery occlusion. They differ not only in terms of invasiveness, but also in terms of the haemodynamics they induce.

Endovascular stenting of the iliac artery is a less invasive procedure. The benefit of this procedure is that it *preserves the native artery and normal flow direction*, which is less likely to have an impact on overall haemodynamics. It *enables physiological, antegrade flow*.

Fem-fem crossover grafting, on the other hand, is a more invasive surgical procedure. Some *retrograde flow is introduced* into the system by this procedure, potentially *increasing shear stress* and *turbulence* and affecting endothelial function and graft patency. Furthermore, the graft can cause a *"steal" phenomenon*, in which blood is diverted away from the native artery, potentially jeopardising flow to areas still served by the native circulation.

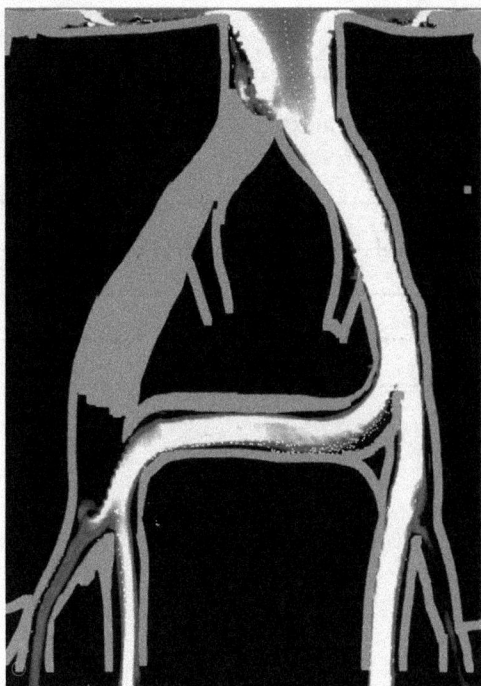

RESEACH INSIGHT

- Due to the successful endovascular treatment of extensive stenoses and occlusions of the iliac arteries, femoral–femoral artery bypass is now uncommonly performed for arterial occlusive disease. Combined iliac artery stenting and femoral–femoral artery bypass is indicated in patients with unilateral long occlusions of the common iliac and/or external iliac artery, with or without involvement of the ipsilateral common femoral artery, and stenosis or relatively focal occlusion of the contralateral (donor) iliac arteries, with or without contralateral (donor) common femoral artery stenosis.

- **REF.**
- (1) Combined Iliac Stenting and Fem-fem Bypass | Thoracic Key. https://thoracickey.com/combined-iliac-stenting-and-fem-fem-bypass/.
- (2) Femorofemoral (Femoral-Femoral) Bypass - Medscape. https://emedicine.medscape.com/article/1830260-overview.

MODEL CASE:	**WATCH LIVE:**	
bilateral internal iliac artery stenting via a 4F access site	https://tinyurl.com/4e68vynh	

NOTES, TIPS AND TRICKS:

ILIAC CASE: 5

A 74-YEAR-OLD PATIENT CAME IN WITH SEVERE INTERMITTENT CLAUDICATION AF-
FECTING THE LEFT LEG AND HAD PREVIOUSLY UNDERGONE A LEFT CFA ENDARTEREC-
TOMY. A DECISION WAS AGREED TO PERFORM AN ANGIOPLASTY ON THE PROXIMAL
LEFT CIA STENOSIS AND SFA OCCLUSION.

READ CAREFULLY ...

Access	Pre Op checklist, supine, GA , cleaned and draped, Retrograde right femoral; then difficult left CFA access to do the iliacs.
Equipments	Standard (Micro-access. J Wire. Glidewire+Cobra. Amplatz+Proglide. Pigtail. contrast+HepSaline) + POBAs and Atrium stent 6x35.
Angiogram Findings	Confirmed proximal left CIA stenosis and left proximal SFA stenosis with midsection occlusion
Procedure	Utilized rim catheter for Terumo passage into left SFA; occlusion intraluminally traversed; wire exchanged to Amplatz; performed SFA angioplasty with 4mm x 20 cm POBA; Wire reveresed into Aorta. challanging Left CFA access but done. Placed two 6mm x 35mm Atrium stents in iliacs; improved appearance via further 6mm x 4cm POBA dilation
Complications	Left femoral access closed. Check angiogram via right access revealed no flow in left EIA and CFA. conducted cutdown; exposed and controlled left CFA/SFA/PFA vessels; removed significant intimal hyperplasia; restored inflow/outflow; closed patch with 5.0 prolene. Further angio: No flow in SFA. Further arteriotomy through patch and fogarty passed and further intima retrieved. Good flow achieved.
Closure	closed incision in layers

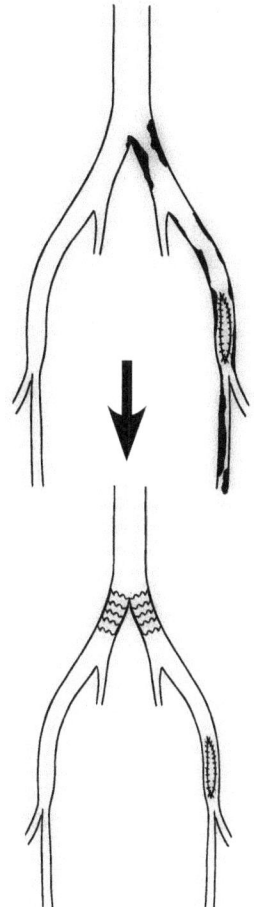

CONCISELY SUMMARIZE THE PROCEDURE USING KEY TERMS (ANSWER BELOW).

CHECK YOUR KNOWLEDGE

Qs ON STRATEGY

In case of bilateral CIA lesions and SFA lesions. Which one should be treated first?

Iliacs (inflow) first usually; but not in a combined case like this.

Qs ON ACCESS

What is the best access path to support this treatment?

Utilizing a contralateral access initially to address the distal (SFA) lesion is recommended, followed by an ipsilateral approach complemented by the deployment of a kissing stent.

Qs ON RECANALIZATION

What complication can occur in accessing a previously patched femoral artery?

Intimal hyperplasia can dislodge and block the artery

Can high dose of heparin prevent patch hyperplasia from dislodging? What can do so?

No. Ensuring meticulous surgical techniques is essential in preventing patch hyperplasia dislodge.

Qs ON COMPLICATIONS

What is the preferred course of action if the CFA/EIA become occluded after angioplasty?

Traditionally, the favoured method has been to undertake an open approach. Another possibility is to try recanalizing the affected area, followed by considering primary stenting as a viable option.

Is utilizing a covering sheath essential while traversing the iliac lesion prior to the placement of a balloon-mounted stent?

It is only deemed necessary in cases where the iliac lesion is extremely tight, creating a risk for the stent to become dislodged before achieving the correct position.

IN-DEPTH ANALYSIS

Procedure : KISSING ILIAC STENTS/SFA POBA PLASTY. COMPLICATED WITH OCCLUDED **CFA.** NEEDED OPEN APPROACH, PATCH AND EMBOLECTOMY TO **SFA**

COMMENTS:

- This case highlights the critical importance of contingency planning and adaptive strategies in interventional procedures. It illustrates the challenges often faced in vascular interventions, specifically when access through a previously repaired and patched CFA is involved. The initial complication, characterized by the absence of flow in the external iliac and common femoral arteries, required a calculated decision to undertake a cutdown and subsequent exposure of the left CFA/SFA/PFA. The substantial volume of intimal hyperplasia discovered highlights the often-unanticipated complexities that can occur even after a successful angioplasty and stenting procedure.
- Furthermore, the follow-up arteriotomy through the patch and the retrieval of further intima underscore the necessity for vigilance and the willingness to address complications iteratively, until a successful outcome is achieved. This sequence of events emphasizes the need for continued diligence, flexibility, and technical skill in interventional medicine.

BIOMECHANICS INSIGHT:

- The significant stenosis in the left CIA and SFA suggests a high degree of arteriosclerosis, which would *increase the rigidity and reduce the elasticity* of the arterial walls. This can complicate both the initial access and the passage of guidewires and catheters, as demonstrated by the difficulties encountered in gaining retrograde access to the left CFA.
- The kissing stents technique employed here would have allowed for a *more uniform and balanced radial force distribution* in the aorta's bifurcation area, helping maintain luminal patency.
- The hyperplastic intima indicates a significant response to previous vascular injury, which *altered the biomechanical behavior* of the vessel. By excising this hyperplastic intima, it was possible *restored a more normal hemodynamic flow,* reducing the likelihood of restenosis.

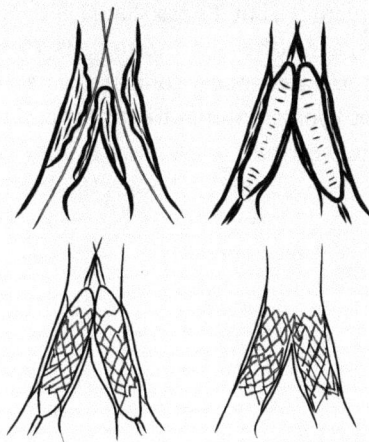

HAEMODYNAMIC INSIGHT:

- The previously patched CFA and subsequent intimal hyperplasia led to reduced luminal diameter, increasing the *resistance to blood flow according to Poiseuille's law*. The resulting *increased shear stress* on the vessel walls can further induce *vascular remodelling*, contributing to the significant intimal hyperplasia encountered. The hyperplasia, in turn, presents another hemodynamic obstacle, as it further reduces luminal diameter and ***disrupts smooth laminar flow,*** leading to ***turbulent flow*** and increased likelihood of thrombosis.

- The unusual Proglide closure on the left and subsequent cutdown showed an occlusion, possibly due to a combination of the residual hyperplastic intima and ***the physical pressure of the closure device*** disrupting the ***delicate hemodynamic balance*** within the vessel.
- The further arteriotomy, intima retrieval, and patch closure demonstrate a good understanding of the importance of achieving optimal hemodynamics. This follow-up intervention was essential to restore streamlined flow, thereby reducing the risk of turbulent flow patterns that could precipitate further complications such as stent occlusion.

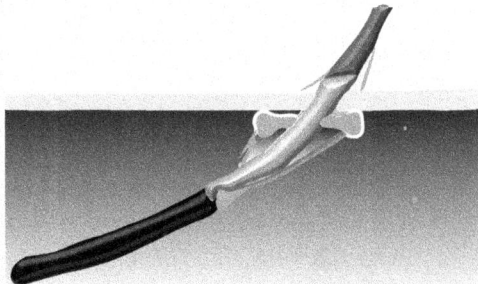

EVIDENCE INSIGHT:

- Historically, open repair was the go-to treatment for aortoiliac disease, boasting patency rates of 72–90% over 10 years for aortobifemoral grafting. Current guidelines still consider this approach optimal for multi-segment diseases and occlusions. However, advancements in technical skill and endovascular equipment are starting to challenge this. Evidence of this shift includes an 850% increase in angioplasty and stenting for aortoiliac occlusive disease, concurrent with a 15.5% decrease in aortobifemoral grafting.
- Open bypass maintains superior long-term primary patency rates compared to endovascular intervention, but it's associated with higher operative morbidity, mortality, longer hospital stays, and higher short-term costs. Further complicating the choice of treatment, secondary patency rates appear comparable between open and endovascular procedures. Extra-anatomic bypass, another treatment option, is typically reserved for patients unable to undergo anatomic bypass or endovascular therapy, but its clinical outcomes are inferior to both.
- REF. Mo Med. 2021 Jul-Aug;118(4):381-386.

ILIAC CASE: 6

An 81-year-old patient presented with severe intermittent claudication in the right leg. Duplex scan showed significant disease and occluded right iliacs. A decision was agreed to perform iliac recanalisation.

READ CAREFULLY ...

Access	Pre Op checklist, supine, LA , cleaned and draped, Retrograde right femoral; Terumo wire navigation with a sheathless CXI catheter used due to sheath advancement difficulty, followed by an Amplatz wire change and 7F bright tip sheath insertion. On the left side, a 7F bright tip sheath was placed without complication.
Equipments	Standard (Micro-access. J Wire. Glidewire+Cobra. Amplatz+Proglide. Pigtail. contrast+HepSaline) + V12 stent 10x59. Zilver Flex
Angiogram Findings	Initial angiogram from left showed occluded right CIA.
Procedure	Bilateral iliac stents (right: 10mmx59mm v12, left: 10mmx38 v12) placed at the aortic bifurcation. Right-side stent delivered through a 7F destination sheath and further extended with an additional 8mmx59mm v12 stent and a Zilver Flex. Angiogram revealed a proximal shelf right side. Proximal extension of the kissing iliac stents with 2x 10x59mm v12 done.
Complications	Satisfactory bilateral CFA perfusion.
Closure	Standard

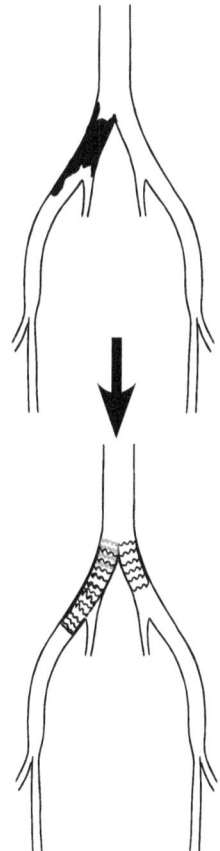

CONCISELY SUMMARIZE THE PROCEDURE USING KEY TERMS (ANSWER BELOW).

CHECK YOUR KNOWLEDGE

Qs ON ACCESS

If advancing the entry sheath proves impossible, what alternatives are available?

Options include manoeuvring with a terumo and utilizing a small (CXI) catheter, or attempting access from the opposite side.

Qs ON STENTING

What can be done in the case of discovering a proximal shelf post-kissing stent implementation?

One strategy could be to extend it from the other side.

Is utilizing a V12 mandatory when extending a kissing stent shelf?

Yes

IN-DEPTH ANALYSIS

Procedure : KISSING ILIAC STENTS. DIFFICULT ACCESS RIGHT FEMORAL. NEEDED **CXI** SHEATH-LESS AND TERUMOR. ILIAC STENT NEEDED 2 EXTENSIONS **V12** AND ZILVER FLEX

COMMENTS:

- The initial difficulty with sheath advancement on the right CFA demonstrates the need for alternative tools and methods, such as the terumo wire with a sheathless CXI catheter in this instance. The challenge was appropriately managed without converting to a more invasive procedure, maintaining patient safety.
- The second complication, identification of a proximal shelf during the angiogram, highlights the importance of intraprocedural imaging for quality control and ensuring optimal outcomes. The ability to identify and immediately address this issue by extending the kissing iliac stents proximally prevented potential post-procedure complications like stent thrombosis or occlusion, ultimately enhancing patient prognosis.

BIOMECHANICS INSIGHT:

- The procedural adaptability demonstrated here – using a terumo wire in conjunction with a sheathless CXI catheter – is crucial when dealing with complex vascular anatomies or calcified vessels that may provide resistance. The manipulation of the wire and catheter navigation would be impacted by vascular resistance, tortuosity, and pressure gradients.
- The insertion and extension of the iliac stents (kissing stents) highlight the need to consider the forces exerted on these devices. Notably, radial force (which maintains the stent's patency), longitudinal force (which may lead to stent deformation or migration), and external forces from the pulsatile nature of blood flow or movements of the surrounding tissues.
- The use of 'kissing stents' in the aortic bifurcation also brings up biomechanical considerations related to ensuring parallel stent placement, managing potential device-device interaction, and maintaining proper scaffolding to allow physiological splitting of blood flow into the iliac arteries.

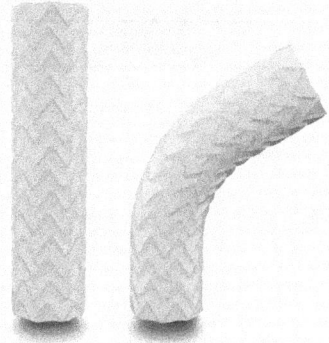

HAEMODYNAMIC INSIGHT:

- The discovery and management of the proximal shelf highlight the essential role of *shear stress* in endothelial function and thrombus formation. A shelf could cause *local disruptions in laminar blood flow*, leading to an area of <u>low</u> shear stress, which is associated with platelet <u>activation</u> and coagulation cascade <u>initiation</u>, potentially resulting in thrombosis. The proactive decision to extend the stents proximally to cover this shelf would restore laminar flow, reducing thrombogenic risk.
- Proper placement of kissing stents is crucial to maintain the Y-shaped bifurcation flow dynamics, ensuring a balanced flow distribution to the iliac arteries and reducing the risk of stent thrombosis or restenosis.

EVIDENCE INSIGHT:
- A meta-analysis to evaluate the technical and clinical outcomes of aortoiliac occlusive disease (AIOD) treatment using the kissing stent technique included 605 patients from a subset of 22 suitable studies, showed an overall primary patency rate of 81% at 24 months. Age being a significant predictor of sustained primary patency.
- REF: J Endovasc Ther. 2019 Feb;26(1):31-40.

MODEL CASE:	WATCH LIVE:	
Right common iliac artery stenosis and heavy calcified complex popliteal lesion	https://tinyurl. com/3srahs6n	

NOTES, TIPS AND TRICKS:

ILIAC CASE: 7

A 79-year-old patient presented with a short distance claudication in the left leg. Duplex scan showed significant disease in left iliacs. A decision was agreed to perform a left iliac angioplasty.

READ CAREFULLY ...

Access	Pre Op checklist, supine, LA , cleaned and draped, retrograde left CFA micropuncture with ultrasound guidance, utilizing a 7 Fr sheath.
Equipments	Standard (Micro-access. J Wire. Glidewire+Cobra. Amplatz+Proglide. Pigtail. contrast+HepSaline) + BeGraft 9mm x 30mm balloon expandable covered stent
Angiogram Findings	severe proximal stenosis in a short segment of the proximal left common iliac.
Procedure	Placement of a 9mm x 30mm BeGraft balloon-expandable covered stent. Achieved positive post-procedural angiographic outcomes with preserved three-vessel runoff below the knee.
Complications	No immediate complications observed post-procedure.
Closure	6/7Fr Mynx for hemostasis.

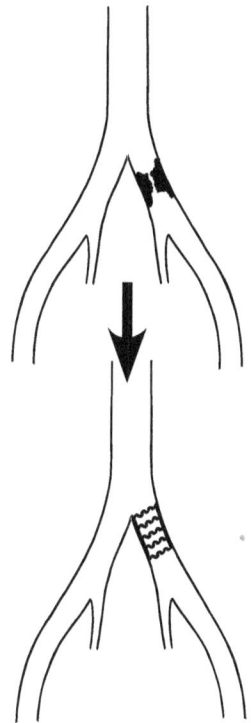

CONCISELY SUMMARIZE THE PROCEDURE USING KEY TERMS (ANSWER BELOW).

CHECK YOUR KNOWLEDGE

Qs ON RECANALISATION

Does the path of the wire alter in the presence of a severe stenotic lesion?

Yes, this can be observed in the angiography.

Qs ON BALLOONING

In the case of an isolated severe iliac stenosis, does POBA offer advantages compared to a primary stenting strategy?

A covered primary stenting approach is generally safer and potentially more effective.

Qs ON STENTING

Is the Bentley BeGraft appropriate for use in the iliac system?

Yes

How does BeGraft diameter relate to inflation pressure and size?

There is a positive correlation between diameter and pressure, and a negative correlation between diameter and length. Refer to the specific chart for detailed information.

IN-DEPTH ANALYSIS

PROCEDURE : ILIAC STENT. LEFT STANDARD RETROGRADE. SUCCESSFUL

COMMENTS:

- Iliac stenting is a commonly used procedure to treat aortoiliac occlusive disease. Covered balloon-expandable (CBE) stents are a viable treatment option for patients with complex aortoiliac lesions because of their high rates of technical success and favorable patency across all devices at 12 months.

- One such CBE stent is the BeGraft balloon expandable covered stent. It has mainly been used as a proximal extension to an iliac branch device (IBD) for endovascular repair of isolated common iliac artery aneurysms, but can also be used for a different indication such as the case in here. The BeGraft covered stent is deployed and a second balloon is used to further dilate the proximal part of the stent to allow adequate sealing in the proximal common iliac artery.

- REF:

- A systematic review of covered balloon-expandable stents for treating .... https://www.sciencedirect.com/science/article/pii/S0741521420310818.

- The BeGraft Balloon Expandable Covered Stent as a Proximal Extension to .... https://ris.utwente.nl/ws/portalfiles/portal/84392460/BeGraft.pdf.

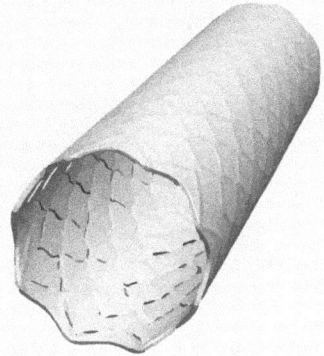

BIOMECHANICS INSIGHT:

- The BeGraft and BeGraft+ stent-grafts are made of a cobalt-chromium alloy covered in expanded polytetrafluoroethylene (ePTFE). Cobalt-chromium alloys have enabled a *reduction in stent strut thickness* while retaining modest radiopacity.

- The alloy also offers *superior radial force*, ensuring optimal luminal gain and resisting vascular recoil. The radial force is crucial in a *high-pressure environment* like the iliac artery, and the stent's *high mechanical durability* ensures it maintains its structural integrity over time.

- The balloon-expandable nature of this stent is crucial in *accurate deployment* and attaining the precise fit within the stenotic area. This not only maximizes the immediate luminal diameter but also *minimizes geographical miss*, an important factor in reducing restenosis risk.

- *Geographic miss (GM) is a term* used to describe a poorly deployed stent (mainly coronary) or a stent missing (part of) a lesion. GM includes longitudinal mismatches, where the injured or diseased segment is not covered by the stent, and axial mismatches, where the balloon-artery size ratio is either less than 0.9 or greater than 1.3. IVUS has been shown to decrease the incidence of GM.

HAEMODYNAMIC INSIGHT:

- The stent placement in the common iliac artery has restored a more physiological flow pattern, relieving the previously increased pressure gradient across the lesion.

- The BeGraft balloon-expandable covered stent and its capability to adapt to the diameter of the lesion due to its balloon-expandability, provides an optimal diameter for laminar flow.

Laminar flow is crucial to avoid turbulent flow that can lead to increased shear stress on the vessel wall. The PTFE covered stent offers a smooth luminal surface reducing the wall shear stress and endothelial cell activation.

- The appropriate sizing of the stent (9mm x 30mm) contribute to preventing flow disturbances, such as the creation of a flow jet (if stent is smaller) or the development of post-stenotic turbulence (if stent is bigger), both of which could incite endothelial dysfunction and neointimal proliferation.

ILIAC CASE: 8

A 79-year-old patient with uncontrolled AF presented with an acute ischaemic legs. CTA scan showed extensive embolus in both iliacs and SFAs. A decision was agreed to perform bilateral embolectomy and angiography +/- proceed.

READ CAREFULLY ...

Access	Pre Op checklist, supine, GA , cleaned and draped, Bilateral CFA/SFA/PFA exposure and control of vessels.
Equipments	Standard (Micro-access. J Wire. Glidewire+Cobra. Amplatz+Proglide. Pigtail. Contrast+HepSaline) + POBA
Angiogram Findings	Efficient flow through left iliac system, Right EIA exhibits stenosis
Procedure	Bilateral proximal and distal femoral embolectomies, Bovine pericardial patch plasty done bilaterally, Retrograde access via right patch with aortic pigtail, Right EIA POBA with 7mm x 40mm balloon
Complications	No immediate complications observed
Closure	sutures

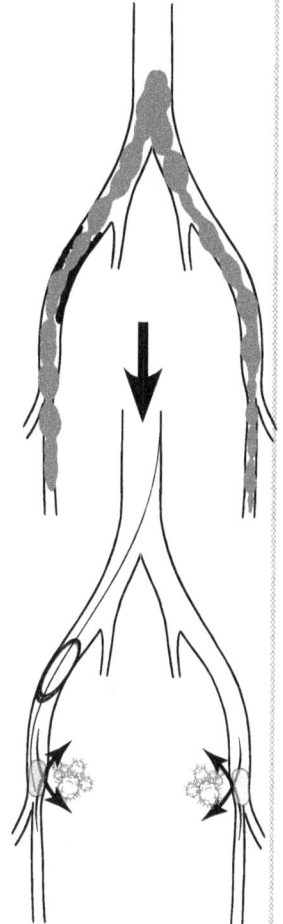

CONCISELY SUMMARIZE THE PROCEDURE USING KEY TERMS (ANSWER BELOW).

CHECK YOUR KNOWLEDGE

Qs ON RECANALISATION

Should the CFAE be extended further proximally in the presence of EIA occlusion?

Yes, it should encompass the region beneath the inguinal ligament because a patch in this area is anticipated to better resist repeated compressions from the inguinal ligament compared to a stent.

How much mobility is observed in the EIA-femoral region?

The EIA-femoral area maintains relative stability between the branches, including the IIA and PFA. However, hip flexion can induce bending effects on the CIA.

IN-DEPTH ANALYSIS

PROCEDURE : ILIAC STENT. LEFT STANDARD RETROGRADE. SUCCESSFUL

COMMENTS:
- Notice the dual-stage approach to the restoration of blood flow. Firstly, the embolectomies were performed, followed by a patch plasty bilaterally, which is a robust, time-tested technique to restore arterial integrity and re-establish flow.
- Secondly, the focal point of the procedure is the treatment of the right EIA stenosis. The use of Percutaneous Transluminal Angioplasty (POBA) with a 7mm x 40mm balloon is a well-planned, targeted intervention. Such a procedure is generally associated with a good success rate. However, the inherent risk of recurrence of restenosis after POBA is worth noting. If this complication arises, a repeat angioplasty or alternative methods such as stenting may be necessary to maintain an open and functional EIA.

BIOMECHANICS INSIGHT:
- The femoral patches applied bilaterally are in close proximity to the inguinal ligament, a crucial anatomical landmark separating the femoral and external iliac arteries. The inguinal ligament's potential effect on the patch can be considerable due to the dynamic nature of the ligament, given its role in hip flexion and its position across the anterior aspect of the hip joint. The inguinal ligament during hip flexion could induce strain on the patch, potentially leading to its deformation, and compensatory thickening and intimal hyperplasia over time. This makes the material selection and the securement of the patch critically important.
- Treating the EIA stenosis located near the inguinal ligament is essential, as the biomechanical stresses associated with hip flexion could exacerbate the hemodynamic impact of this stenosis. Specifically, the dynamic compressive forces of the ligament on the EIA during hip flexion might potentially reduce the effective lumen of the artery, resulting in a critical hemodynamic compromise, especially during periods of increased lower limb demand.

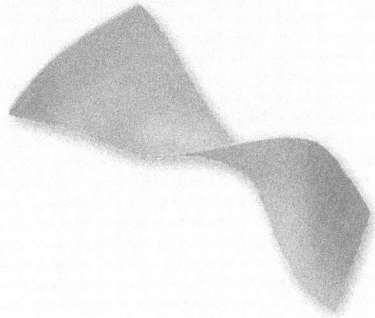

HAEMODYNAMIC INSIGHT:
- The goal of patch plasty procedure is not only to repair the arteriotomy site but also to ensure the maintenance of an *optimal lumen diameter* post-embolectomy, which directly influences the haemodynamics through the modified Hagen-Poiseuille equation*. An appropriately sized lumen will facilitate laminar blood flow and minimise turbulent flow, thus reducing vascular resistance and enhancing tissue perfusion downstream.
- The stenosis in the right EIA poses a significant haemodynamic challenge. Stenosis *increases resistance* to blood flow, governed by the principles of the Bernoulli's equation, leading to

a *higher pressure gradient across* the narrowed segment of the artery. This could result in *decreased downstream perfusion*, ischaemia and, ultimately, claudication symptoms.

- * A physical law that gives the pressure drop in an incompressible and Newtonian fluid in laminar flow flowing through a long cylindrical pipe of constant cross section.

EVIDENCE INSIGHT:

- Surgical arterial thromboembolectomy remains a cornerstone treatment for acute limb ischemia (ALLI) due to its efficiency and simplicity, even providing a training opportunity for less experienced personnel. Catheter-directed thrombolysis, while initially fraught with complications, has evolved into a less invasive alternative with wider clinical applications. Recently, endovascular interventions, particularly percutaneous mechanical thrombectomy devices, are gaining prominence, although the quest for optimally effective systems without unwanted complications continues.

ILIAC CASE: 9

A 65-year-old patient presented with a non-healing ulcer on left foot. The patient has had radiotherapy to prostate cancer. Duplex scan showed occluded Rt EIA, with small and diseased iliac tree. A decision was agreed to proceed to iliac angioplasty +/- stenting.

READ CAREFULLY ...

Access	Pre Op checklist, supine, GA , cleaned and draped, Bilateral CFAs micropunctured via ultrasound. Sheaths: 4Fr, later upsized to 6Fr..
Equipments	Standard (Micro-access. J Wire. Glidewire+Cobra. Amplatz+Proglide. Pigtail. contrast+HepSaline). Mustang balloon. Zilver flex stents.
Angiogram Findings	Reduced arterial tree diameter in pelvis, likely due to prior radiotherapy. Right EIA shows ~8cm occlusion and disease and disease at iliac bifurcation. Moderate stenosis in left EIA.
Procedure	Subintimal wire and catheter manipulation across stenosis. Retrograde lumen crossing unsuccessful, antegrade re-entry achieved from the left with a standard Terumo, exchanged to a stiff wire. Right EIA stented with 6mm x 8cm and 6mm x 6cm Zilver flex stents. Angioplasty of right and left EIA with 4mm x 8cm Mustang balloon and 5mm x 4cm standard angioplasty balloon respectively.
Complications	Dissection observed at left EIA site. 6mm x 6cm Zilver flex stent placed in left EIA.
Closure	Hemostasis via manual compression.

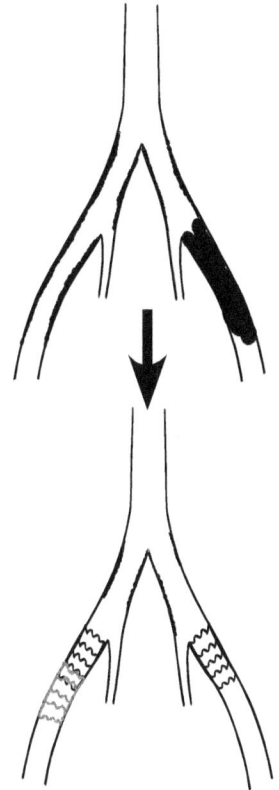

CONCISELY SUMMARIZE THE PROCEDURE USING KEY TERMS (ANSWER BELOW).

CHECK YOUR KNOWLEDGE

Qs ON STRATEGY

What impact does radiotherapy have on iliac arteries?

Radiotherapy can cause iliac arteries to become smaller and more rigid.

Qs ON RECANALISATION

Is utilizing subintimal access appropriate for iliac arteries impacted by radiotherapy?

Yes

Qs ON BALLOONING

Is angioplasty an appropriate treatment for iliac arteries that have been impacted by radiotherapy?

Yes

Qs ON STENTING

Is stenting an appropriate approach for iliac arteries affected by radiotherapy?

Yes

IN-DEPTH ANALYSIS

PROCEDURE : EIA OCCLUSION. FAILED SUBINTIMAL. SUCCESSFUL UP AND OVER FROM LEFT. STENTING. COMPLICATION: DISSECTION. ZILVER FLEX.

COMMENTS:
- This case presented a challenging one of bilateral external iliac artery (EIA) disease, likely complicated by prior pelvic radiotherapy. The right EIA featured a significant occlusion and additional disease at the iliac bifurcation, while the left EIA showed moderate stenosis.
- The successful antegrade re-entry on the left side after failing to cross retrograde into the lumen was essential. The use of Zilver flex stents and angioplasty resulted in an improved arterial flow. The observed dissection at the left EIA site, while a notable complication demonstrates the inherent risks of these procedures.

BIOMECHANICS INSIGHT:
- This case demonstrates a complex interplay of haemodynamics and tissue mechanics, particularly with respect to vascular elasticity, compliance, and fluid dynamics.
- In this case, the initial findings of a small calibre arterial tree in the pelvis may suggest altered vascular compliance due to previous radiotherapy.
- The dissection noted in the left EIA site represents an escalation in the biomechanical complexity. Dissection involves mechanical disruption of the arterial wall layers, altering its biomechanical characteristics and leading to potential destabilisation. Careful management is crucial to prevent worsening of the dissection and maintain hemodynamic stability.

HAEMODYNAMIC INSIGHT:
- The smaller than typical arterial tree within the pelvis, likely secondary to the effects of prior radiotherapy, have significant hemodynamic implications, such as potentially increasing vascular resistance, altering blood flow dynamics, and contributing to regions of low wall shear stress that may promote further atherosclerotic disease development.
- The affected left EIA regions were likely areas of disturbed and turbulent flow, leading to increased vascular resistance, impaired perfusion downstream, and potentially contributing to symptoms.
- The use of stents would act as scaffolding to maintain the patency of the rather unpredictable vessel, decrease vascular resistance, and reinstate laminar flow conditions.

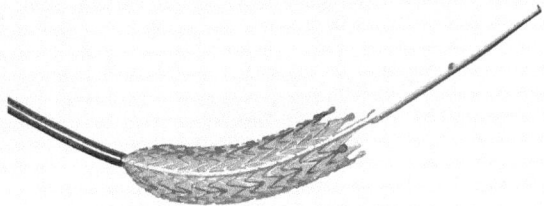

EVIDENCE INSIGHT:
- Radiation arteritis, a not so uncommon condition given nearly half of cancer patients undergo radiotherapy, presents unique clinical and radiological characteristics due

to its non-specific radiation effects and variable late tissue injury manifestations. The disease can complicate further with coexisting radiation-induced iliac vein disease and small vessel disease when it affects the iliac segment. Therefore, a comprehensive approach to diagnosing and treating all potential late radiation effects is crucial. Though the disease process may be intricate and pose diagnostic challenges, effective planning can streamline the treatment. Failing to do so can quickly lead to serious consequences such as limb loss or life-threatening complications. REF. Vascular & Endovascular Review 2020;3:e06 DOI: https://doi.org/10.15420/ver.2019.07

ILIAC CASE: 10

A 65-year-old patient presented with a left foot tissue loss. The patient had previous left EIA stenting. Duplex scan showed in-stent stenosis in the left EIA. A decision was agreed to proceed to iliac angioplasty +/- stenting.

READ CAREFULLY ...

Access	Pre Op checklist, supine, LA , cleaned and draped, CFA retrograde micropuncture. Gradual dilatation over the wire and increased to a 6Fr sheath.
Equipments	Standard (Micro-access. J Wire. Glidewire+Cobra. Amplatz+Proglide. Pigtail. contrast+HepSaline). Zilver flex stents.
Angiogram Findings	A brief segment stenosis at the proximal segment of the left CIA and a brief segment of in-stent stenosis within the left EIA.
Procedure	Stenting of the left CIA/EIA performed primarily using 7mm x 8cm, 8mm x 6cm, and 9mm x 6cm (Cook Zilver) stents. Subsequent balloon dilatation done using 7mm x 8cm and 8mm x 8cm standard balloons.
Complications	Post-procedure angiograms showed satisfactory results.
Closure	Achieved haemostasis through manual compression to the groin

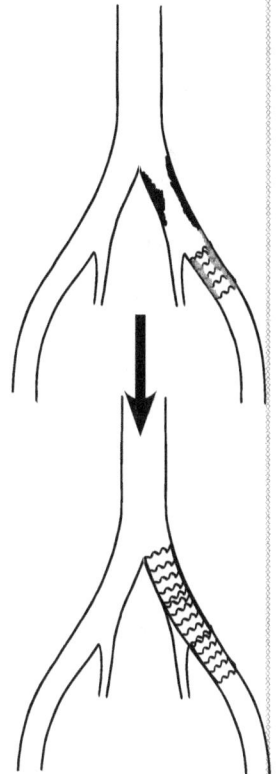

CONCISELY SUMMARIZE THE PROCEDURE USING KEY TERMS (ANSWER BELOW).

CHECK YOUR KNOWLEDGE

Qs ON STRATEGY

What is presently considered the most effective treatment for in-stent stenosis?

Balloon Angioplasty: Including the utilization of drug-coated balloons to mitigate the risk of restenosis.

Atherectomy: Employed to excise plaque accumulation directly.

Stent Placement: Potentially involving drug-eluting stents to prevent recurrent narrowing.

Pharmacotherapy: Leveraging drugs to manage contributory factors like high cholesterol and hypertension.

Bypass Surgery: Considered in severe cases to facilitate an alternative pathway for blood circulation.

What is the recommended course of action for a small AAA aneurysm in this context?

Leave it alone.

Qs ON BALLOONING

Should the balloon have the same dimensions as the stent?

No, utilizing a smaller balloon is acceptable, as seen in this second case.

IN-DEPTH ANALYSIS

PROCEDURE : LEFT ILIAC IN-STENT PLASTY AND RE-ALIGNMENT.

COMMENTS:

- Remarkably, the target here were both a de novo stenosis in the proximal CIA and a recurrent in-stent stenosis in the EIA. Recurrent in-stent stenosis is a common complication associated with the use of stents. This suggests the primary stent placement did not fully achieve the desired outcome of patency, leading to a second treatment need. Repeat interventions, like in this case, highlights the importance of careful monitoring.

BIOMECHANICS INSIGHT:

- A critical factor contributing to the in-stent restenosis is the arterial response to the mechanical *injury inflicted during the stent placement*. The ensuing neointimal hyperplasia, exacerbated by hemodynamic forces such as *shear stress*, often precipitates a restenosis within the stent.
- The Cook Zilver stent's radial force, *scaffolding* ability, and *flexibility* can influence both the acute procedural outcome and the propensity for in-stent restenosis.
- The post-dilatation strategy, utilizing standard balloons with defined dimensions, aims to optimize stent expansion, *enhancing the stent-artery interaction*. This step is vital to minimize *malapposition*, which can be a nidus for stent thrombosis and neointimal hyperplasia, again leading to in-stent restenosis.

HAEMODYNAMIC INSIGHT:

- Stenotic lesions create a considerable perturbation in the haemodynamics of the vessel. The decreased lumen diameter *increases local fluid velocity* according to the principles of the Bernoulli effect and the continuity equation. This elevated velocity at the site of stenosis results in *increased shear stress* on the vessel walls, potentially exacerbating the inflammatory and proliferative processes leading to further arterial wall remodeling and restenosis.
- Additionally, *post-stenotic regions* often experience *turbulent flow*, which not only lowers the efficiency of blood delivery distally but also can contribute to the pathogenesis of downstream vascular disease by inducing endothelial dysfunction.

EVIDENCE INSIGHT:

- A meta-analysis and systematic review aimed to evaluate the long-term clinical safety and effectiveness of drug-coated balloons (DCBs) in treating in-stent restenosis (ISR). The study included 18 trials involving 3,782 patients and examined a variety of cardiovascular outcomes. DCB treatment significantly reduced the late lumen loss (LLL) (MD: -0.13; p = .01). No difference was found for minimum luminal diameter and diameter stenosis (DS)%. The safety and efficacy of DCBs and drug-eluting stents in treating ISR were similar for up to three years of follow-up. REF.

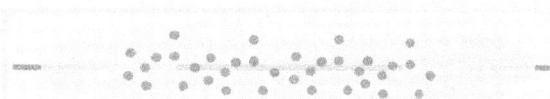

Catheter Cardiovasc Interv. 2020 Aug;96(2):E129-E141.

ILIAC CASE: 11

A 54-year-old patient presented with a right leg short distance claudication. Duplex scan showed narrowing of the proximal CIA bilaterally and occlusion of the popliteal artery from the adductor hiatus with multiple collaterals, some well-established. A decision was agreed to proceed to iliac angioplasty +/- stenting.

READ CAREFULLY ...

Access	Pre Op checklist, supine, LA , cleaned and draped, 6Fr (later 7Fr) sheath puncture. Ultrasound-assisted right CFA puncture using 7Fr sheath	
Equipments	Standard (Micro-access. J Wire. Glidewire+Cobra. Amplatz+Proglide. Pigtail. contrast+HepSaline). V12 stents.	
Angiogram Findings	Aortic distal aneurysmal enlargement noted. Bilateral proximal iliac arteries show significant constriction. Patency in right and left CFA and SFA. Popliteal artery occluded from adductor hiatus with collaterals. Popliteal occlusion to P3 level. Bifurcation reconstitution with three-vessel run-off. Only posterior tibial foot supply; distal peroneal and ATA occluded	
Procedure	Bilateral proximal CIA balloon mounted stents 10mm x 38mm stents	
Complications	None immediate	
Closure	6Fr Angioseal	

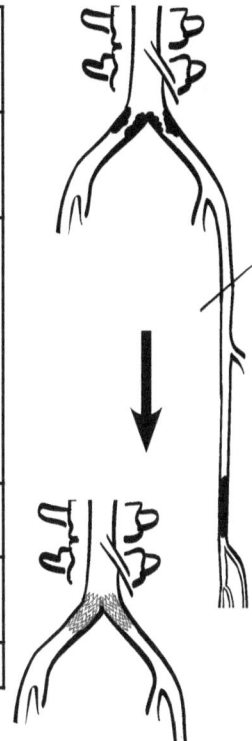

CONCISELY SUMMARIZE THE PROCEDURE USING KEY TERMS (ANSWER BELOW).

CHECK YOUR KNOWLEDGE

Qs ON STRATEGY

What potential complications may arise during a straightforward kissing stent procedure?

Possible issues include the rupture of the iliacs at or beyond the stent site, the occurrence of dissection, and the formation of a stent shelf.

Is addressing a popliteal occlusion mandatory when implementing iliac kissing stents?

Not necessarily; in the absence of critical ischemia, as in this scenario, it is not essential to treat a popliteal occlusion concurrently with iliac kissing stents.

Qs ON STENTING

Is it more favorable to opt for primary stenting in the case of iliacs?

Yes, particularly if the lesion is extremely proximal and/or involves the aorta, as demonstrated in this case where the contralateral iliac is also diseased

What type of stent is generally preferred in iliac kissing stent procedures?

The balloon-mounted covered stent, such as the V12, is usually preferred.

What can assist in the precise placement of a kissing stent?

Utilizing Mag x2 can be beneficial in achieving accurate placement.

IN-DEPTH ANALYSIS

PROCEDURE : ILIAC STENTING. STRAIGHTFORWARD. KISSING STENT. 6FR THEN 7FR ACCESS AND **V12** BALLOON MOUNTED STENT **10x38.**

COMMENTS:
- This case presents a compelling intersection of multiple vascular pathologies, namely the distal aortic aneurysmal change and bilateral iliac artery stenosis necessitating the deployment of kissing stents. This combination creates a unique challenge from both the anatomical and hemodynamic perspectives.
- The distal aortic aneurysm presents a potential source of altered flow dynamics that may influence downstream perfusion. Aneurysms, by nature of their enlarged, irregular lumen, can create abnormal blood flow patterns, such as areas of turbulence or recirculation. This can lead to increased wall shear stress and hemodynamic strain on the arterial walls, potentially exacerbating the disease progression in the common iliac arteries, and even influencing the stent's performance after implantation.
- The placement of kissing stents in the iliac arteries adjacent to an aneurysmal aorta necessitates a heightened consideration of hemodynamic and biomechanical factors. It is crucial to carefully balance the desire to re-establish optimal blood flow and relieve stenosis with the need to minimize turbulence that could propagate adverse effects on the aortic aneurysm or stent patency.
- Furthermore, the aneurysm itself may be a sign of a systemic arterial disease, suggesting a more generalized predisposition to arterial dilatation and rupture. As a result, a patient with an aortic aneurysm and peripheral arterial disease could carry a heightened risk of complications, warranting comprehensive, vigilant follow-up.

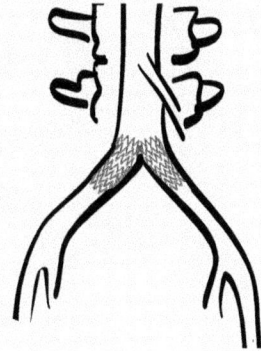

BIOMECHANICS AND HAEMODYNAMIC INSIGHT:
- In this context, the distal aortic aneurysmal change carries significant implications for the successful placement and durability of bilateral iliac "kissing" stents. The ***aortic-iliac junction is a high-flow, high-stress area*** subject to both ***shear and circumferential*** stress due to pulsatile blood flow. Furthermore, the presence of an aneurysm can create ***turbulent flow patterns*** that may increase these stresses.
- When kissing stents are placed in the iliac arteries, they can alter these haemodynamics, ***potentially exacerbating any turbulent flow into the aneurysm***. This turbulent flow can contribute to further aneurysmal growth and potentially rupture due to increased wall stress if the aneurysm size is considerable (not in this case). Moreover, these hemodynamic changes can also affect the ***stent stability*** and lead to ***stent migration***, particularly if the aneurysmal aorta's distal fixation zone is compromised.
- Biomechanically, the placement of the kissing stents must also take into consideration the ***"bird-beaking" effect***, where the close approximation of the stents in the distal aorta can

result in a gap or "beak" at the apex. This effect can ***expose the aortic wall to mechanical stress*** and jeopardize the stent's seal, increasing the risk of endoleaks, stent migration, or the development of an aorto-iliac ***dissection***.

EVIDENCE INSIGHT:

- Some interesting studies demonstrated that mice with iliac artery stenosis exhibited rapid early growth and predominantly rightward AAA expansion, resulting in slightly larger and asymmetric AAAs compared to the standard group. These groups also showed a significant increase in TGFβ1 and cellular infiltration. This was somewhat mirrored in human AAA patients with stenosed iliac arteries, although observations were variable. The study concluded that moderate iliac stenosis at the time of aneurysm induction can lead to faster AAA growth, aneurysm asymmetry, and increased vascular inflammation after 8 weeks, suggesting possible upstream effects of iliac stenosis on AAA progression. REF: J Vasc Res. 2019;56(5):217-229.

ILIAC CASE: 12

A 74-year-old patient presented with a right leg short distance claudication. Duplex scan showed CIA stenosis. A decision was agreed to proceed to iliac angioplasty +/- stenting.

READ CAREFULLY ...

Access	Pre Op checklist, supine, LA , cleaned and draped, Bilateral ultrasound-assisted retrograde femoral artery punctures. 7-French sheaths insertion.
Equipments	Standard (Micro-access. J Wire. Glidewire+Cobra. Amplatz+Proglide. Pigtail. contrast+HepSaline). V12 stents.
Angiogram Findings	Severe stenosis in right CIA. Left CIA and other observed arteries showed no significant pathology.
Procedure	8 x 40 mm and 8 x 30 mm covered balloon expandable stents Deployed in right and left CIAs respectively.
Complications	None immediate
Closure	6Fr Angio-Seal device in left groin and compression in right groin.

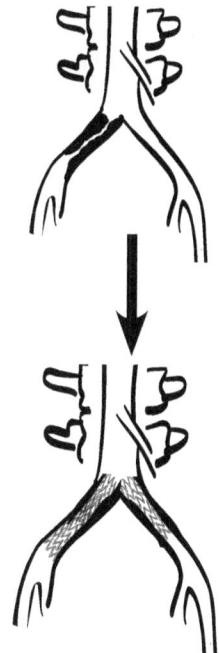

CONCISELY SUMMARIZE THE PROCEDURE USING KEY TERMS (ANSWER BELOW).

CHECK YOUR KNOWLEDGE

Qs ON STRATEGY

Is it justified to use a stent to treat a contralateral iliac that is not diseased?

Yes, particularly if treating the diseased iliac could negatively impact the non-diseased one.

Does the necessity to treat the contralateral side depend on the iliac lesion extending very proximally or into the aorta?

No, addressing the other side is warranted in cases involving a large bulky lesion, regardless of its proximity to the aorta.

What are the medicolegal ramifications if the now-asymptomatic, treated limb experiences occlusion leading to limb loss, and what should be included in the proper consenting process with the patient?

The patient needs to be adequately informed and understand the potential necessity of deploying a stent in the other leg to prevent severe consequences such as limb loss.

IN-DEPTH ANALYSIS

PROCEDURE : KISSING ILIAC STENTS. RIGHT DISEASED BUT NOT LEFT..

COMMENTS:
- In this case, the placement of stents in both the right and left common iliac arteries, despite the absence of significant disease in the left artery, is reflective of the "kissing stent" technique. This method is often utilized to ensure the patency of both vessels when one is affected, particularly in aortic or iliac bifurcation lesions.
- The rationale behind treating the non-diseased iliac artery with stenting, even when it's not presenting any significant disease, is to prevent potential complications such as contralateral occlusion or compromised blood flow caused by stent protrusion into the aortic lumen. Moreover, this approach helps maintain the appropriate anatomical configuration and ensures the maximum possible blood flow through both arteries.

BIOMECHANICS INSIGHT:
- In a "kissing stent" technique like this, two balloon-expandable stents are simultaneously deployed within the bifurcation of a vessel, in this case, the right and left common iliac arteries. This approach is not only adopted to treat the lesion on the diseased side (right common iliac artery in this case) but also, crucially, to maintain the structural integrity of the vasculature at the bifurcation.
- The placement of a stent in the non-diseased left iliac artery, despite it presenting no significant pathology, is a strategy used to **prevent** stent protruding into the aorta that may compromise the lumen of the contralateral side, leading to reduced blood flow, and potential thrombosis or occlusion.
- Moreover, the kissing stent technique **assists in resisting the radial forces** exerted by the aortic blood flow, which could potentially **cause deformation or displacement** of a solitary stent. By applying a counteracting radial force, the stents **ensure maintenance of the bifurcated architecture** of the common iliac artery, while **distributing shear stress and strain more evenly** across the vessel wall.
- This biomechanical **harmony** in the vascular system achieved by the kissing stent technique can **enhance the longevity of the procedure's success** by reducing the risk of restenosis or stent fracture.

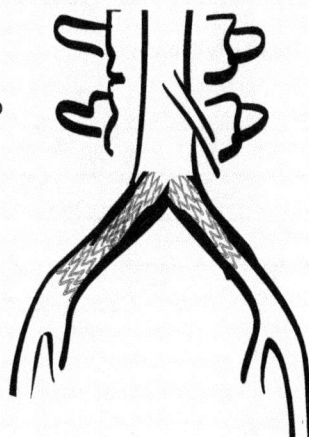

HAEMODYNAMIC INSIGHT:
- The primary haemodynamic consideration here pertains to the **maintenance of unimpeded bilateral flow** at the site of the aortic bifurcation. In the absence of a stent in the non-diseased artery (the left common iliac artery in this instance), the stent in the contralateral artery can cause flow disturbances, potentially leading to reduced perfusion or thrombosis in

the non-stented artery.

- By implementing stents in both arteries, the 'kissing' configuration helps *maintain laminar flow* at the bifurcation, *minimizing areas of flow stagnation or low wall shear stress* that could precipitate thrombus formation. The parallel placement of the stents helps *distribute the pressure gradients* more evenly, thus mitigating the risks of stent migration or deformation due to high-velocity aortic flow.

Furthermore, this bilateral approach can also *prevent the development of a 'steal' phenomenon*, where the stent in the diseased artery could *potentially divert blood flow* from the non-stented artery.

MODEL CASE:
Challenges of performing endovascular interventions on complex lesions and preventing restenosis

WATCH LIVE:
https://tinyurl.com/4swbrj6h

NOTES, TIPS AND TRICKS:

ILIAC CASE: 13

A 60-year-old patient with a history of Bilateral debilitating IC, on wheelchair, pushed by his wife. He has a previous Rt EIA Plasty and stent. Duplex showed a degree of in-stent stenosis. A decision was agreed to proceed to Rt iliac angiogram/angioplasty +/- proceed.

READ CAREFULLY ...

Access	Pre Op checklist, supine, LA , cleaned and draped, ultrasound-guided Left CFA retrograde puncture, with a 5 French 45 cm sheath positioned within the left CFA.
Equipments	Standard (Micro-access. J Wire. Glidewire+Cobra. Amplatz+Proglide. Pigtail. contrast+HepSaline).
Angiogram Findings	CO_2 angiography revealed patent left EIA with very mild stensis in the stent, CFA, and profunda, with significant stenosis in the proximal SFA segment and a patent stented mid SFA. Three-vessel distal run-off and a distal calf peroneal artery with reduced calibre were noted
Procedure	Glide wire navigation across proximal SFA stenosis, and plain balloon angioplasty with 5 mm and 6 mm balloons sequentially.
Complications	None immediate
Closure	standard

CONCISELY SUMMARIZE THE PROCEDURE USING KEY TERMS (ANSWER BELOW).

CHECK YOUR KNOWLEDGE

Qs ON STRATEGY

Qs ON ACCESS

If it is not feasible to access EIA lesion from I/L or C/L femorals, what other options are there?

Brachial or distal CFA or SFA (micro needle)

Qs ON RECANALISATION

Qs ON BALLONING

Does POBA usually provides enough angioplasty in such cases?

Not usually a good result

Qs ON STENTING

IN-DEPTH ANALYSIS

PROCEDURE : POBA FOR SFA STENOSIS. DUPLEX POST SHOWING PFA NOW STENOTIC AND SFA 50% STENOTIC.

COMMENTS:
- In this case, the prolonged plain balloon angioplasty (POBA) approach presents a possible concern for the development of postoperative profunda stenosis due to its potential impact on vessel compliance and the subsequent risk of elastic recoil or neointimal hyperplasia.
- The utilization of CO_2 as a contrast medium helps to mitigate the nephrotoxicity associated with iodinated contrast agents.
- Despite these considerations, the overall outcome of the procedure appears satisfactory, and the hemodynamic significance of the distal run-off remaining unchanged.

BIOMECHANICS INSIGHT:
- In this case, the angioplasty performed on the stenotic proximal segment of the SFA presents interesting biomechanical considerations. The application of the plain old balloon angioplasty (POBA) in the stenotic area induces mechanical stresses in the arterial wall, such as shear, circumferential, and axial stress, which can influence the endothelial function and vascular response.
- The vessel wall compliance is altered due to the balloon-induced radial expansion, which could precipitate vascular injury, barotrauma, and potentially stimulate the pathway for intimal hyperplasia. The interaction of mechanical stimuli and vascular remodeling following angioplasty is a complex interplay of various molecular and cellular mechanisms, including endothelial dysfunction, inflammation, smooth muscle cell proliferation, and extracellular matrix reorganization.
- In this context, the risk for post-procedural profunda femoris artery (PFA) stenosis might be related to the direct mechanical impact of the angioplasty or hemodynamic changes in the bifurcation region, affecting the shear stress distribution, which is known to influence local vascular remodeling.

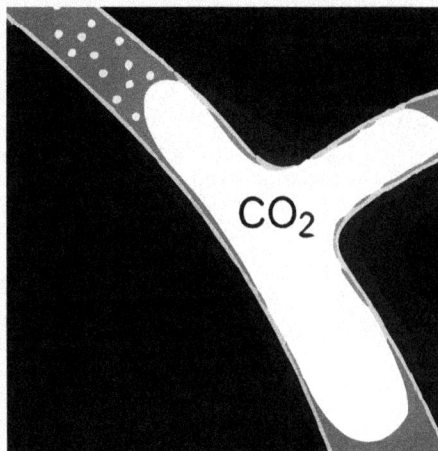

- The alternative contrast medium (CO_2) is less nephrotoxic and mitigates the potential for contrast-induced nephropathy. Nevertheless, CO_2 has a lower viscosity than iodinated contrast, which could affect the clarity during the procedure.

HAEMODYNAMIC INSIGHT:
- Stenosis in the proximal segment of the SFA significantly alters the hemodynamics by increasing resistance to flow, reducing shear stress downstream and potentially causing turbulent flow proximally. This can lead to endothelial dysfunction, platelet activation, and atherosclerotic progression.

- The angioplasty performed would have restored more normal flow conditions in the SFA, rectifying the high resistance, and ameliorating ischemic symptoms. However, this intervention comes with its own potential hemodynamic implications. For instance, balloon angioplasty can cause dissection or barotrauma, leading to local turbulent flow and increased wall shear stress, promoting platelet aggregation and thrombus formation, which could precipitate acute closure of the artery.
- The impact on the profunda femoris artery (PFA) after angioplasty in the SFA is another noteworthy consideration. Hemodynamics at the bifurcation regions are complex due to flow separation, and angioplasty in one branch might alter the flow patterns and shear stress distribution in the other.

EVIDENCE INSIGHT:
- A Meta-Analysis from Cochrane Database Syst Rev (2019) showed that drug-eluting balloons (DEBs) were associated with a lower risk of target lesion revascularization (TLR) and binary restenosis at 6 and 24 months compared to uncoated balloon angioplasty (POBA). However, the study included a small number of participants and the quality of the included studies was low. More research is needed to confirm these findings. REF. Cochrane Database Syst Rev. 2019 Jan 26;1(1):CD012510.

ILIAC CASE: 14

A 60-year-old patient with a history of right Ilio-profunda bypass presented with an acute occlusion. A decision was agreed to proceed to Rt iliac bypass thrombolysis +/- stenting.

READ CAREFULLY ...

Access	Pre Op checklist, supine, LA , cleaned and draped, Ultrasound-guided 6-French left CFA puncture.
Equipments	Standard (Micro-access. J Wire. Glidewire+Cobra. Amplatz+Proglide. Pigtail. contrast+HepSaline).
Angiogram Findings	>75% stenosis in right external iliac artery, occluded left Ilio-profunda bypass graft. Collateral vessels at left calf proximal, single vessel runoff right
Procedure	Stenting of right external iliac artery with 7 mm x 40 mm and 6 mm x 60 mm self-expandable stents. SIM-1 catheter placed across aortic bifurcation. Alteplase bolus (5 mg) administered.
Complications	None immediate
Closure	6-French sheath secured to right groin with sutures and dressings

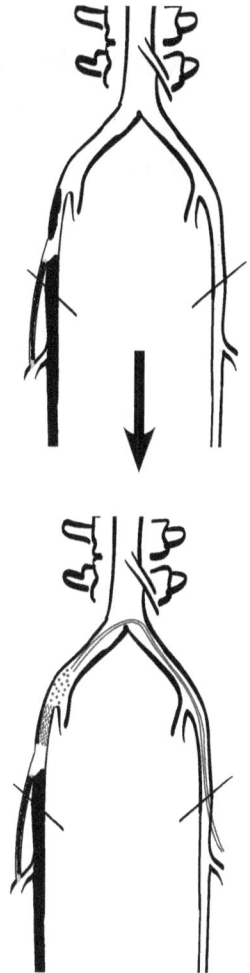

CONCISELY SUMMARIZE THE PROCEDURE USING KEY TERMS (ANSWER BELOW).

CHECK YOUR KNOWLEDGE

Qs ON RECANALISATION

Where should the catheter tip be positioned for thrombolysis in the case of an acutely occluded ilio-femoral bypass?

In the proximal CIA.

Qs ON CATHETER

What kind of catheters are beneficial for thrombolysis procedures?

In this instance, a SIM-1 catheter was utilized.

Qs ON BALOONING

Is it necessary to address an asymptomatic side during the revascularization of the other side?

Yes, especially if it is significantly impacted and could potentially be affected by the treatment of the other side, at least in terms of access.

IN-DEPTH ANALYSIS

PROCEDURE : BYPASS THROMBOLYSIS + EIA STENTING.

COMMENTS:
- The use of alteplase as a thrombolytic agent illustrates the integration of medical and endo-vascular therapy in maintaining patency and function of the lower limb bypass. Thrombolysis was employed to dissolve the occlusive thrombus, enabling a more effective stenting process.
- It's important to remember that this hybrid approach requires careful patient selection, considering factors such as comorbidities, anatomy, and thrombus characteristics.

BIOMECHANICS INSIGHT:
- The fibrinolysis catalyzed by alteplase alters the biomechanical landscape of the occluded vessel, transitioning it from an occluded to a semi-patent state. This BIOMECHANICALly driven modulation is essential but should be supported by the subsequent mechanical intervention, i.e., stenting.
- Following thrombolysis, self-expandable stents, which leverage the principle of radial force, provide mechanical scaffolding in the stenosed right external iliac artery. These stents serve to reestablish and maintain luminal diameter and facilitate hemodynamic improvement.
- It's important to recognize the intricate interplay between these BIOMECHANICAL and biomechanical processes, and their critical role in restoring and optimizing vascular integrity and perfusion. Nonetheless, careful patient selection remains paramount given the complexity of the procedure and the potential for varying patient-specific responses to this type of intervention.

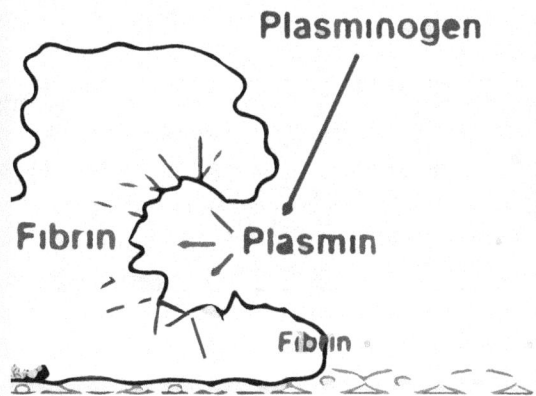

HAEMODYNAMIC INSIGHT:
- The placement of self-expandable stents in the right external iliac artery with severe stenosis represents a profound hemodynamic intervention. By applying radial force to the stenosed arterial wall, the stents mechanically widen the narrowed vessel, thus significantly reducing vascular resistance in accordance with the principles of Poiseuille's Law.
- The introduction of alteplase, a potent fibrinolytic, initiates a hemodynamic shift by inducing thrombolysis within the occluded left Ilio-profunda bypass graft. This enzymatic dissolution of the occlusive thrombus not only improves local blood flow by re-establishing luminal patency, but also primes the system for the stenting intervention.

EVIDENCE INSIGHT:

- A study published in ScienceDirect investigated the results of thrombolytic therapy in the management of acute bypass graft occlusion and identified risk factors for technical failure and amputation.
- Another study published in the Journal of Vascular Surgery assessed the technical and short- and long-term clinical outcomes of catheter-directed thrombolysis (CDT) with urokinase for occluded infrainguinal bypass grafts. The study found that clinical success after CDT was observed in 62% of procedures with an associated complication rate of 36%. Patent outflow vessels before and after CDT are factors associated with long-term limb salvage. Amputation-free survival after 5 years is 71.3%
- REF:
- Thrombolysis for lower extremity bypass graft occlusion. https://www.sciencedirect.com/science/article/pii/S0741521411010755.
- A comprehensive report of long-term outcomes after catheter-directed .... https://www.jvascsurg.org/article/S0741-5214%2819%2930178-8/fulltext.

MODEL CASE:	**WATCH LIVE:**	
Complex iliofemoral lesion recanalization complicated by arteriovenous fistula, partial thrombosis of the DFA, and small intramuscular hematoma	https://tinyurl.com/4aw8ffx6	

NOTES, TIPS AND TRICKS:

ILIAC CASE: 15

A 79-year-old patient with a history of a left 5th toe necrosis. Duplex scan showed occluded left EIA and SFA. A decision was agreed to proceed for recanalisation.

READ CAREFULLY ...

Access	Pre Op checklist, supine, LA , cleaned and draped, ultrasound-guided 6-French retrograde puncture of left CFA.
Equipments	Standard (Micro-access. J Wire. Glidewire+Cobra. Amplatz+Proglide. Pigtail. contrast+HepSaline).
Angiogram Findings	Left EIA fully occluded. Multisegment disease and long-segment occlusion in proximal and mid-to-distal SFA.
Procedure	Left iliac artery occlusion addressed with 9 mm x 5 cm stent. SFA disease and occlusion treated with 5 mm x 20 cm and 5 mm x 4 cm balloons.
Complications	On completion angio: Occlusive thrombus in proximal PTA. Reduced flow at distal AT; DP patent. The occluding thrombus in the proximal posterior tibial artery was managed with a 9 mg dose of TPA, a 2.5 mm x 10 cm & a short 3 mm x 4 cm balloon angioplasty and thrombus extraction with a Pat-Rat aspiration device. Completion angio: peroneal artery did not fully fill with contrast, however, a two-vessel runoff was maintained at the feet.
Closure	6-French angioseal closure device

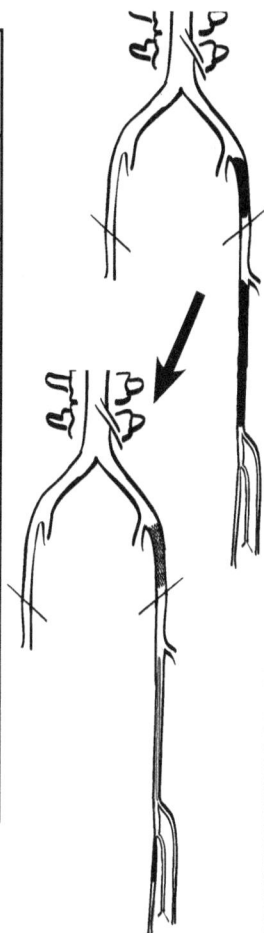

CONCISELY SUMMARIZE THE PROCEDURE USING KEY TERMS (ANSWER BELOW).

CHECK YOUR KNOWLEDGE

Qs ON ACCESS

Can both EIA and SFA disease be managed from an ipsilateral position?

While it is not the advised course of action, it may be possible if the sheath can be adjusted to an antegrade position

Qs ON CATHETER

Which kind of catheter should be utilized for thrombolysis in this instance?

Pat-Rat aspiration device

Qs ON COMPLICATIONS

What is the initial treatment approach for a lesion that has experienced embolization affecting the distal runoff?

Suction
or angiopasty balloon
or thrombolysis (this case)

Is it imperative to secure a fully patent runoff post-thrombolysis?

No, if satisfactory runoff is present.

IN-DEPTH ANALYSIS

PROCEDURE : EIA PLASTY - COMPLICATED WITH DISTAL EMBOLISATION TO PT. NOT FULLY RESPONDED TO TPA AND PLASTY.

COMMENTS:
- Distal embolization typically occurs when fragments of the thrombus or atheromatous plaque dislodge and migrate to smaller, distal vessels, leading to their occlusion and potentially causing ischemia.
- The treatment using a combination of thrombolytic therapy with tissue plasminogen activator (TPA), balloon angioplasty, and thrombus aspiration can make a major difference as in this case.
- The sluggish flow in the distal anterior tibial artery and the peroneal artery's incomplete opacification following TPA administration indicate that some degree of microvascular obstruction might remain. Given the patent dorsalis pedis and the observed dual vessel runoff to the feet, the risk for significant limb-threatening ischemia appears mitigated for now, but continued surveillance for signs of critical limb ischemia is recommended.

BIOMECHANICS INSIGHT:
- Distal embolization is a complex biomechanical process that is influenced by several key factors, including the characteristics of the plaque or thrombus, the hemodynamic forces at play, and the intervention techniques utilized.
- In terms of plaque characteristics, more friable or unstable atheromatous plaques are prone to dislodgement, especially under the mechanical stresses induced by an intervention. The process of angioplasty or stenting, with its accompanying balloon inflation or stent deployment, can create significant radial forces and disrupt the plaque's integrity, leading to fragmentation and subsequent distal embolization. Similarly, the mechanical disruption of a thrombus can lead to clot fragmentation and embolization.

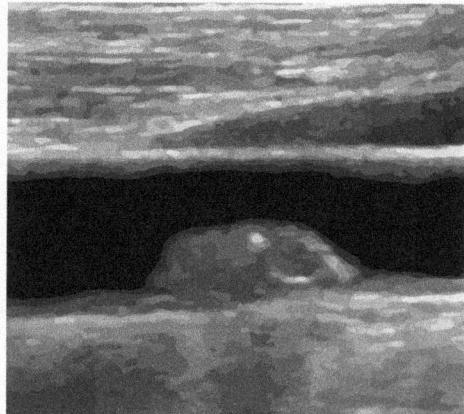

- High-pressure balloon inflations or oversized stents can increase the radial force applied to the vessel wall and potentially disrupt unstable plaques. Furthermore, the use of catheter-directed thrombolysis can cause thrombus dissolution and potentially the release of small emboli.

HAEMODYNAMIC INSIGHT:
- Vulnerable or 'soft' plaques with a lipid-rich core and thin fibrous cap are more prone to rupture during intervention, releasing their contents into the bloodstream.
- The interventional procedures can also disrupt the steady laminar flow within the vessel, creating turbulent flow and associated shear stresses that can further dislodge plaque or

thrombus components. Additionally, the sudden restoration of flow in an occluded or stenotic vessel following intervention can produce a 'washout' phenomenon, with abrupt increases in flow velocity leading to distal embolization of loosened material.

- Post-intervention, oscillatory wall shear stress (a reversal in the direction of shear forces), often observed in stented segments due to altered flow dynamics, can trigger the release of emboli from the arterial wall or stent strut. This could explain the occlusive thrombus in the proximal posterior tibial artery, and sluggish flow and incomplete opacification in distal vessels observed in this case.

EVIDENCE INSIGHT:

- In a review article by Marques t al (2014), distal embolization, characterized by the migration of detached debris or thrombus, was shown to pose a serious threat to cause limb amputation or even mortality. The incidence of limb loss or death following distal embolization is approximately 0.6% and 0.2% of all procedures, respectively. It's crucial to assess patients with lesions that have a higher predisposition for distal embolization as the application of Embolic Protection Devices (EPDs) could be key in averting Acute Limb Ischemia (ALI) during these lower limb interventions. Conversely, the indiscriminate and unregulated deployment of such devices should be cautioned against as it can inflict injury to the vessel wall, paradoxically escalating the risk of distal embolization in certain circumstances.
- REF: Endovascular Today May 2014

MODEL CASE:	WATCH LIVE:	
Supera external iliac and common femoral artery	https://tinyurl. com/2ubn5ann	

NOTES, TIPS AND TRICKS:

ILIAC CASE: 16

A 58-year-old patient with a history of acute ischaemic right leg. Duplex scan showed occluded iliac and sfa on right side. A decision was agreed to proceed for embolectomy +/- proceed (hybrid approach).

READ CAREFULLY ...

Access	Pre Op checklist, supine, GA , cleaned and draped, CFA access and sloupes used.
Equipments	Standard (Micro-access. J Wire. Glidewire+Cobra. Amplatz+Proglide. Pigtail. contrast+HepSaline).
Angiogram Findings	Post iliac embolectomy, angiogram showed EIA stenosis, patent SFA, pop, TPT, AT origin occlusion, AT and PT to foot.
Procedure	Heparin use. Transverse arteriotomy. Iliac embolectomy (4F Fogarty), thrombus removal, inflow initiation. SFA distal embolectomy, thrombus retrieval, backflow restoration. Vessel flushing. Arteriotomy closure (5.0 prolene). 6F sheath angiogram. EIA stenting (10x80 Zilver).
Complications	Not specified
Closure	Arteriotomy and puncture site (5.0 prolene), subcutaneous (vicryl), skin (monocryl)

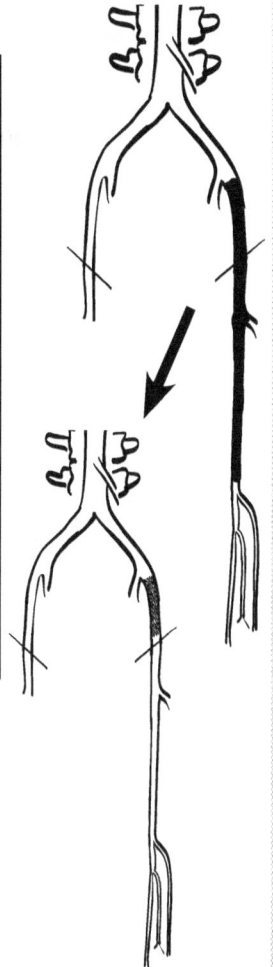

CONCISELY SUMMARIZE THE PROCEDURE USING KEY TERMS (ANSWER BELOW).

CHECK YOUR KNOWLEDGE

Qs ON STRATEGY

How might a hybrid strategy be implemented in an acute embolectomy?

Open thrombectomy succeeded by EIA plasty and stenting

In what situations would this be considered?

In immediately threatened limb

Qs ON STENTING

In an acute scenario, would utilizing a covered stent or an uncovered stent be more appropriate (if a stent is to be used at all)?

In this situation, uncovered.

Qs ON COMPLICATIONS

Is it reasonable to allow occlusion of distal runoffs to persist after an embolectomy?

Yes, since the patient should now be optimized, addressing this issue can be more effectively tackled in the future.

IN-DEPTH ANALYSIS

PROCEDURE : OPEN EMBOLECTOMY AND ILIAC STENTING. TPT STILL OCCLUDED.

COMMENTS:
- This case represents a complex intervention, where the management of a stenotic external iliac artery (EIA) was necessitated amidst the performance of an embolectomy. The simultaneous treatment of both conditions highlights the multifaceted approach often required in vascular surgeries.
- Treating EIA stenosis in this context shows the critical role of ensuring optimum blood flow to lower extremities, which is crucial for patient recovery post-embolectomy.
- The insertion of a Zilver stent into the EIA serves to address the stenosis, facilitating enhanced blood flow while potentially reducing the risk of re-embolization.

BIOMECHANICS INSIGHT:
- The embolectomy procedure aimed to mechanically remove the thrombus, thereby re-establishing perfusion and mitigating the potential ischemic effects in the lower extremity. Meanwhile, the stenotic EIA presented an additional hemodynamic challenge. Stenosis in arterial vessels creates a significant pressure gradient across the lesion and leading to sub-optimal perfusion. Addressing this stenotic lesion was critical to maintain distal flow.
- The Zilver stent, a tubular structure typically made from a metal alloy, is designed to be both flexible and sturdy. It supports the arterial wall, preventing the vessel from collapsing and ensuring a consistently patent lumen. Upon deployment, the stent undergoes a biomechanical transformation – a radial expansion – exerting an outward force on the arterial wall and overcoming the inherent stenosis. This improves blood flow dynamics, reducing the shear stress on endothelial cells, and mitigating thrombogenic conditions despite being a foreign body in this high flow area.

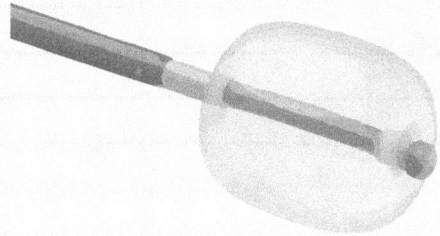

HAEMODYNAMIC INSIGHT:
- The thromboembolic occlusion in the iliac and superficial femoral arteries (SFA) disrupted normal laminar flow, which not only reduced perfusion to the lower limb but also exacerbated local thrombogenic conditions. Stasis of blood, a component of Virchow's triad, promotes clot formation and further thrombus propagation. Simultaneously, the presence of stenosis in the external iliac artery (EIA) presented a significant hemodynamic challenge. The narrowed lumen increased resistance to flow as per Poiseuille's law, which can dramatically alter pressure and velocity distributions within the vessel. The stenotic EIA caused a pressure gradient leading to impaired distal perfusion and potential for turbulent flow at the site of stenosis, both of which can trigger further thromboembolic events.
- The restored flow dynamics can positively impact endothelial function. Endothelial cells, which are sensitive to shear stress, play a pivotal role in vasodilation, inflammation, and thrombosis regulation. By rectifying turbulent flow and promoting laminar flow, the interven-

tion helps maintain a healthier endothelium and, thus, a reduced risk of future thrombotic events.

MODEL CASE:
Mechanical thrombectomy for recurrent thrombotic occlusion of the left common femoral artery

WATCH LIVE:
https://tinyurl.
com/34j3bjkz

NOTES, TIPS AND TRICKS:

Iliac Case: 17

A 68-year-old patient with a history of numbness in right foot. CTA showed right EIA occlusion. A decision was agreed to proceed for a Right iliac recanalisation.

READ CAREFULLY ...

Access	Pre Op checklist, supine, LA , cleaned and draped, - Left CFA accessed via US-guided retrograde puncture with 6Fr sheath. Right CFA accessed via US-guided micropuncture proximal to bifurcation using 6Fr sheath.
Equipments	Standard (Micro-access. J Wire. Glidewire+Cobra. Amplatz+Proglide. Pigtail. contrast+HepSaline).
Angiogram Findings	Extensive right EIA occlusion from iliac bifurcation to inguinal ligament. Collateral-facilitated retrograde filling to CFA. Notable right CFA stenosis partially occluded by sheath. Patent SFA, popliteal, and proximal crural vessels without significant stenosis
Procedure	Subintimal manipulation of wire and catheter across the occlusion from the right femoral access, with reentry at the proximal EIA stump.Primary stent placement within the occlusion using overlapping 7x40mm and 6 x 40mm Zilver Flex stents. Post-stent placement balloon angioplasty with a 7 x 80mm balloon. Final angiography depicts successful EIA recanalisation. The sheath's presence in the CFA partially occludes it, leading to less than ideal run-off, but post-procedure patency of the CFA, SFA, popliteal and proximal crural vessels is maintained. Post-sheath removal, swift flow into the CFA and SFA is reestablished.
Complications	Small volume of extravasation observed on final angiogram after sheath removal. - Ultrasonography reveals minor hematoma at the right groin. No signs of pseudoaneurysm.
Closure	Right groin: manual compression- Left groin: 6-French Angio-Seal closure device.

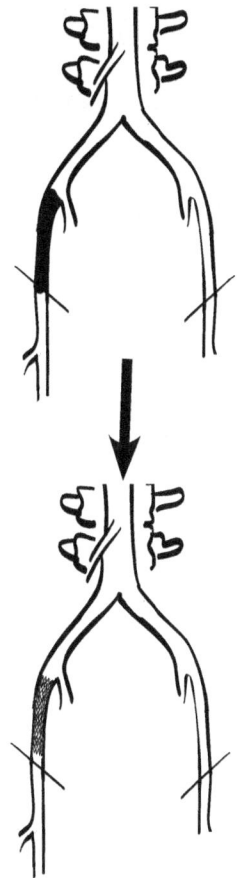

CONCISELY SUMMARIZE THE PROCEDURE USING KEY TERMS (ANSWER BELOW).

CHECK YOUR KNOWLEDGE

Qs ON ACCESS

In the case of EIA occlusion, is it preferable to administer treatment from an ipsilateral or contralateral position?

Either approach can be suitable provided there is sufficient space to operate; in this instance, the ipsilateral approach was utilized.

Qs ON RECANALISATION

When intraluminal navigation is not feasible in the EIA, what should the operator remain cautious of?

They should avoid dissecting into the aorta; in this situation, they reverted to a previous strategy.

Qs ON STENTING

Which stent is suitable for use in the EIA near the inguinal ligament?

The Zilver Flex is a good option, potentially requiring the use of two overlapping stents.

What else should one be cautious of?

Avoid positioning the stent below the inguinal ligament.

IN-DEPTH ANALYSIS

PROCEDURE :   EIA STENTING. SUBINTIMAL I/L (ANGIO FROM C/L). ZILVER FLEX STENT.

COMMENTS:

- This case demonstrates a complex vascular intervention involving a challenging, long-segment occlusion of the external iliac artery (EIA). The use of a subintimal recanalisation approach, while technically demanding, was particularly beneficial in this scenario. This method allowed the restoration of flow across the occluded segment by creating a new pathway within the layers of the arterial wall, essentially bypassing the obstruction.

- However, it's important to note the inherent risk associated with the subintimal technique. This technique can be hazardous due to potential perforation or dissection risks, leading to possible complications such as acute limb ischemia or the need for further invasive procedures. In this case, though, the procedure was carried out successfully without immediate complications.

- The deployment of Zilver Flex stents within the EIA is noteworthy. The flexibility and durability of these self-expanding stents make them ideal for use in the EIA, which requires hardware capable of withstanding high degrees of mechanical stress due to its location and constant exposure to significant blood flow while bending. The overlapping technique utilized here is commonly used to treat long lesions and ensure complete and accurate coverage of the occluded segment.

- A point of concern, however, was the presence of the sheath causing partial occlusion of the common femoral artery (CFA), which could lead to suboptimal distal flow. However, this issue was resolved after sheath removal, which restored swift flow into the CFA and SFA.

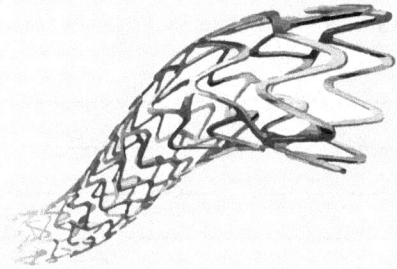

-

BIOMECHANICS AND HAEMODYNAMIC INSIGHT:

- The use of the Zilver Flex stent in the EIA speaks to several biomechanical considerations. The *self-expanding property* of these stents plays a critical role in adapting to the vessel's contour and diameter, maintaining luminal patency. The radial force exerted by the stent *must strike a delicate balance*: it must be sufficiently robust to resist the *inward recoil* and external compressive forces associated with the arterial wall and surrounding tissue, but not so aggressive that it damages the vessel. Furthermore, the *stent's flexibility* is crucial *in a dynamic environment* like the EIA, where the stent *must tolerate* the biomechanical forces of pulsatile blood flow and body movements.

- Hemodynamically, the objective of the procedure was to restore blood flow through the occluded EIA, reducing the overall vascular resistance and improving distal perfusion. *The presence of the sheath*, however, caused a transient *increase in resistance* due to partial occlusion of the common femoral artery (CFA). This is a critical factor as it could have led to decreased shear stress in the vessel, predisposing to thrombogenesis. However, the restoration of a swift flow into the CFA and SFA post-sheath removal likely reestablished favorable hemodynamic conditions.

- Lastly, the ***choice of overlapping stents*** requires consideration of blood flow dynamics. Overlapping stents might potentially ***disrupt laminar flow***, leading to areas of ***low wall shear stress*** that could promote ***intimal hyperplasia*** and restenosis. However, careful stent placement can help mitigate this, and the success of the recanalisation seen in the completion angiogram suggests this was achieved.

MODEL CASE:
Can new endovascular tools change common femoral artery (CFA) treatment?

WATCH LIVE:
https://tinyurl.
com/2p9atnbu

NOTES, TIPS AND TRICKS:

ILIAC CASE: 18

A 66-year-old patient with a history of left leg rest pain. The patient had a previous Left CFA endarterectomy and Left EIA angio. CTA showed Multi-level stenoses in the SFA. A decision was agreed to proceed for a left sfa and iliac angio.

READ CAREFULLY ...

Access	Pre Op checklist, supine, LA , cleaned and draped, Retrograde right CFA access achieved under ultrasound; transitioned from 6Fr sheath to 6Fr Destination sheath..
Equipments	Standard (Micro-access. J Wire. Glidewire+Cobra. Amplatz+Proglide. Pigtail. contrast+HepSaline).
Angiogram Findings	Patent left CIA, IIA, post-endarterectomy CFA, PFA, PopA, TPT, and main run-off via PA. Moderate stenoses in mid and distal EIA, severe in SFA. ATA occlusion past-origin, PTA occlusion from origin with distal reconstitution from collaterals. Incomplete pedal arch.
Procedure	Crossed left EIA, SFA with 0.035" catheter/guidewire manipulation. 6mm POBA to EIA stenoses, 5mm POBA throughout SFA .
Complications	A non-flow limiting dissection noted in proximal SFA. Further balooning showed marginal improvement post-repeat inflation.
Closure	6Fr AngioSeal implemented for hemostasis; minor oozing resolved post-prolonged compression.

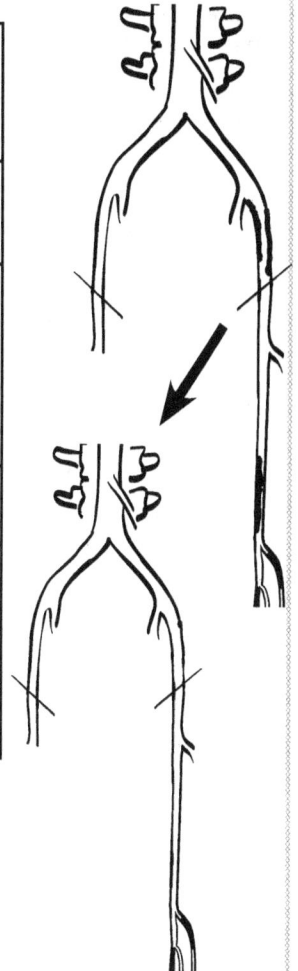

CONCISELY SUMMARIZE THE PROCEDURE USING KEY TERMS (ANSWER BELOW).

CHECK YOUR KNOWLEDGE

Qs ON STENTING

If two stents are placed separately in the iliac, does the intervening area have a heightened risk for early stenosis? Moreover, do the stents have a hemodynamic impact on this region?

See long answer in the In-Depth Analysis

Qs ON COMPLICATIONS

What initial measure can be taken in response to an SFA dissection?

Conducting a prolonged repeat angioplasty can be a solution.

How can the risk of dissection be minimized following angioplasty?

Implementing a prolonged balloon angioplasty utilizing a long balloon can help in reducing the risk.

IN-DEPTH ANALYSIS

PROCEDURE : EIA AND SFA PLASTY. COMPLICATED WITH DISSECTION. NO STENT.

COMMENTS:

- A non-flow limiting dissection following angioplasty, while not uncommon, can become a precarious condition if not resolved appropriately. While the absence of immediate flow limitation may seem reassuring, the long-term patency could be jeopardized. Unresolved dissections can lead to intraluminal thrombus formation, which may subsequently precipitate acute limb ischemia, or contribute to restenosis and late lumen loss.

- The marginal improvement after repeat balloon inflations in this case raises concerns about the possible progression or worsening of the dissection. Therefore, ongoing close surveillance of the patient will be essential to ensure early detection of any potential complications. This scenario may also necessitate further intervention like stenting, if the dissection evolves to become flow-limiting or if symptoms persist, balancing the risks and benefits with the individual patient's overall health status and comorbid conditions.

- However, these decisions should ideally be guided by the patient's symptoms, hemodynamic significance of the lesion, and evidence of flow limitation or ischemia. In the absence of these, conservative management with antithrombotic therapy and close surveillance might be the more prudent approach.

BIOMECHANICS AND HAEMODYNAMIC INSIGHT:

- The vascular system inherently presents a *viscoelastic nature*, meaning its *mechanical properties vary depending* on the direction of applied force and the degree of deformation over time. This unique biomechanical characteristic is crucial in understanding the propensity for dissection after balloon angioplasty, especially in atherosclerotic vessels with compromised structural integrity.

- The development of non-flow limiting dissections after angioplasty indicates a degree of *arterial wall disruption*. It essentially represents a communication between the true lumen and the false lumen created by delamination of intima-media layers of the arterial wall. While the *initial hemodynamic impact* may be minimal, potentially explaining the lack of flow limitation, the long-term consequences can be significant. Persistent dissections can *disrupt laminar flow*, increasing *turbulence* and *shear stress* on the vessel wall. This elevated shear stress can *stimulate platelet activation* and thrombogenesis, leading to subacute thrombotic occlusions.

- Furthermore, the disturbed flow dynamics can *exacerbate neointimal hyperplasia* and contribute to restenosis. This is mediated through *mechanotransduction mechanisms* where endothelial cells translate the altered shear stress into intracellular BIOMECHANICAL signals promoting cellular proliferation and extracellular matrix production.

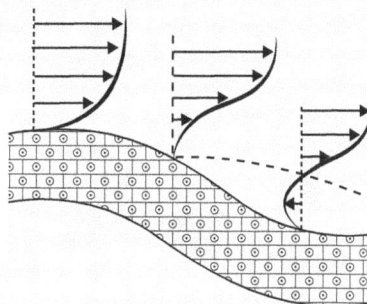

- The marginal improvement in this case, despite repeated and prolonged balloon inflation, suggests a *degree of vessel wall resilience or elasticity* that may reflect underlying *fibrocalcific changes* due to advanced atherosclerosis.
- Thus, a thoughtful management strategy is warranted here, incorporating the potential for downstream complications, the likely hemodynamic impact of incomplete resolution, and the potential need for adjunctive stenting versus atherectomy. At the same time, consideration should be given to medical optimization focusing on aggressive antiplatelet and antithrombotic strategies to mitigate thrombogenic risks. This case emphasizes the importance of an integrated understanding of vascular biology, biomechanics, and haemodynamics in managing such vascular complexities.

ILIAC CASE: 19

A 82-year-old patient with a history of Rt Short distance claudication <50 yards. Previous EVAR. CTA Rt EIA and IIA stenosis. A decision was agreed to proceed for a Rt iliac angio.

READ CAREFULLY ...

Access	Pre Op checklist, supine, LA , cleaned and draped, ultrasound-guided retrograde R CFA access and placed 6-Fr sheath.
Equipments	Standard (Micro-access. J Wire. Glidewire+Cobra. Amplatz+Proglide. Pigtail. contrast+HepSaline).
Angiogram Findings	Severe R EIA stenosis with calcified plaque into R IIA and sluggish R IIA flow. Noted minor, non-flow-limiting dissection flap in distal R EIA.
Procedure	Used 7 mm x 2 cm Formula balloon-expandable stent to address R EIA origin stenosis post vessel prep with 7 mm x 4 cm balloon. R IIA treatment was complex due to ostial disease, possible embolic event post-stenting. Noted patent profunda.
Complications	Reduced R IIA flow post-stenting, suggesting possible embolic event due to complex R IIA treatment.
Closure	Manual compression

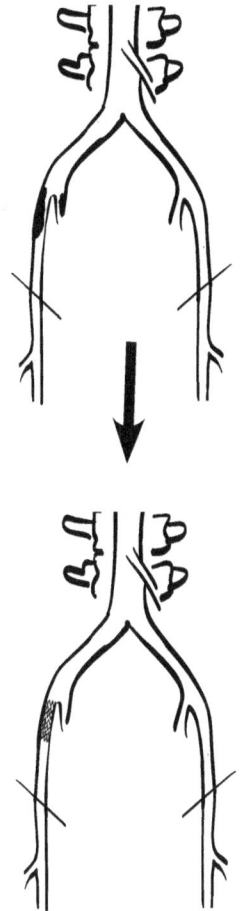

CONCISELY SUMMARIZE THE PROCEDURE USING KEY TERMS (ANSWER BELOW).

CHECK YOUR KNOWLEDGE

Qs ON STRATEGY

What are the available strategies for managing a severe proximal EIA stenosis?

Vessel preparation followed by the deployment of either a covered or uncovered stent.

Qs ON COMPLICATIONS

What complications are not uncommon when treating EIA?

It's not uncommon to encounter plaque dislodgement, which can block the IIA wall.

Is there an opportunity to address a blocked IIA following EIA angioplasty?

Treatment can be attempted, although it is not frequently successful, and the patient should be informed of the high risk of bleeding. Currently, the patient is experiencing severe buttock pain and is recommended to perform exercises to alleviate it.

IN-DEPTH ANALYSIS

PROCEDURE : RT EIA PLASTY AND STENTING BUT AFFECTED IIA.

COMMENTS:

- The case highlights the complexity and potential complications associated with the management of stenosis in the External Iliac Artery (EIA), particularly in the context of an endovascular aneurysm repair (EVAR). Successful EVAR is critically dependent on a patent and robust iliac system for secure device fixation and smooth flow.
- Significant EIA stenosis, as exhibited in this case, can potentially compromise the inflow and outflow dynamics, affect stent placement and ultimately the success of the EVAR short and long term.

BIOMECHNICAL AND HAEMODYNAMIC INSIGHT:

- EIA stenosis may result in an *elevated resistance to blood flow*, thus reducing the *perfusion pressure* downstream. This can cause a significant drop in the distal pressure, compromising the perfusion of lower limbs and increasing the risk of limb ischemia. The consequent reduction in flow could contribute to the risk of thromboembolic complications, including graft thrombosis.
- EIA stenosis can also affect stent-graft deployment during EVAR. Significant stenosis may limit the ability to accurately place and seal the stent-graft, especially in the presence of an angulated or tortuous access route. Furthermore, the *altered arterial wall compliance* due to calcified plaque could impose *additional mechanical stress* on the stent-graft, potentially leading to graft failure. The ongoing biomechanical interaction between the stent-graft and the diseased iliac artery wall may *influence the durability* of the repair.
- The ostial location of the disease could create a hostile sealing zone, affecting the secure fixation of the stent-graft, thereby increasing the risk of Type 1b endoleak.

MODEL CASE:
Multilevel angioplasty with quadruple angioplasty of the external iliac, lower popliteal, peroneal trunk, and anterior tibial arteries

WATCH LIVE:
https://tinyurl.com/25nu6wfk

NOTES, TIPS AND TRICKS:

ILIAC CASE: 20

A 64-year-old patient with a sudden onset of ischaemic leg. The patient had Right EIA stent. Duplex showed occluded right iliac stent. A decision was agreed to proceed for embolectomy and iliac stent recanalisation.

READ CAREFULLY ...

Access	Pre Op checklist, supine, GA , cleaned and draped, Right groin incised and CFA, PFA, SFA exposed. Vessels slung and clamped post 5000 IU heparin. Transverse arteriotomy performed..
Equipments	Standard (Micro-access. J Wire. Glidewire+Cobra. Amplatz+Proglide. Pigtail. contrast+HepSaline).
Angiogram Findings	Thrombus found in stent. PT occluded proximally and distally, reconstituting mid-leg. Significant distal thrombus in AT and Peroneal artery occlusion mid-leg.
Procedure	Stent relined with 10x59 V12 atrium stent. PT crossed with command wire and underwent PTA with 2x10 cm balloon. 5 mg Actilase used in AT and PTA performed with 3x10 cm balloon.
Complications	Failure to cross Peroneal artery.
Closure	Arteriotomy closed with 6/0 prolene. Wound sealed in three layers, followed by 20 ml of 0.25% chirocaine application.

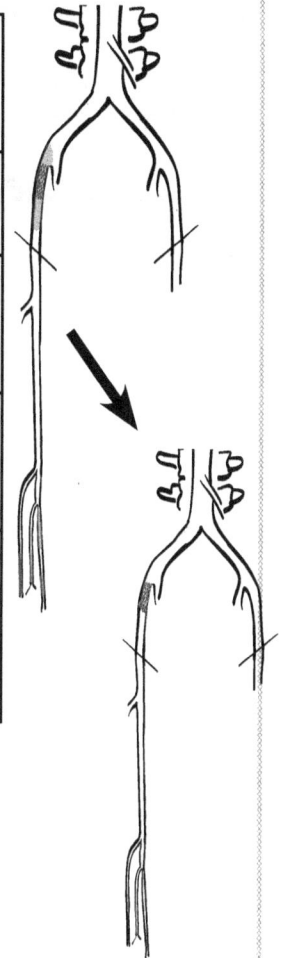

CONCISELY SUMMARIZE THE PROCEDURE USING KEY TERMS (ANSWER BELOW).

CHECK YOUR KNOWLEDGE

Qs ON STRATEGY

What measures should be taken to prevent clot migration to the distal part in the realigned iliac stent?

One strategy is to "sling the vessels" and employ a large sheath to remove the clot; in this case, a 7Fr sheath was used, although a 20Fr has been utilized in previous procedures.

Qs ON RECANALISATION

Is suction thrombectomy a requirement for addressing distal clots?

Not necessarily; in this case, a simple balloon angioplasty, which is a common approach, coupled with the use of actilase was employed.

Qs ON BALLOONING

Is utilizing a long balloon necessary for treating a localized blocked runoff artery?

Yes, it might be beneficial to avoid dissection and to facilitate even distribution of the clot along the arterial wall.

Qs ON COMPLICATIONS

What factors can impede the flow in the CFA, potentially leading to cessation?

Causes can include complications from a previous patch and the development of intimal hyperplasia, among others.

IN-DEPTH ANALYSIS

PROCEDURE : SUCTION THROMBECTOMY FROM OCCLUDED STENT + EIA STENTING + PT AND AT PLASTY AND LOCAL THROMBOLYSIS.

COMMENTS:

- Stent thrombosis was managed in this case using stent relining rather than direct suction thrombectomy. Suction thrombectomy could have potentially offered a more immediate and robust response to the thrombus within the stent. It allows for removal of thrombus material, rapidly restoring blood flow, and reducing the thrombus burden before stent relining, which could minimize the risk of distal embolization. However, the chosen method may have been dictated by the specifics of the case, including the location and extent of the thrombus, or available resources and expertise.

- The use of local thrombolysis with Actilase in the AT was a necessary step given the significant distal thrombus observed. This could facilitate thrombus breakdown and may improve downstream flow in the presence of such severe peripheral arterial occlusions.

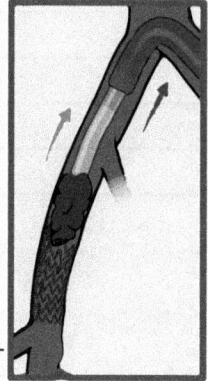

BIOMECHNICAL AND HAEMODYNAMIC INSIGHT:

- The thrombus within the stent *disrupts the laminar flow* of blood, leading to turbulent flow, which increases the risk of *further thrombus formation* and propagates a vicious cycle of thrombogenesis. Turbulence contributes to increased shear stress on the arterial walls and can *perpetuate endothelial dysfunction* and injury, instigating further platelet aggregation and thrombus formation.

- Stent relining is an important strategy to reinforce the vessel's biomechanical properties and maintain patency. The choice to employ a 10x59 V12 atrium stent provides both *radial strength and flexibility*, crucial to counteract the vessel's intrinsic and extrinsic forces, and ensure a balance between conformity and support.

- The administration of local thrombolysis would instigate fibrinolysis, breaking down the thrombus, thereby improving distal flow and reducing the ischemic risk. However, it's essential to consider the fibrin-specificity and half-life of the thrombolytic agent, which would influence the resolution rate of the thrombus and the risk of bleeding complications.

MODEL CASE:
Recanalization for limb salvage

WATCH LIVE:
https://tinyurl.com/
yth3bv8n

NOTES, TIPS AND TRICKS:

SIMPOD™ TRAINING CASES

https://www.vssmasterclass.co.uk

SIMPOD™ ILIAC 1

LESION: Lt EIA. 23mm long. 90% stenosis. Sim EIA diameter: 12.5mm
YOUR TASK: Angioplasty +/- stenting via Rt femoral

Notes:

SIMPOD™ ILIAC 2

LESION: Rt EIA. 40mm long. 95% stenosis. Sim EIA diameter: 12.5mm
YOUR TASK: Angioplasty +/- stenting via Lt femoral

Notes:

SIMPOD™ ILIAC 3

LESION: Rt IIA. 21mm long. 99% stenosis. Sim IIA diameter: 8.1mm
YOUR TASK: Angioplasty +/- stenting via Lt femoral

Notes:

SIMPOD™ ILIAC 4

LESION: Lt EIA. 45mm long. 75% stenosis. Sim EIA diameter: 6.5mm
YOUR TASK: Angioplasty +/- stenting via Rt femoral

Notes:

SIMPOD™ ILIAC 5

LESION: Rt EIA. 33mm long. 95% stenosis. Sim EIA diameter: 6.3mm
YOUR TASK: Angioplasty +/- stenting via Lt femoral

Notes:

SIMPOD™ ILIAC 6

LESION: Rt CIA. 65mm long. 80% stenosis. Sim EIA diameter: 12.4 to 6.3mm
YOUR TASK: Angioplasty +/- stenting via Rt femoral

Notes:

SIMPOD™ ILIAC 7

LESION: Lt EIA. 140mm long. 70% stenosis. Sim EIA diameter: 6.5mm
YOUR TASK: Angioplasty +/- stenting via Rt femoral

Notes:

SIMPOD™ ILIAC 8

LESION: Lt EIA. 68mm long. 85% stenosis. Sim EIA diameter: 7.7mm
YOUR TASK: Angioplasty +/- stenting via Rt femoral

Notes:

SIMPOD™ ILIAC 9

LESION: Lt EIA: 40x 85% in 5.8mm+ Rt CIA and EIA: 15 & 30mm; 90% &70%; 15 & 7.4
YOUR TASK: Angioplasty +/- stenting via Lt femoral

Notes:

SIMPOD™ ILIAC 10

LESION: Rt IIA. 38mm long. 80% stenosis. Sim EIA diameter: 6.3mm
YOUR TASK: Angioplasty +/- stenting via Lt femoral

Notes:

SIMPOD™ ILIAC 11

LESION: Lt EIA. 18mm long. 85% stenosis. Sim EIA diameter: 6.7mm
YOUR TASK: Angioplasty +/- stenting via Rt femoral

Notes:

SIMPOD™ ILIAC 12

LESION: Rt CIA. 22mm long. 90% stenosis. Sim EIA diameter: 15mm
YOUR TASK: Angioplasty +/- stenting via Lt femoral

Notes:

SIMPOD™ ILIAC 13

LESION: Lt EIA. 48mm long. 90% stenosis. Sim EIA diameter: 6.5mm YOUR TASK: Angioplasty +/- stenting via Rt femoral		
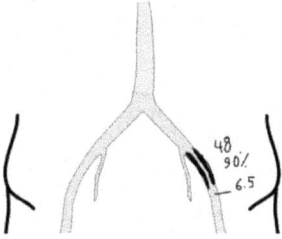		
Notes:		

CHAPTER 3
SFA ENDOVASCULAR THERAPIES Q&A

SFA CASE: 1

A 67-year-old patient presented with a left leg severe claudication. Duplex scan showed 90% stenosis in left CFA and a blocked SFA. A decision was agreed to do a CFA endartrectomy and SFA angioplasty.

READ CAREFULLY ...

STAGE 1	
Access	following a CFA endarterectomy, a 6 Fr sheath in the CFA introduced.
Complication	Damage to posterior wall of artery and CFA bifurcation, potential narrowing of proximal PFA
Closure	Multiple sutures

STAGE 2	
Access	6 Fr sheath in the SFA
Angiogram	Heavily calcified artery with multiple stenoses and short occlusions
Procedure	Attempt to pass wire through calcified artery unsuccessful
Complications	Wire passage not successful
Closure	Decision to stop. 6-0 prolene for sheath entry site

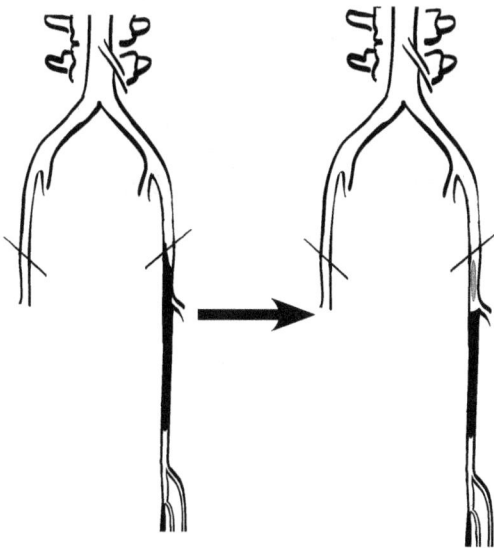

CONCISELY SUMMARIZE THE PROCEDURE USING KEY TERMS (ANSWER BELOW).

CHECK YOUR KNOWLEDGE

Qs ON ACCESS

What should be the subsequent course of action if SFA plasty fails after CFA endarterectomy?

Discontinue if the perfusion is satisfactory, otherwise, a bypass may be contemplated.

Qs ON RECANALISATION

If the wire cannot successfully pass, what are the typical considerations?

Subintimal or using a retrograde approach from a more distant point of access are potential strategies.

What are optimal strategies for canalizing the SFA in CTO scenarios where other strategies such as subintimal angioplasty have not succeeded?

- Retrograde approach: In some cases, a retrograde approach may be attempted where the occlusion is crossed from a distal puncture site and re-entering the true lumen of the SFA. This can be challenging and may require specialized techniques and equipment.
- Use of a dedicated CTO device: Some dedicated CTO devices such as the Crosser catheter, Outback re-entry device, or Tornus catheter may be considered for crossing the occlusion and re-entering the true lumen.
- Re-entry techniques: Re-entry techniques such as the Outback re-entry system, the Frontrunner catheter, or the Stingray balloon can be used to create a new channel within the occlusion and re-enter the true lumen.
- Hybrid techniques: Hybrid techniques that combine both antegrade and retrograde approaches may be considered for complex CTOs that are difficult to cross with a single approach.

IN-DEPTH ANALYSIS

PROCEDURE : SUCCESSFUL **CFA** ENDARTERECTOMY AND **BOVINE** PATCH. ATTEMPTED **SFA** RECANALISATION FOLLOWING **CFA**E. FAILED AS WIRE WENT INTO POSTERIOR WALL. THEN UNABLE TO PASS WIRE THROUGH **SFA** OCCLUSION

COMMENTS:

- In this case, the patient underwent an open CFA endarterectomy and an attempt SFA plasty. An endarterectomized artery wall has become l more vulnerable to damage. This might resuly in an arterial dissection, whereby the forceful manipulation of the wire or catheter can lead to a tear in the arterial wall, creating a false lumen through which blood flows, potentially leading to further complications such as vessel occlusion or aneurysm formation.
- The Excessive force or incorrect placement of the catheter or wire can cause a perforation in the artery wall, which may result in bleeding, hematoma formation, or even retroperitoneal hemorrhage.

BIOMECHEMICAL INSIGHT:
- Key biomechanical aspects to consider in this case include:
- Vascular wall stress: When manipulating a catheter or guidewire, it is essential to consider the stress exerted on the arterial wall. Excessive stress can lead to intimal injury, medial dissection, or even perforation. Factors contributing to vascular wall stress include intraluminal pressure, vessel diameter, and wall thickness.

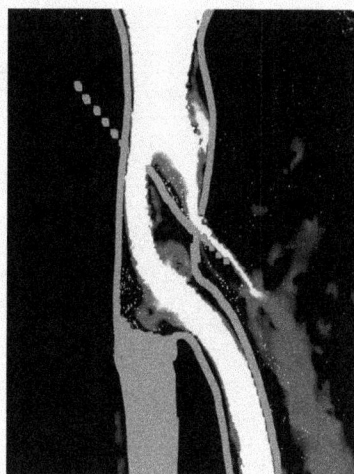

- Catheter and guidewire characteristics: The mechanical properties of catheters and guidewires, such as stiffness, flexibility, and torque response, can significantly impact the forces transmitted to the arterial wall. Understanding the interplay between these characteristics is essential to optimize device selection and minimize the risk of arterial damage.
- Calcification and plaque morphology: Heterogeneous plaque composition, particularly in the presence of heavily calcified lesions, can create irregular stress distributions and make the arterial wall more susceptible to injury. Utilizing intravascular imaging modalities like intravascular ultrasound (IVUS) or optical coherence tomography (OCT) can provide better visualization of plaque morphology and facilitate safer device manipulation.
- Hemodynamic forces: Blood flow exerts shear stress on the endothelial surface, which can

influence the endothelial response to injury and the propensity for restenosis. Understanding the impact of local hemodynamic conditions and their interplay with device manipulation is critical for minimizing the risk of endothelial injury and subsequent complications.

- Material fatigue: Repeated mechanical stress on the arterial wall, particularly at the site of previous endarterectomy, can lead to material fatigue and increased susceptibility to injury. This highlights the importance of gentle and precise manipulation of catheters and guidewires to reduce cumulative stress on the vascular wall.

MODEL CASE:
Tandem lesions of high-grade stenosis in the proximal superficial femoral artery and total occlusion of the popliteal artery, treated with Ranger drug-coated balloon (DCB)

WATCH LIVE:
https://tinyurl.com/y2kuyc8k

NOTES, TIPS AND TRICKS:

SFA CASE: 2

A 65-year-old patient presented with a non-healing ulcer on left foot. Duplex scan showed severe stenosis in left SFA and at. A decision was agreed to proceed to SFA +/- AT angioplasty.

READ CAREFULLY ...

Access	Pre Op checklist, supine, GA , cleaned and draped, ultrasound antegrade left CFA access, noted variant profunda anatomy. Used 6Fr sheath..
Equipments	Standard (Micro-access. J Wire. Glidewire+Cobra. Amplatz+Proglide. Pigtail. contrast+HepSaline).
Angiogram Findings	CFA patent, PFA anatomy variant. Focal severe stenosis in mid SFA, rest patent. PopA, TPT patent with two-vessel runoff via PA and PTA. Multiple severe stenoses in mid-ATA. Pedal arch patent.
Procedure	Intraluminal crossing of SFA and ATA stenoses. 6mm and 3mm POBA applied to SFA and ATA stenoses, respectively.Post-procedure angiogram showed patent SFA and brisk flow via ATA, preserved PA, PTA, and patent pedal arch.
Complications	No immediate post-procedure complications.
Closure	Employed 6Fr MynxControl for haemostasis during closure.

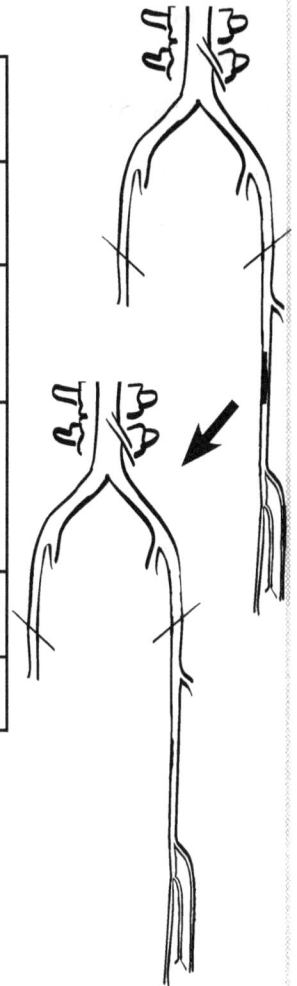

CONCISELY SUMMARIZE THE PROCEDURE USING KEY TERMS (ANSWER BELOW).

CHECK YOUR KNOWLEDGE

Qs ON STRATEGY

Is it necessary to treat runoff disease if the proximal region has been addressed and two other runoffs are functioning properly?

Establishing a comprehensive pedal/plantar loop enhances oxygen pressure readings (from 42 to 59 mmHg) and notably increases the amputation-free rate as evidenced in the RENDEZVOUS Registry. Moreover, the 12-month wound healing rate was considerably higher in the PAA group compared to the no-PAA group, a trend that held true irrespective of the severity of the inframalleolar disease (severe cases: 59.6% vs 33.2%).

What is the effect of a complete vs incomplete foot arch?

Effect on wound healing rate, amputation site healing, and patency of proximal vessels.

Qs ON BALLOONING

Is POBA sufficient for the treatment of SFA stenosis?

Yes, if the check angiogram are exceptionally smooth and brisk.

IN-DEPTH ANALYSIS

PROCEDURE : SFA (6)AND AT (3) POBA PLASTY

COMMENTS:

- This case demonstrates a successful use of Percutaneous Transluminal Angioplasty (POBA) to address the significant stenoses in both the SFA and ATA.
- The balloon exerts a radial force against the arterial wall. This radial expansion, in biomechanical terms, induces a controlled dissection within the intima and media, pushing the atheromatous plaque against the vessel wall and thus re-establishing a more optimal lumen diameter. This dilatation reduces the wall shear stress in accordance with the law of Laplace (which states that wall tension in a vessel is directly proportional to the radius of the vessel), subsequently enhancing blood flow by reducing turbulence and resistance.

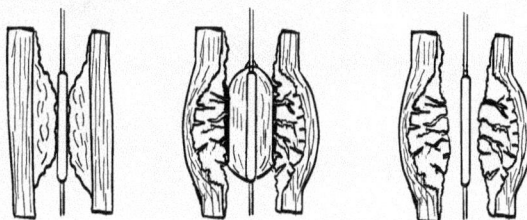

- The impact of POBA on the artery is twofold: acute and chronic. Acutely, it increases the internal diameter and improves the haemodynamics by optimising flow dynamics and diminishing local pressure gradients. Chronically, the arterial injury caused by the balloon dilatation instigates a healing response. This healing process involves remodelling of the arterial wall, involving intimal hyperplasia and neo-atherosclerosis. The balance between the therapeutic benefit of luminal gain and the potential negative remodelling responses is critical in understanding the long-term patency of the artery.

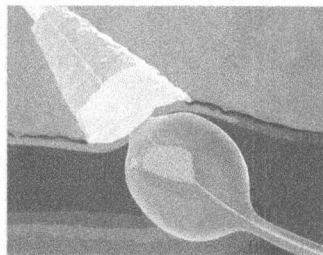

- The use of a 6Fr MynxClosure device for closure is helpful. Its unique extravascular, bioabsorbable, sealant-based design ensures optimal haemostasis without leaving any foreign material permanently in or at the femoral artery puncture site. This reduces the risk of foreign body reactions, infections, arterial occlusion or pseudoaneurysm formation, while providing a secure closure and allowing early mobilisation.

SFA CASE: 3

A 52-year-old patient with a previous left AKA presented with a critical limb ischaemia in the right foot. Duplex scan showed a complete sfa occlusion on right side. A decision was agreed to proceed to SFA/AT angioplasty +/- stenting.

READ CAREFULLY ...

Access	Pre Op checklist, supine, LA , cleaned and draped,Ultrasound-guided antegrade puncture of R CFA with 6Fr sheath and retrograde puncture of R PTA at ankle via 4Fr access.
Equipments	Standard (Micro-access. J Wire. Glidewire+Cobra. Amplatz+Proglide. Pigtail. contrast+HepSaline).
Angiogram Findings	Extensive SFA calcification and proximal stenoses. Mid-distal SFA occlusion, heavily calcified, with reconstitution at adductor hiatus. Patent popliteal artery, three-vessel runoff, DP, and dorsal arch, but PTA occlusion at ankle.
Procedure	SFA occlusion traversed from retrograde access of distal posterior tibial artery using a 0.018 support catheter and guidewire after failed antegrade approach. Pre-dilation of occlusion with 4mm balloon, followed by dilation of SFA with 5mm and 6mm balloons. Deployment of 5.5mm x 200mm and 5.5mm x 80mm Supera stents across mid-distal SFA. Minimal debris at TP trunk bifurcation, dilated proximal PTA and peroneal with 3mm balloon.
Complications	Minimal debris at TP trunk bifurcation, groin and scrotal hematoma occurrence.
Closure	6Fr Angioseal employed with no haemostasis. Prolonged compression for haemostasis of groin and scrotal haematoma. Femstop applied pre-ward transfer.

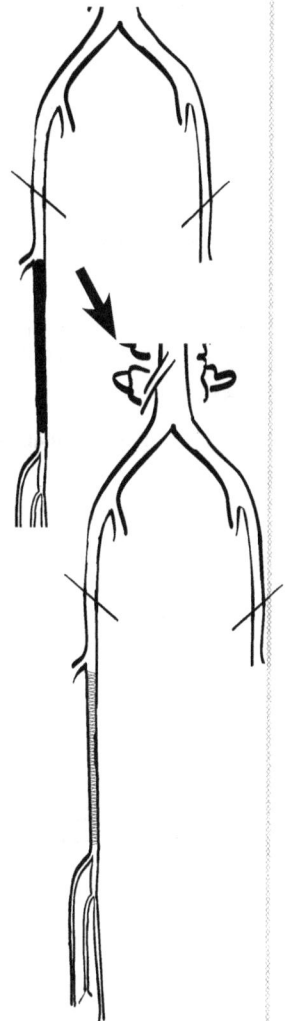

CONCISELY SUMMARIZE THE PROCEDURE USING KEY TERMS (ANSWER BELOW).

CHECK YOUR KNOWLEDGE

Qs ON STRATEGY

Is it justified to use a stent to treat an undiseased contralateral iliac?

Yes, if treating the other iliac could negatively impact it.

Qs ON ACCESS

Does a distal PTA occlusion prevent utilizing it for retrograde access?

No

What alternatives exist when it is impossible to cross the SFA?

Retrograde approach

Can you explain what SAFARI is?

SAFARI, or Subintimal Arterial Flossing with Antegrade-Retrograde Intervention, is a dual-access technique utilized in complex peripheral artery CTO interventions to facilitate recanalization by navigating through the subintimal space and stabilizing the true lumen, enhancing the success rate in difficult cases.

Qs ON RECANALISATION

Why opt for utilizing the diseased PT artery in SAFARI procedures addressing SFA occlusions?

It presents the most straightforward choice for securing through-and-through access.

Qs ON BALLONING

Can ballooning effectively eliminate dislodged debris?

It can to a certain degree, but not completely.

Is it possible to predict lesions which will end up in dislodged debris?

Predicting which lesions will result in dislodged debris can be challenging as it depends on a variety of factors including the nature of the lesion, the technique used, and the individual patient's circumstances. It is always recommended to approach each case with a comprehensive assessment to mitigate potential risks.

Qs ON STENTING

Is primary stenting of SFA useful in in cases where accessing the SFA/Safari is challenging?

yes

What might occur with the occluding lesion in the SFA following a Sarafi procedure?

It can dislodge and cause distal occlusions.

Qs ON COMPLICATIONS

What steps should be taken if debris is discovered in the tibials after a challenging SFA crossing?

Could employing a primary covered stent lessen the likelihood of debris becoming dislodged?

Ballooning can be a partial solution, as demonstrated in this instance.

Potentially, yes.

IN-DEPTH ANALYSIS

PROCEDURE : SFA SAFARI APPROACH (CFA/PT). NOT CROSSABLE ANTEGRADE. WIRE SNARED. SUPERA STENT USED.

COMMENTS:

- The SAFARI (Subintimal Antegrade Flossing with an Antegrade-Retrograde Intervention) technique was employed for this procedure, taking advantage of the unique characteristics of the superficial femoral artery (SFA) to navigate its calcified and occluded segments. Here, both antegrade (from the common femoral artery, CFA) and retrograde (from the posterior tibial artery, PTA) accesses were used to enable guidewire and catheter negotiation of the obstructed SFA.
- This approach capitalizes on the biomechanical properties of the vasculature, exploiting the less tortuous anatomy of the SFA and the presence of collateral vessels around the occlusion to create a subintimal plane that can be dilated and stented. While antegrade access provides an ideal approach to proximal lesions, retrograde access from the distal posterior tibial artery offers a *supplemental point of control*, allowing more complex manipulations in *highly calcified vessels*.
- Crossing of the SFA occlusion proved challenging but was ultimately successful, involving both intraluminal and subintimal traversal with a 0.018 support catheter and guidewire. The act of wire 'flossing' or snaring from the antegrade sheath, a hallmark of the SAFARI technique, facilitated the wire exchange and stenting.
- Supera stents, known for their superior radial force and flexibility, were used across the heavily calcified mid-distal SFA. This device is *engineered for mechanical durability,* providing superior resistance to external compression and *extreme bending*, while *preserving luminal diameter* and haemodynamics, thereby maintaining perfusion and patency.
- The haemodynamic impact of successful revascularization of the SFA was evident by the

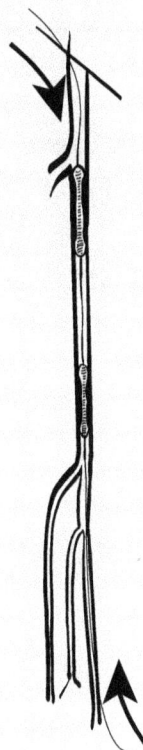

re-established flow in the SFA and beyond.

MODEL CASE:
sfa angioplasty

WATCH LIVE:
https://tinyurl.com/
bd7mc5xv

NOTES, TIPS AND TRICKS:

SFA CASE: 4

A 67-year-old patient with a history of multiple angioplasties and recoiling. Presented with Bilateral claudication < 80 yards with night pain. Duplex scan showed 75% right and left SFA stenosis. Duplex scan showed a complete SFA occlusion on right side. A decision was agreed to proceed to right SFA angioplasty +/- stenting.

READ CAREFULLY ...

Access	Pre Op checklist, supine, LA , cleaned and draped, Ultrasound-guided antegrade right CFA micropuncture and 4 French sheath used.	
Equipments	Standard (Micro-access. J Wire. Glidewire+Cobra. Amplatz+Proglide. Pigtail. contrast+HepSaline).	
Angiogram Findings	Widespread femoropopliteal disease with moderate stenoses in both the mid and distal segments of the SFA as well as the above-knee portion of the popliteal artery. A single vessel provides below-knee perfusion through the peroneal artery.	
Procedure	Glidewire and catheter navigated to popliteal artery below the knee. Using an Amplatz wire as support, multiple rounds of 5mm balloon angioplasty were executed.	
Complications	Despite the appearance of several short non-flow-limiting dissections, the angiographic outcome was satisfactory. The distal run-off maintained its pre-procedure appearance.	
Closure	6 French angio seal	

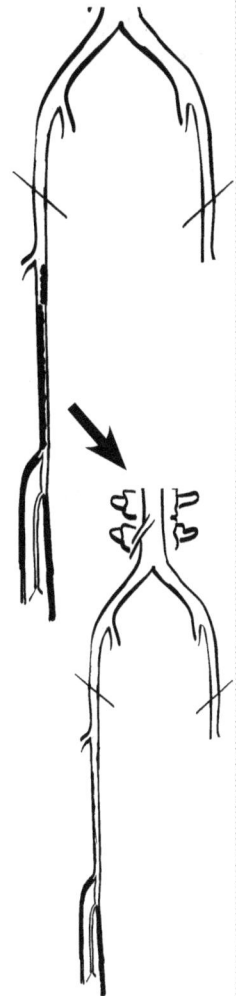

CONCISELY SUMMARIZE THE PROCEDURE USING KEY TERMS (ANSWER BELOW).

CHECK YOUR KNOWLEDGE

Qs ON STRATEGY

What treatment options would you explore for persistent SFA stenosis despite numerous POBA interventions?

DCB

Under what circumstances would you think about addressing runoffs if the SFA has been managed?

In cases of critical limb ischemia or symptoms associated with runoff disease. It should be noted that the PTA and ATA were not addressed in this case.

Qs ON COMPLICATIONS

When is it appropriate to address a dissection occurring post SFA POBA?

If it is limiting the flow.

IN-DEPTH ANALYSIS

PROCEDURE : SFA REPEATED ANGIOPLASTY (POBA) WITH NON-FLOW LIMITING DISSECTION

COMMENTS:

- The repeated use of POBA indicates that the stenoses were significant and resistant to initial interventions. It shows a persistent attempt at resolving the issue non-surgically, however, such an approach can increase the risk of dissection, as was noted in this case.
- The presence of non-flow limiting dissections post-angioplasty, while not immediately detrimental to blood flow, is nonetheless noteworthy. Although these dissections did not limit the flow immediately following the intervention, they could potentially contribute to restenosis or occlusion in the future. Careful follow-up will be crucial in this case to ensure that these dissections do not evolve into more significant complications over time.

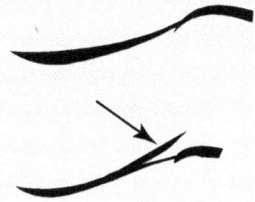

SFA Case: 5

A 59-year-old patient with a history of significant LEFT IC. Duplex showed a severe peri and in-stent stenosis with severely reduced PSV. A decision was agreed to proceed to left sfa stent angioplasty +/- stenting.

READ CAREFULLY ...

Access	Pre Op checklist, supine, GA , cleaned and draped, Right CFA puncture with ultrasound guidance. Retrograde approach.
Equipments	Standard (Micro-access. J Wire. Glidewire+Cobra. Amplatz+Proglide. Pigtail. contrast+HepSaline).
Angiogram Findings	Patent left iliac artery, CFA, profunda, mid SFA; stenosis in proximal SFA stent; 3-vessel runoff to ankle; attenuated peroneal artery in distal calf
Procedure	5 French 45 cm sheath advancement, CO2 angiography, 5000 IU heparin administration IA, glide wire and catheter negotiation across stenosis, 5 mm and 6 mm balloon angioplasty
Complications	None immediate
Closure	Haemostasis via manual pressure to right groin site

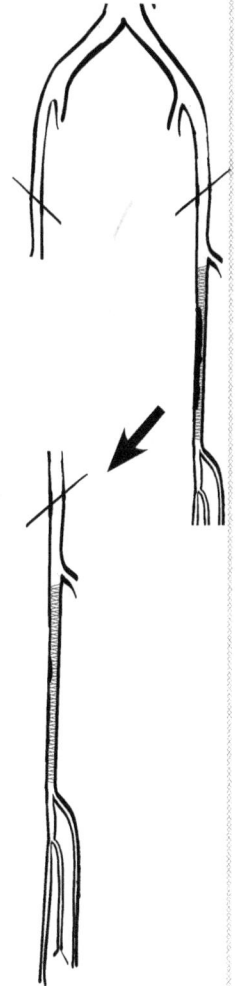

CONCISELY SUMMARIZE THE PROCEDURE USING KEY TERMS (ANSWER BELOW).

CHECK YOUR KNOWLEDGE

Qs ON BALLONING

Does POBA work well for in-stent stenosis?

In this instance, it successfully reduced the stenosis from a critical level (75%) to a non-critical one (50%).

Can performing a POBA on the proximal SFA have repercussions on the profunda?

Yes, it can, as demonstrated in this and other observed cases; it is akin to the effect seen with iliac kissing stents. A notable concern is that inserting a balloon in the PFA may lead to easy dissection, although this risk might be mitigated by using a long balloon that is only minimally inflated.

IN-DEPTH ANALYSIS

PROCEDURE : POBA FOR IN-STENT STENOSIS. DUPLEX POST SHOWING PFA NOW STENOTIC AND SFA 50% STENTED

COMMENTS:

- The POBA technique was employed to manage the in-stent stenosis. It involves inflation of a balloon within the stenotic segment, creating a mechanical force that disrupts the stenosis and pushes the plaque against the vessel wall, thereby improving lumen diameter and blood flow. Whilst straightforward, this method remains generally suboptimal in treating effectively the in-stent stenosis to provide a long term good patency and freedom from re-intervention.
- The biomechanical and hemodynamic implications of treating the SFA stenosis can also impact the profunda femoris artery (PFA), given it bifurcates from the common femoral artery (CFA) at the same level as the SFA. The therapeutic intervention on the proximal SFA could inadvertently alter the local flow dynamics at the level of the bifurcation, which could affect the hemodynamics in the PFA. Embolic debris dislodged during the intervention on the SFA could migrate into the PFA, leading to microvascular occlusion.

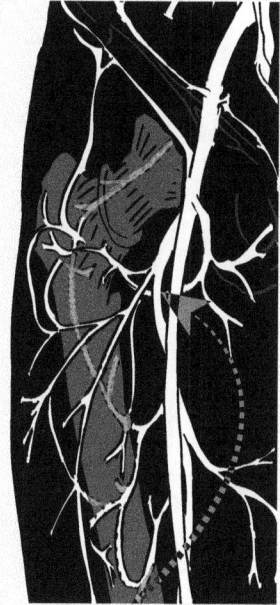

MODEL CASE:
recanalization for limb salvage

WATCH LIVE:
https://tinyurl.com/
yth3bv8n

NOTES, TIPS AND TRICKS:

SFA Case: 6

A 61-year-old patient with a history of significant IC in the RIGHT leg. Duplex showed a severe diseased CFA and blocked SFA. A decision was agreed to proceed to ?RIGHT CFA endartrectomy and SFA angioplasty +/- stenting.

READ CAREFULLY ...

Access	Pre Op checklist, supine, GA , cleaned and draped, Patched 6 French sheath puncture.
Equipments	Standard (Micro-access. J Wire. Glidewire+Cobra. Amplatz+Proglide. Pigtail. contrast+HepSaline).
Angiogram Findings	Severe calcification observed in the superficial femoral artery (SFA) with a tight stenosis in the middle of the SFA and adductor canal
Procedure	- SFA crossed using V18 and CXI/Navicross guidewires.Attempted to pass a 7x100 mm balloon through the adductor stenosis, but unsuccessful. Managed to cross the stenosis using a 4x60mm Serenity balloon.Performed angioplasty, resulting in an improved appearance of the affected area. Subsequently, performed angioplasty of the entire SFA using a 7mm balloon.
Complications	No complications reported.
Closure	Puncture site closed using a 5/0 prolene suture.

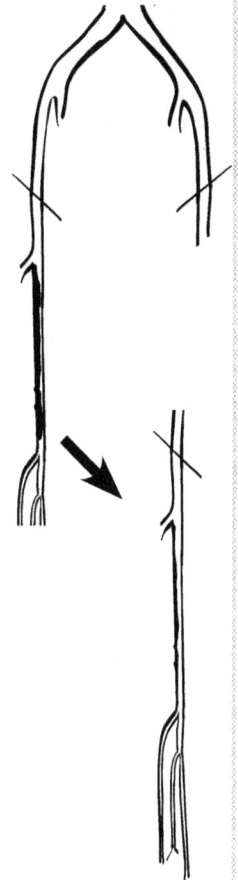

CONCISELY SUMMARIZE THE PROCEDURE USING KEY TERMS (ANSWER BELOW).

CHECK YOUR KNOWLEDGE

Qs ON BALLONING

What approach should be taken if the angioplasty balloon couldn't pass through the lesion despite the wire managing to do so?

Decrease the size of the balloon.

Which variety of angioplasty balloons are well-suited for tight lesions?

Serenity balloon.

IN-DEPTH ANALYSIS

PROCEDURE :SFA v18 / CXI/NAVICROSS. INITIALLY NOT PASSED THEN BALLOONED AND PASSED.

COMMENTS:

- During the procedure, the superficial femoral artery (SFA) was accessed using the Navicross and CXI wires, which are commonly employed for their excellent manoeuvrability and trackability. These wires were chosen due to their unique design and characteristics, allowing for precise control and navigation within the complex vascular anatomy of the SFA.
- The SFA presented with severe calcification, resulting in a tight stenosis located in the mid-SFA and adductor canal. This calcification posed a challenge to the advancement of the balloons initially attempted for angioplasty. However, by employing the 4x60mm Serenity

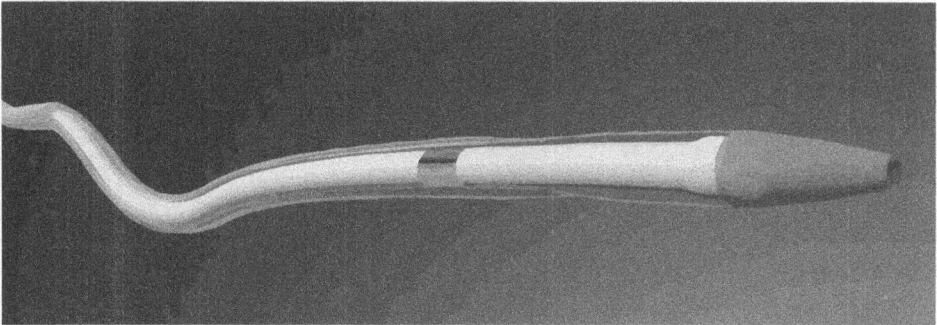

balloon, the adductor stenosis was eventually crossed successfully.
- From a biomechanical perspective, the use of the Navicross and CXI wires/catheters facilitated controlled and targeted forward force application, enabling successful navigation through the calcified and stenotic segments of the SFA. The wires' exceptional trackability and support were vital in ensuring precise positioning and minimizing the risk of vessel injury or dissection during the procedure.

SFA CASE: 7

A 77-year-old patient with a history of ulcers in the right leg. Duplex showed near occlusion of left CFA and tight stenosis in left CIA. A decision was agreed to proceed to left CFA endartrectomy and CIA angioplasty +/- stenting.

READ CAREFULLY ...

STAGE 1	
Access	Pre Op checklist, supine, GA , cleaned and draped, left CFA endarterectomy and patch done. Access retrogradely via puncturing the patch.
Result	Initial angiogram: tight mid left CIA not feasible to cross easily from left femoral access

STAGE 2	
Access	USS-guided rigth CFA puncture. Pig tail in aorta
Angiogram	Tight mid left CIA stenosis.
Procedure	Stenosis crossed. 10x59mm atrium stent to left CIA. Good angio and IVUS check
Complic.	Left SFA appeared occluded now.

STAGE 3	
Access	Up-and-over from right to left. Destination 6Fr sheath secured. terumo wire into SFA and CXI catheter Angio
Angio	Occlusion mid SFA to AK popliteal.
Procedure	terumo wire cxi, then navicross catheter to cross. 6x200mm angioplasty to the whole SFA.
Angio	Good inflow through CIA, Patent IIA SFA and 2 vessel run off into foot with ATA dominant
Closure	femseal to right

CONCISELY SUMMARIZE THE PROCEDURE USING KEY TERMS (ANSWER BELOW).

CHECK YOUR KNOWLEDGE

Qs ON RECANALISATION

Can IVUS fully substitute for contrast angiography in iliac angioplasty?

It didn't in this case; a run was still performed after verifying the tightness with IVUS.

What constitutes a suitable wire/catheter pairing for dealing with complete occlusions?

The Terumo wire CXI followed by a Navicross catheter.

Qs ON BALLONING

Is it mandatory to address the proximal lesion prior to tackling the distal one?

No, not if the proximal lesion is on the contralateral side. In this scenario, the right iliac was treated first, followed by the left SFA.

When encountering an extremely tight stenosis in a 6mm SFA artery, what kind of balloon is advisable to initiate with?

It is recommended to start with a smaller (4mm) low-profile balloon initially for predilation.

Is it advised to transition directly from predilation to a full-sized balloon?

No, it is better to progress gradually, moving from a 5mm balloon to a 6mm one.

Qs ON STENTING

Is it generally a good choice to primarily stent an opened SFA occlusion?

No. Despite what is suggested by "published" data, many are trying to avoid this approach.

If a remaining 50% stenosis is observed in the SFA despite multiple plastic surgeries, would inserting a stent be a consideration?

No, provided that the flow through the area remains satisfactory.

IN-DEPTH ANALYSIS

PROCEDURE :IVUS. ILIAC STENTING FIRST THEN UP-AND-OVER SHEATH AND SFA PLASTY.

COMMENTS:

- The complexity of this case can be appreciated when we unravel the intricate choreography of decision-making, steeped in a deep understanding of anatomy, haemodynamics, and the principles of interventional radiology. The sagacity of each decision is highlighted by the potential risks associated with alternative paths.

- The initial decision to switch the access from the left to the right Common Femoral Artery (CFA) is a crucial element that hinges on a profound appreciation of the complications of attempting to cross a severely stenotic left Common Iliac Artery (CIA). A forceful attempt at crossing the lesion from the left might have led to a hazardous subintimal passage with an ominous possibility of failing to re-enter the true arterial lumen, increasing the risk of aortic dissection. Therefore, the right-sided access exemplifies a tactically astute and safer approach in the context of this difficult anatomy.

- The discovery of the occlusion of the left Superficial Femoral Artery (SFA) after the angioplasty of the left CIA highlights the vigilant surveillance required during these interventions. The stenting procedure, despite being highly beneficial for the patency of the CIA, inherently carries a risk of embolic events downstream, possibly aggravated by the new application of the left CFA bovine patch. The angioplasty of the CIA may dislodge plaque or thrombus material, which can then migrate to the SFA causing acute occlusion. Alternatively, the thrombus could form de novo over the CFA area and initiate a cascade of thrombosis in the SFA. The detection and immediate addressing of this complication highlights the indispensability of continuous imaging guidance and the preparedness to manage such acute events.

- Upon identifying the SFA occlusion, the entire length of the SFA was subjected to angioplasty. This decision should not be viewed merely as a reactionary measure to the occlusion, but rather as a strategic move in its own right. The rationale here is that the angioplasty of the full length of the SFA, even in the face of acute occlusion, can improve the long-term patency of the vessel, which appears diseased especially at the adductor hiatus.

- In essence, this case magnifies the complexity and nuance involved in vascular interventions. Each decision has been made with a deep understanding of the associated biomechanical and hemodynamic implications and a commitment to patient safety and successful outcomes.

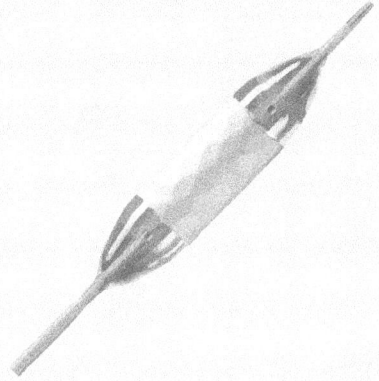

MODEL CASE:
Recanalization of recent superficial femoral artery occlusion under filter protection and tibial artery angioplasty

WATCH LIVE:
https://tinyurl.com/mp6jtdcv

NOTES, TIPS AND TRICKS:

SFA Case: 8

A 49-year-old patient with a history of Left leg gangrene. Duplex showed a multifocal diseased SFA with occlusion of the mid/distal SFA and significant stenosis popliteal artery. A decision was agreed to proceed to left SFA and tibial angioplasty +/- stenting.

READ CAREFULLY ...

Access	Pre Op checklist, supine, GA , cleaned and draped, Left CFA accessed using ultrasound-guided ante-grade micropuncture. 6Fr sheath.
Equipments	Standard (Micro-access. J Wire. Glidewire+Cobra. Amplatz+Proglide. Pigtail. contrast+HepSaline).
Angiogram Findings	Multifocal SFA disease with mid/distal SFA occlusion. Left P1 stenosis. Single-vessel runoff to foot via PT with incomplete plantar arch. Abnormal right CFV filling suggestive of AVF (prior varicose vein stripping history).
Procedure	Wire and catheter manipulation across occlusion into TP trunk. Overlapping 5mm x 14cm POBA angioplasties performed. Good post-procedure angiographic results.
Complications	Small non-flow limiting mid-SFA dissection.
Closure	6Fr Mynx

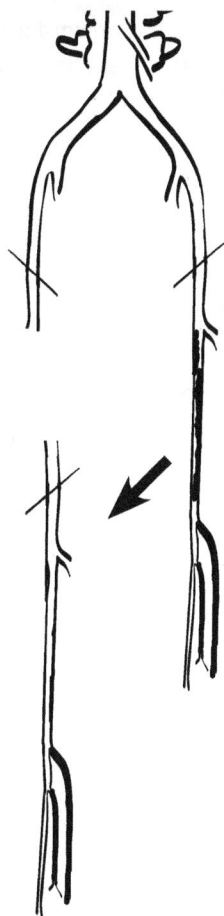

CONCISELY SUMMARIZE THE PROCEDURE USING KEY TERMS (ANSWER BELOW).

CHECK YOUR KNOWLEDGE

Qs ON STRATEGY

In situations where there is an incomplete foot arch accompanied by severe proximal disease, would undertaking an ultra-distal plasty be considered after addressing the more proximal issue?

No. Initially, addressing the severely diseased proximal lesions should suffice.

Qs ON STENTING

Under what circumstances would you manage a post-angiography dissection using a stent?

Only if it is restricting flow and not amenable to repeated angioplasty treatments.

IN-DEPTH ANALYSIS

PROCEDURE :SFA-TPT- PLASTY. COMPLICATION WITH DISSECTION. NO STENTS

COMMENTS:

- This case demonstrates the remarkable achievement of successful intraluminal recanalization throughout the entire occluded SFA, POP and TPT, despite its considerable length. This significant accomplishment not only restores blood flow but also streamlines the procedural approach.

- The ability to cross intraluminally without the need for stenting in the superficial femoral artery (SFA) and popliteal artery can offer significant advantages from biomechanical and hemodynamic perspectives. By successfully navigating through the occluded segment intraluminally, the natural arterial lumen is preserved, minimizing the risks associated with stenting in such delicate anatomical areas, such as stent fracture, restenosis, and thrombosis.

- This tactic is particularly beneficial in maintaining the biomechanical properties of the artery, including its compliance and vessel wall integrity. Preserving the natural lumen allows for physiological vessel dilation and contraction in response to hemodynamic changes, ensuring appropriate blood flow regulation. It also minimizes alterations to the arterial wall structure, preserving its mechanical strength and reducing the risk of long-term complications.

- When attempting to cross an occlusion intraluminally, advanced techniques and tools play a crucial role. The use of specialized wires with high flexibility and steerability enables precise navigation through tortuous vessels, allowing the wire to follow the natural course of the vessel without causing damage or perforation.

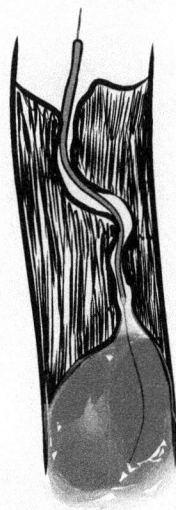

SFA CASE: 9

A 53-year-old patient with a history of Left leg gangrene. Duplex showed severe peri and in-stent stenosis with severely reduced PSV. A decision was agreed to proceed to left SFA angioplasty +/- stenting.

READ CAREFULLY ...

Access	Pre Op checklist, supine, LA , cleaned and draped, Ultrasound-guided retrograde puncture of Right Common Femoral Artery (CFA).
Equipments	Standard (Micro-access. J Wire. Glidewire+Cobra. Amplatz+Proglide. Pigtail. contrast+HepSaline).
Angiogram Findings	Patent left external iliac artery, left CFA, and pro-funda. Significant stenosis in proximal Superficial Femoral Artery (SFA) segment. Mid SFA stent patent with no in-stent stenosis. Three-vessel distal run-off to ankle; peroneal artery diminishes in distal calf.
Procedure	Glide wire and catheter traversed stenotic proximal SFA segment. Performed balloon angioplasty (5mm, then 6mm) across stenosis.
Complications	none
Closure	Manual pressure

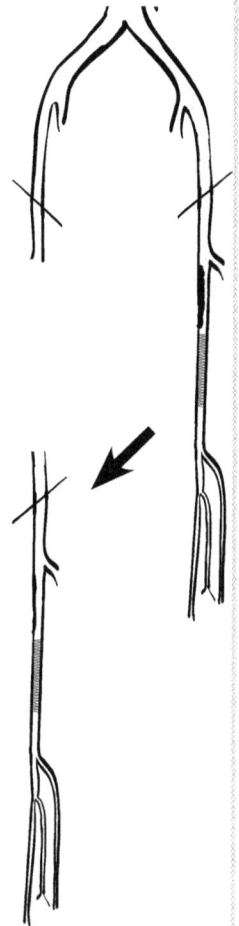

CONCISELY SUMMARIZE THE PROCEDURE USING KEY TERMS (ANSWER BELOW).

CHECK YOUR KNOWLEDGE

Qs ON BALLONING

If the SFA opened reasonably well with POBA, is there a possibility to explore other treatment options?

Yes, the appropriate approach can vary depending on the individual patient and the intended long-term results. Using DCB or atherectomy, for example, can always be considered.

Is there a necessity for employing DCB in addressing the moderate SFA stent stenosis located within a previously placed stent?

It seems logical to consider it, although it was not utilized in this particular instance.

IN-DEPTH ANALYSIS

PROCEDURE :SFA STENOSIS ABOVE A STENT. CO2 ANGIO. TREATED WITH POBA

COMMENTS:

- This case presents a significant, proximal Superficial Femoral Artery (SFA) stenosis, a challenging vascular territory due to its biomechanical and hemodynamic peculiarities. The SFA undergoes substantial mechanical stress owing to its location in the adductor canal where it's subjected to kinking, stretching, and compressional forces during leg movement. This biomechanical stress impacts the longevity and patency of interventions in this region.

- The stenosis in this case is situated proximally to a previously positioned stent, thus its treatment is critical to ensure adequate blood flow and maintain the patency of the downstream stent. If left untreated, this upstream lesion could compromise inflow, leading to an increased risk of stent thrombosis, and hence, a need for further revascularization procedures.

- From a hemodynamic perspective, the proximal lesion can cause turbulent blood flow, potentially inducing hyperplasia, leading to in-stent stenosis, a common cause of stent failure. Although in-stent stenosis was not detected on angiogram, regular monitoring is recommended. This is because signficant in-stent stenosis, if it occurs, needs to be promptly treated to prevent hazardous clinical complications.

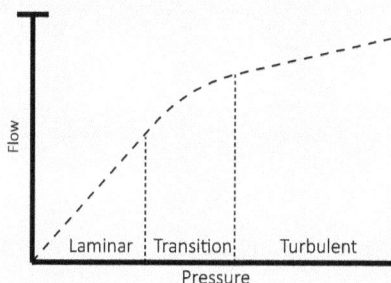

- The successful balloon angioplasty, in this case, has not only re-established a streamlined blood flow but also optimally preserved the functionality of the pre-existing stent. The absence of immediate complications and the achievement of satisfactory haemostasis further highlights the success of the intervention.

MODEL CASE:
High-grade in-stent restenosis of the right superficial femoral artery treated with Ranger stent.

WATCH LIVE:
https://tinyurl.com/2zr4r28j

NOTES, TIPS AND TRICKS:

SFA CASE: 10

A 57-year-old patient with a history of a non healing ulcer at the Base of left first toe. Duplex shows an SFA stenosis. A decision was agreed to proceed to left SFA angioplasty +/- stenting.

READ CAREFULLY ...

Access	Pre Op checklist, supine, LA , cleaned and draped, Ultrasound-aided retrograde right CFA access with 45cm 7Fr Destination sheath. Retrograde left PTA access with 4Fr pedal access sheath, also ultrasound-guided.
Equipments	Standard (Micro-access. J Wire. Glidewire+Cobra. Amplatz+Proglide. Pigtail. contrast+HepSaline).
Angiogram Findings	Patent left CFA and PFA with proximal stenoses. SFA occlusion. Patent PopA, TPT stenosis, proximal PTA stenosis. Patent proximal ATA (distally occluded), occluded DP, incomplete pedal arch.
Procedure	Antegrade SFA occlusion crossing attempts unsuccessful; retrograde PTA access used instead. Unable to advance nav6 filterwire past occlusion. Prox-mid SFA occlusion treated with rotational atherectomy. Angioplasty conducted with both POBA and DEB.
Complications	No immediate post-procedure complications.
Closure	Right CFA closed with 6Fr AngioSeal haemostasis; left distal PTA with manual pressure haemostasis. Patient well-tolerated the procedure.

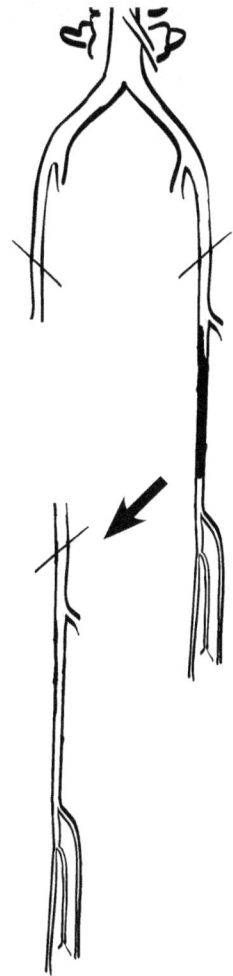

CONCISELY SUMMARIZE THE PROCEDURE USING KEY TERMS (ANSWER BELOW).

Qs ON ACCESS

Is dual proximal and distal access always necessary in atherectomy cases?

No, but it becomes necessary if passing through an intraluminal location is not possible.

Qs ON RECANALISATION

How would you proceed if the filter couldn't pass through to a distal location?

Continue without utilizing the filter.

Qs ON ATHERECTOMY

When performing an atherectomy, do you initiate the procedure from a proximal or distal location?

Proximally

If atherectomy couldn't address the distal portion, what would be your next step?

Utilize POBA and DCB.

IN-DEPTH ANALYSIS

PROCEDURE :LEFT SFA RECANALISATION WITH IVUS & ROTATIONAL ATHERECTOMY. POBA AND DCB TO LEFT SFA, POPA, TPT AND PTA.

COMMENTS:

- This case represents a multifaceted and challenging scenario of peripheral arterial disease, specifically focusing on the long segment superficial femoral artery (SFA) occlusion.
- The SAFARI (Subintimal Arterial Flossing with Antegrade-Retrograde Intervention) technique was utilized in this case as a robust method to manage the challenging long-segment SFA occlusion, highlighting the benefits of dual (both proximal and distal) access strategies in peripheral arterial interventions.
- The SAFARI technique permits a bidirectional approach to the occlusion which is an advantage in lengthy and complex lesions as seen in this case. Proximally, antegrade access aids in the initial attempts to cross the occlusion, while distally, retrograde access provides an alternative route when antegrade attempts are unsuccessful, which was exactly the scenario encountered in this case. Biomechanically, it is often easier to puncture and cross chronic total occlusions (CTOs) from the distal end, where the occlusion tends to be softer and the subintimal space is frequently broader. This is due to the natural tapering of arteries and the direction of blood flow which often pushes dislodged plaque towards the distal end of the occlusion. Additionally, the distal access provides a 'way out' for the guidewire, minimizing the risk of perforation or dissection, while also allowing for the guidewire to be 'externalized' and forming a continuous 'monorail' from the proximal to the distal access sites, providing a firm platform for subsequent balloon angioplasty or stenting.
- Rotational atherectomy of the proximal-mid SFA occlusion enabled effective plaque modification, preparing the lesion for further treatment. This is a significant step in managing complex occlusive disease and was imperative for the successful passage and expansion of the DCB.
- Following atherectomy, the extensive use of DCB angioplasty throughout the SFA and popliteal arteries capitalized on the antiproliferative properties of the paclitaxel coating. It aimed to reduce the risk of restenosis by inhibiting neointimal hyperplasia, a common issue in patients with such peripheral arterial disease.
- There appear to be some limitations with the atherectomy device not advancing into the distal SFA occlusion. This challenge highlights the complexity of the occlusive disease and the anatomical difficulties encountered in endovascular therapies.

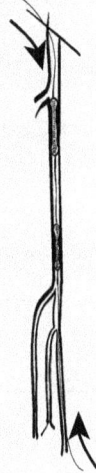

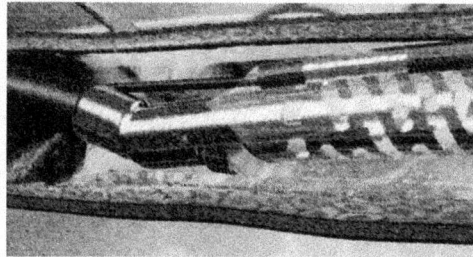

MODEL CASE:
Nothing Left Behind Strategy Long Stent
Graft Lesion Directional Atherectomy
Drug-Coated Balloon

WATCH LIVE:
https://tinyurl.
com/2dkrbmfj

NOTES, TIPS AND TRICKS:

SIMPOD™ TRAINING CASES

https://www.vssmasterclass.co.uk

SIMPOD™ SFA 1

LESION: Lt SFA. 60mm long. 90% stenosis. Sim SFA diameter: 6.1mm
YOUR TASK: Angioplasty +/- stenting via Lt femoral

Notes:

SIMPOD™ SFA 2

LESION: Rt SFA. 90mm long. 85% stenosis. Sim SFA diameter: 6.5mm
YOUR TASK: Angioplasty +/- stenting via Lt femoral

Notes:

SIMPOD™ SFA 3

LESION: Lt SFA. 40mm long. 85% stenosis. Sim EIA diameter: 6.1mm
YOUR TASK: Angioplasty +/- stenting via Rt femoral

Notes:

SIMPOD™ SFA 4

LESION: Lt SFA. 120mm long. 85% stenosis. Sim SFA diameter: 6.5mm
YOUR TASK: Angioplasty +/- stenting via Lt femoral

Notes:

SIMPOD™ SFA 5

LESION: Rt SFA. 60mm long. 80% stenosis. Sim EIA diameter: 7.7mm
YOUR TASK: Angioplasty +/- stenting via Rt femoral

Notes:

SIMPOD™ SFA 6

LESION: Rt SFA. 60mm long. 85% stenosis. Sim EIA diameter: 6.2mm
YOUR TASK: Angioplasty +/- stenting via Rt femoral

Notes:

SIMPOD™ SFA 7

LESION: Lt SFA. 48mm long. 90% stenosis. Sim EIA diameter: 6.4mm
YOUR TASK: Angioplasty +/- stenting via Lt femoral

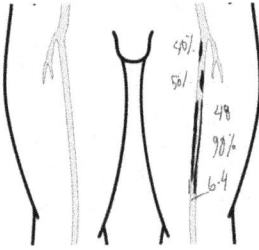

Notes:

SIMPOD™ SFA 8

LESION: Rt SFA. 70mm long. 85% stenosis. Sim EIA diameter: 6.3mm
YOUR TASK: Angioplasty +/- stenting via Rt femoral

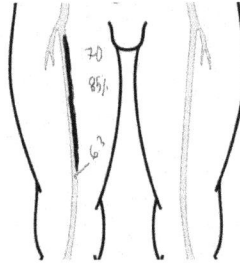

Notes:

SIMPOD™ SFA 9

LESION: Lt SFA. 200mm long. 80% stenosis. Sim EIA diameter: 6.9mm
YOUR TASK: Angioplasty +/- stenting via Rt femoral

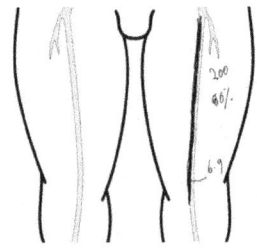

Notes:

SIMPOD™ SFA 10

LESION: Lt SFA. 31mm long. 85% stenosis. Sim EIA diameter: 7.8mm
YOUR TASK: Angioplasty +/- stenting via Lt femoral

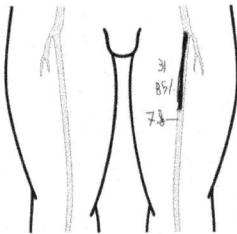

Notes:

SIMPOD™ SFA 11

LESION: Lt SFA. 27mm long. 85% stenosis. Sim EIA diameter: 6.6mm
YOUR TASK: Angioplasty +/- stenting via Lt femoral

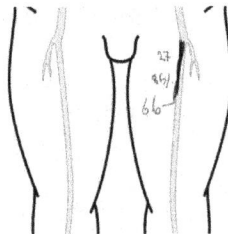

Notes:

SIMPOD™ SFA 12

LESION: Rt SFA. 85mm long. 85% stenosis. Sim EIA diameter: 6.3mm
YOUR TASK: Angioplasty +/- stenting via Rt femoral

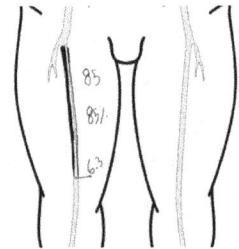

Notes:

CHAPTER 4 POPLITEAL (+/- SFA AND/OR TIBIALS) ENDOVASCULAR THERAPIES Q&A

POP CASE: 1

A 71-year-old diabetic patient presented with a toe gangrene. Duplex scan showed an SFA occlusion and severe popliteal and TPT disease. A decision was agreed to perform angioplasty of SFA, popliteal and below the knee tibials.

READ CAREFULLY ...

Access	Pre Op checklist, supine, GA , cleaned and draped, Successful puncture of left CFA (below injection sinus area) under ultrasound guidance. Antegrade right CFA access with 6Fr sheath. Retrograde distal right ATA pedal access
Equipments	Standard (Micro-access. J Wire. Glidewire+Cobra. Amplatz+Proglide. Pigtail. contrast+HepSaline) + POBAs and DEBs (IN.PACT Admiral Paclitaxel-coated). No stents
Angiogram Findings	CFA and PFA are patent. Focal moderate stenosis at origin of SFA. Focal distal occlusion of SFA. Popliteal artery segments P1 and P2 are patent, with moderate stenosis in segment P3. ATA occlusion at its origin, with reconstitution at mid-calf level. Significant stenosis within TPT, multiple occlusions in the peroneal artery (PA), and complete occlusion of PT. Incomplete plantar arterial arch
Procedure	Subintimal crossing of distal SFA occlusion. Multiple antegrade attempts to traverse ATA were unsuccessful. Decision made for retrograde distal ATA access, successfully crossing proximal ATA occlusion via intraluminal technique 5mm POBA of proximal SFA stenosis and distal SFA occlusion. 5mm DEB applied to distal SFA occlusion. 3mm POBA of P3 PopA and along ATA, 3.5mm prolonged high-pressure POBA addressing moderate stenosis in proximal ATA.
Complications	None. Rapid flow via widely patent SFA, PopA, and ATA. Improved filling of pedal arch
Closure	Manual pressure haemostasis to right CFA and ATA access sites.

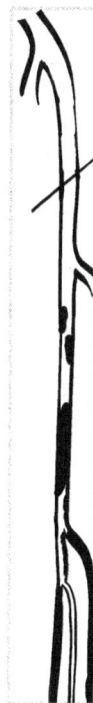

CONCISELY SUMMARIZE THE PROCEDURE USING KEY TERMS (ANSWER BELOW).

CHECK YOUR KNOWLEDGE

Qs ON ACESS

What is the optimal initial approach for this case, and what should be the alternative strategy if it does not yield the expected result?

The preferred starting point is an antegrade CFA puncture with an attempt to cross the SFA downward, either through the luminal or subintimal pathway. Should this be unsuccessful, the fallback plan should be to employ a retrograde approach through the AT.

What aspects rendered the AT cannulation exceptionally challenging or even unfeasible in this scenario?

In this case, the difficulties arose from the presence of a proximal tight lesion, the adoption of a less-than-ideal pathway to reach the affected region, and a complete occlusion of the AT at a point flush with the surface.

If the antegrade cannulation of the AT falls short, given that the AT is the solitary artery extending distally to the DP and foot arch, what constitutes the best secondary choice?

Consider attempting Pop/TPT cannulation directly.

Qs ON BALLOONING

What can you do to a poorly responding tibial stenosis following balloon angioplasty?

Just re-plasty with possibly larger and high pressure. See what happened to AT in this case.

IN-DEPTH ANALYSIS

PROCEDURE SUMMARY : SFA (5), POP(3), AND ATA(3 THEN 3.5) OCCLUSION PLASTY. NO STENT. UNSUCCESSFUL 1ST THEN SUCCESS. DCB. SUBINTIMAL.

COMMENTS:

- The subintimal revascularization employed for the distal SFA occlusion required adept manipulation of guidewires and catheters, capitalizing on the arterial wall's inherent viscoelasticity and the subintimal space's pliability for optimal negotiation.
- The DEB combines controlled radial force application with sustained circumferential wall stress modulation to minimize vessel recoil and ensure luminal patency. The antiproliferative agents delivered by the DEB mitigate neointimal hyperplasia, thereby counteracting biomechanical and cellular responses that contribute to restenosis.
- The biomechanical difference between drug-eluting balloon (DEB) and plain old balloon angioplasty (POBA) balloons is that DEB balloons have a coating of antiproliferative drugs (such as paclitaxel or sirolimus) that are released into the vessel wall during inflation, while POBA balloons have no drug coating.
- - A study by Tepe et al. 1 evaluated the mechanical characteristics and drug delivery of four different DEB balloons (In.Pact Pacific, Lutonix, SeQuent Please, and Passeo-18 Lux) and one POBA balloon (Admiral Xtreme). They found that all DEB balloons had lower compliance and higher burst pressure than the POBA balloon, and that the drug delivery varied among the DEB balloons depending on the coating technology and balloon material.
- - A study by Werk et al. 2 compared the mechanical performance and drug release of two DEB balloons (SeQuent Please and Paccocath) and one POBA balloon (Mustang). They found that both DEB balloons had similar compliance and burst pressure as the POBA balloon, but higher drug release (90% vs. 0%).
- (1) Comparison Among Drug-Eluting Balloon, Drug-Eluting Stent, and Plain .... https://www.sciencedirect.com/science/article/pii/S193687981401749X.
- (2) Drug-eluting balloon (DEB) versus plain old balloon angioplasty (POBA .... https://journals.sagepub.com/doi/full/10.1177/03000605221081662.

RESEARCH INSIGHT

- - A study by Sallustro et al. [1] compared the 24-month outcomes of a new dual-drug coated balloon (Elutax) versus POBA for femoropopliteal lesions. They found that Elutax was associated with lower restenosis/reocclusion rate, improved primary patency, and lower clinically driven target lesion revascularization (CD-TLR) rate than POBA.
- - A review by Sherif [2] summarized the evidence on angioplasty and stenting for peripheral arterial disease of the lower limbs. He reported that DEB angioplasty showed better primary

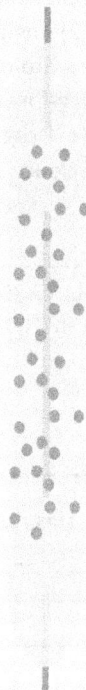

patency and lower CD-TLR rate than POBA for femoropopliteal lesions, especially in short and non-calcified lesions.

- - A review by Scheinert et al. [3] evaluated the efficacy and safety of DEB for treatment of superficial femoral artery (SFA) and popliteal disease. They concluded that DEB angioplasty was superior to POBA in terms of primary patency and CD-TLR rate at 12 and 24 months, with no significant difference in mortality or major adverse events.

- (1) Results of New Dual-Drug Coated Balloon Angioplasty versus POBA for .... https://www.sciencedirect.com/science/article/pii/S0890509622006227.

- (2) Angioplasty and stenting for peripheral arterial disease of the lower limbs. https://www.escardio.org/Journals/E-Journal-of-Cardiology-Practice/Volume-16/Angioplasty-and-stenting-for-peripheral-arterial-disease-of-the-lower-limbs.

- (3) Drug-eluting balloons for treatment of SFA and popliteal disease – A .... https://www.sciencedirect.com/science/article/pii/S0720048X17301158.

MODEL CASE:	**WATCH LIVE:**	
safety in CTO treatment	https://tinyurl.com/366cpsb9	

NOTES, TIPS AND TRICKS:

MODEL CASE:	**WATCH LIVE:**	
Long left fast stenosis with in-stent occlusion of the left popliteal artery	https://tinyurl.com/3vxy2nf4	

NOTES, TIPS AND TRICKS:

POP CASE: 2

A 63-year-old diabetic patient presented with worsening left leg ulcer. A Left SFA and popliteal stents were deployed previously. They were found blocked on Duplex. A decision was agreed to perform angioplasty of SFA and popliteal stent +/- below the knee tibials.

READ CAREFULLY ...

Access	Pre Op checklist, supine, GA , cleaned and draped, Successful puncture of left CFA (below injection sinus area) under ultrasound guidance. A retrograde right CFA access. 45cm 6Fr Destination sheath.
Equipments	Standard (Micro-access. J Wire. Glidewire+Cobra. Amplatz+Proglide. Pigtail. contrast+HepSaline) + POBAs. In.Pact Admiral Paclitaxel DEB. Cook Zilver Flex stent. Abbott Xience Alpine Everolimus Drug-eluting stent.
Angiogram Findings	The CFA and PFA are patent. There is severe stenosis in the proximal SFA, with occlusions in the mid and distal SFA, PopA, and TPT. The PA is filled via collateral circulation, but there is no filling observed in the pedal arch.
Procedure	Crossed long segment occlusion with catheter and guidewire. 6mm POBA in SFA and P1 PopA, followed by DEB. Flow-limiting dissection within proximal SFA and mid-SFA (in between two previous stents). Moderate to severe stenoses remained within the P3 PopA, TPT, and proximal PA. Placement of multiple stents in proximal and mid-SFA. 5mm POBA in P2-P3 PopA stent, 3mm POBA in proximal TPT and PA. Placement of stents in P3 PopA and TPT.
Complications	No immediate post-procedure complication.
Closure	6Fr AngioSeal haemostasis.

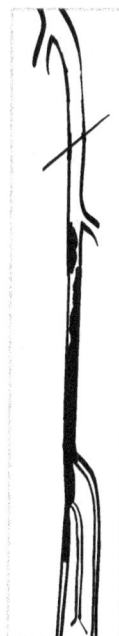

CONCISELY SUMMARIZE THE PROCEDURE USING KEY TERMS (ANSWER BELOW).

CHECK YOUR KNOWLEDGE

Qs ON ACCESS

What is the most suitable initial approach for this case, and what should be the backup plan if the first strategy doesn't lead to the anticipated result?

The best initial strategy would be a retrograde CFA puncture, aimed at comfortably accessing the proximal SFA lesion. However, a drawback to this approach is the potential requirement for a long sheath if the tibials are not easily accessible.

Qs ON CANNULATION

What does the ease of cannulating the obstructed SFA stent indicate?

It suggests the presence of a relatively recent clot.

Qs ON BALLOONING

In treating a blocked stent, which is preferable: initially utilizing a covered stent or initiating with extended ballooning?

The data is insufficient to definitively choose one, which is why DCB is frequently utilized.

How effective is a POBA angioplasty in addressing in-stent stenosis?

While POBA angioplasty can be employed to manage in-stent stenosis, its efficacy may be limited in intricate or resistant lesions characterized by calcification or fibrosis. It also carries a risk of complications such as dissection, rupture, slippage, or restenosis. Consequently, alternatives such as drug-coated balloons (DCB) or drug-eluting stents (DES) might be favoured.

What role does the Abbott Xience Alpine Everolimus Drug-eluting stent play in the treatment of the TPT trunk?

While not commonly used in TPT trunk treatments, some studies have documented positive outcomes with the Abbott Xience Alpine Everolimus DES, highlighting its safety and effectiveness, including high patency and low amputation rates. When compared to bare-metal stents and balloon angioplasty, it demonstrated superior patency and fewer revascularization occurrences, albeit without significant differences in amputation or mortality rates.

IN-DEPTH ANALYSIS

PROCEDURE : SFA Pop stent occlusion. Complication with dissection. Stents down to TPT. Supera. DCB.

COMMENTS:

In this complex case, the patient presented with thrombosed stents affecting multiple segments, including the SFA, PopA, and TPT. The successful navigation and treatment with the use of further multiple stenting and angioplasty procedures demonstrate the importance of adaptable interventional approach. Despite some residual stenosis and patient discomfort, the restoration of in-line flow to the foot indicates a positive outcome, which could significantly improve the patient's quality of life and limb prognosis.

BIOMECHANICAL INSIGHT:
- The comprehensive treatment strategy employed a combination of percutaneous transluminal angioplasty (PTA) and drug-eluting balloon (DEB) angioplasty, as well as the deployment of self-expanding nitinol stents with differing designs (Cook Zilver Flex, Abbott Supera) and a drug-eluting stent (Abbott Xience Alpine Everolimus) to address the heterogeneous nature of the lesions.
- When deploying multiple over-lapping stents in the superficial femoral artery (SFA), several biomechanical factors come into play, which can impact the long-term patency and clinical outcomes. Understanding these factors is crucial for optimizing the treatment strategy in complex peripheral vascular interventions.

  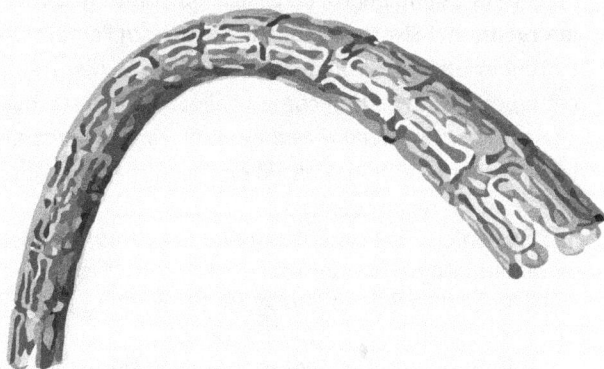

  - Stent configuration: Overlapping stents create a unique, multi-layered stent configuration that affects local hemodynamics and alters the biomechanical forces acting on the stented arterial segment. This configuration may lead to increased radial strength and rigidity, potentially improving vessel scaffolding but also increasing the risk of stent fracture or arterial injury due to excessive radial force.
  - Stent strut apposition and interaction: The interaction between the struts of overlapping stents may result in non-uniform distribution of mechanical stress and strain within the vessel wall. This non-homogeneous distribution could predispose the treated segment to neointimal hyperplasia, in-stent restenosis, and stent thrombosis.
  - Stent material and design: The choice of stent materials and designs, such as the self-expanding nitinol stents used in this case, is essential to ensure adequate flexibility, conformability, and fatigue resistance in the dynamically challenging SFA environment. However, multiple overlapping stents with varying designs may lead to heterogeneous mechanical properties and potentially impact the long-term durability and effectiveness of intervention.

- Drug delivery and elution kinetics: When using drug-eluting stents (DES) or drug-eluting bal-loons (DEB) in combination with overlapping stents, the drug distribution and elution profile may be affected by the complex stent geometry. This could result in uneven drug concentrations within the vessel wall and potentially influence the antiproliferative effect, thereby affecting restenosis rates.
- In conclusion, deploying multiple overlapping stents in the SFA introduces complex biomechanical interactions that can influence the success of endovascular interventions. Careful consideration of stent materials, designs, and drug-elution technologies, along with meticulous procedural techniques, is vital to maximize the potential benefits and minimize potential complications in such intricate cases.

RESEARCH INSIGHT

- **Superficial femoral artery stenting: Impact of stent design and overlapping on the local haemodynamics**[**1]: This study investigated the effect of different stent designs and overlapping configurations on the blood flow and wall shear stress in SFAs using computational fluid dynamics. The results showed that stent design and overlapping influenced the hemodynamics and might have implications for ISR development.
- **The United States StuDy for EvalUating EndovasculaR TreAtments of Lesions in the Superficial Femoral Artery and Proximal Popliteal By usIng the Protégé EverfLex NitInol STent SYstem II (DURABILITY II)**[**2]: This study evaluated the safety and efficacy of a single self-expanding stent up to 20 cm in length in patients with atherosclerotic disease of the SFA and proximal popliteal artery. The results showed that the stent was safe and effective, with high patency rates and improved clinical outcomes at 1 year.
- **Interventional Strategies for the Superficial Femoral Artery**[**3]: This chapter reviewed the current evidence and guidelines for endovascular treatment of SFA lesions, including different types of stents, drug-coated balloons, atherectomy devices, and bioresorbable scaffolds. The authors concluded that there is no single best strategy for SFA intervention, and that individualized treatment based on lesion characteristics, patient preferences, and operator experience is recommended.

  (1) Superficial femoral artery stenting: Impact of stent design and .... https://pubmed.ncbi.nlm.nih.gov/35124437/.

  (2) The United States StuDy for EvalUating EndovasculaR TreAtments of .... https://pubmed.ncbi.nlm.nih.gov/23642924/.

  (3) Interventional Strategies for the Superficial Femoral Artery. https://www.in-techopen.com/chapters/62983.

- Abbott Xience Alpine Everolimus Drug-eluting stent (DES) is a type of stent that releases a drug called everolimus, which inhibits the growth of smooth muscle cells and reduces the risk of in-stent restenosis (ISR). Abbott Xience Alpine Everolimus DES is approved for the treatment of coronary artery disease and peripheral arterial disease, including tibial artery lesions.

MODEL CASE:
Popliteal artery angioplasty and posterior
tibial recanalization

WATCH LIVE:
https://tinyurl.
com/25nu6wfk

NOTES, TIPS AND TRICKS:

POP CASE: 3

A 71-year-old patient presented with a right leg hallux ulcer on a background of Burger's disease and a previous left BKA. Duplex scan showed severely diseased popliteal and tibial arteries. A decision was agreed to perform angiogram and possible angioplasty to popliteal and tibial arteries.

READ CAREFULLY ...

Access	Pre Op checklist, supine, GA , cleaned and draped, Successful puncture of left CFA (below injection sinus area) under ultrasound guidance. Antegrade right CFA micropuncture with a 6Fr sheath.
Equipments	Standard (Micro-access. J Wire. Glidewire+Cobra. Amplatz+Proglide. Pigtail. contrast+HepSaline) + POBAs and DEBs (IN.PACT Admiral Paclitaxel-coated). No stents
Angiogram Findings	CFA, PFA, and proximal SFA are all patent; extensive blockage in distal SFA, popliteal artery, and tibioperitoneal trunk with sizable medial collateral vessel; single vessel runoff through posterior tibial artery; plantar arch remains patent.
Procedure	The femoropopliteal and tibioperitoneal trunk occlusion were traversed using a 0.035" catheter and guidewire combination. The distal SFA and popliteal long segment occlusion were dilated with a 3mm POBA followed by a 5mm balloon. The completion angiogram revealed successful recanalization and swift blood flow through the patent popliteal artery.
Complications	None immediately post-procedure.
Closure	6Fr MynxControl haemostasis.

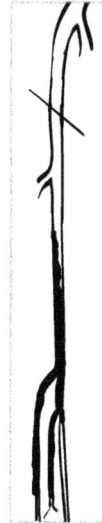

CONCISELY SUMMARIZE THE PROCEDURE USING KEY TERMS (ANSWER BELOW).

CHECK YOUR KNOWLEDGE

Once the wire crosses distally, whuich lesion should be treated first?

Proximal lesion first

IN-DEPTH ANALYSIS

PROCEDURE : POPLITEAL TPT PLASTY. CROSSED WITH 035 WIRE! BALLOONED 3 THEN 5. SUCCESSFUL.

COMMENTS:

- Popliteal angioplasty can be challenging due to the artery's anatomical location, tortuosity, and biomechanical forces, making the procedure technically demanding. Moreover, the presence of a single vessel run-off via the posterior tibial artery highlights the importance of the intervention, as it was the only remaining route for blood supply to the foot. This limited run-off may put the patient at higher risk for future ischemic events, emphasizing the need for vigilant follow-up and optimal medical management.

BIOMECHANICAL INSIGHT:

- The popliteal artery's biomechanical environment presents unique challenges during angioplasty due to its exposure to multiple forces, such as compression, torsion, and shear stress. These forces arise from the artery's location behind the knee joint, where it is subjected to complex, multidirectional movements during flexion, extension, and rotation. The dynamic nature of this region can lead to increased vessel tortuosity, calcification, and higher restenosis rates following endovascular interventions.
- The successful dilation using 3mm and 5mm percutaneous transluminal angioplasty balloons mitigated the the need for stent insertion with its associated risks, which may arise from the biomechanical forces in the popliteal region. A vigilant follow-up are crucial for minimizing restenosis and maintaining long-term patency in such complex cases.

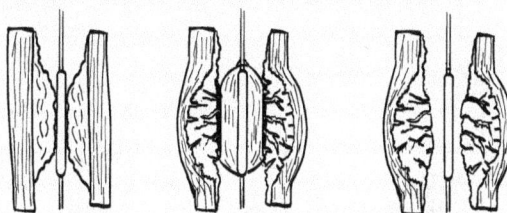

HAEMODYNAMIC INSIGHT:

- The presence of a long segment occlusion in the distal SFA and popliteal artery led to compromised blood flow, thereby placing an increased reliance on the single-vessel run-off via the posterior tibial artery for perfusion. This situation created a high-resistance, low-flow state, leading to potential ischemia and tissue damage in the affected limb. Following the successful recanalization of the occluded segment, the hemodynamic parameters improved significantly, with the angiogram revealing rapid flow via the patent popliteal artery. This restoration of blood flow decreased the resistance and increased the perfusion pressure in the distal vasculature, providing improved oxygen and nutrient delivery to the tissues.
- Nevertheless, the presence of a single run-off vessel may still predispose the patient to a higher risk of future ischemic events due to limited collateral circulation. It is crucial to optimize medical management and ensure a regular follow-up and assessment of the limb's status.

RESEARCH INSIGHT

- One of the best recent studies on the comparison of outcomes for balloon angioplasty, atherectomy, and stenting in the treatment of infrapopliteal disease for chronic limb-threatening ischemia is published in Jan2023. Oh, K. et all (Journal of Vascular Surgery, doi:10.1016) analyzed limb salvage (LS), amputation-free survival (AFS), and target extremity reintervention (TER) outcomes after plain old balloon angioplasty (POBA), stenting, and atherectomy for treating infrapopliteal disease (IPD) with chronic limb-threatening ischemia (CLTI). The researchers used data from the Vascular Quality Initiative registry, and propensity score matching was employed to control for baseline differences between groups. The results showed that the 3-year LS rates for stenting and POBA were 87.6% and 81.9%, respectively, while AFS was superior for stenting (78.1%) compared to POBA (69.5%). LS rates for POBA and atherectomy were similar, as were those for stenting and atherectomy. Stenting demonstrated a significantly longer interval to TER compared to POBA or atherectomy. In conclusion, stenting and atherectomy had comparable LS and AFS outcomes for patients with IPD and CLTI, but stenting offered significant benefits in AFS compared to POBA, and a longer interval to TER than POBA or atherectomy. These factors should be considered when determining the treatment strategy for this challenging anatomic segment.

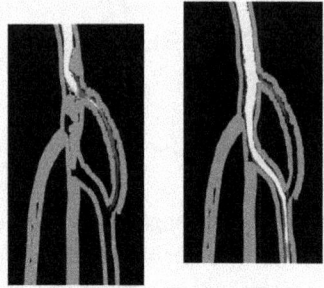

MODEL CASE: Left P1-P2 high-grade stenosis treated with Ranger	**WATCH LIVE:** https://tinyurl. com/4yrbj3ct

NOTES, TIPS AND TRICKS:

POP CASE: 4

A 78-year-old patient presented with severe left intermittent claudication. Duplex scan showed a popliteal occlusion. A decision was agreed to perform angioplasty of popliteal.

READ CAREFULLY ...

Access	Pre Op checklist, supine, LA , cleaned and draped, Ultrasound-assisted retrograde entry to the left common femoral artery, placement of a 6Fr sheath.
Equipments	Standard (Micro-access. J Wire. Glidewire+Cobra. Amplatz+Proglide. Pigtail. contrast+HepSaline) + POBAs and DEBs (IN.PACT Admiral Paclitaxel-coated). No stents
Angiogram Findings	Blockage in the distal section of the left superficial femoral artery. Flow reinstated in the P2 segment of the popliteal artery. Good anterior and posterior tibial artery runoff to the foot.
Procedure	Recanalization of the blocked segment accomplished with a hydrophilic wire. Angioplasty executed using a 5 mm plain balloon.
Complications	None immediately post-procedure.
Closure	6Fr angioseal

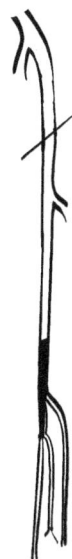

CONCISELY SUMMARIZE THE PROCEDURE USING KEY TERMS (ANSWER BELOW).

CHECK YOUR KNOWLEDGE

Qs ON BALLOONING

How can you determine if the outcomes of the angioplasty are not "fantastic"?

- The appearance of the artery
- Remaining lesions
- TWO VIEWS (Not utilized here)
- IVUS (Not utilized here)
- Collaterals being filled BEFORE the primary 'new' artery

Qs ON STENTING

IF ANGIOPLASTY OUTCOME WAS NOT THAT GREAT BUT FAIRLY ACCEPTABLE IN SFA, IS USING A STENT PROVIDES A BETTER LONG TERM OPTION?

IN-DEPTH ANALYSIS

PROCEDURE : SFA OCCLUSION. STANDARD. POBA..

COMMENTS:

- This case exemplifies the principle of 'simplicity is the ultimate sophistication' in medical practice. This case was managed by keeping the process streamlined yet effective, enabling the successful recanalization of the occluded segment of the left superficial femoral artery and P1. This approach highlights the importance of not over-complicating medical procedures when straightforward strategies are effective. It's a testament to the idea that complexity does not necessarily equate to better outcomes.

BIOMECHANICAL INSIGHT:

- Plain Old Balloon Angioplasty (POBA) employed here plays a critical role in physically opening up the occlusion in the SFA and improving blood flow.
- The success of angioplasty is not only about restoring the lumen but also maintaining it. The recanalized artery is under constant hemodynamic and biomechanical stress due to blood flow and limb movement, which may lead to restenosis. The site of this occlusion, at the adductor hiatus, is a common spot for lesion development due to mechanical stress and flexion and extension movements of the lower limb. These movements can cause the already diseased artery in a high risk patient, to kink, leading to turbulent blood flow and eventual stenosis.
- When considering stenting in this case, there are clear pros and cons. A stent can act as a physical scaffold to keep the vessel open, improving the durability of the angioplasty and reducing the risk of restenosis. However, in areas of high mechanical stress such as the adductor hiatus, the rigidity of a stent can potentially lead to biomechanical complications including fracture or deformation. Additionally, in-stent restenosis or stent thrombosis are possible adverse events.
- Finally, stent placement also limits future treatment options, as repeat endovascular procedures become more complex in a stented segment. A simpler approach of balloon angioplasty with intensive follow-up and targeted secondary interventions might indeed be preferable in this case, balancing biomechanical and hemodynamic factors for optimal patient outcome.

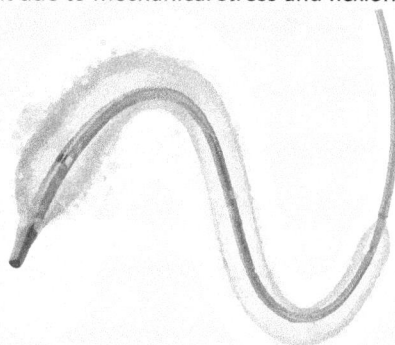

MODEL CASE:
Right popliteal artery occlusion

WATCH LIVE:
https://tinyurl.
com/547w37pj

NOTES, TIPS AND TRICKS:

POP CASE: 5

A 72-year-old patient with a ulcers left leg. Previous Right AKA with prosthetic fitting. The patient had a previous LEFT distal SFA/P1-2 Pop stent. Duplex shows Left POP in-stent stenosis. A decision was agreed to proceed to left Pop angioplasty +/- stenting.

READ CAREFULLY ...

Access	Pre Op checklist, supine, LA , cleaned and draped, Left CFA accessed with ultrasound-guided antegrade micropuncture and a 7Fr bright tip sheath.
Equipments	Standard (Micro-access. J Wire. Glidewire+Cobra. Amplatz+Proglide. Pigtail. contrast+Hep-Saline) + POBAs and DEBs (IN.PACT Admiral Paclitaxel-coated). No stents
Angiogram Findings	CFA and SFA are widely patent. Occlusion observed from P2 across P3 into trifurcation of the popliteal stent. Thin opacification seen in diseased proximal ATA to ankle. Occlusion in TPT and proximal Peroneal, recanalized through large collateral vessels.
Procedure	Stent occlusion to proximal ATA recanalized intraluminally using 0.018 platform and 0.035 half-stiff terumo wire. 5mm Nav6 filter deployed in proximal ATA. Atherectomy of occluded stent and P3 using Jetstream. Nav6 and Jetstream catheter en bloc removal after device snagging. Lesions re-crossed successfully. DEB angioplasty of stent (6 x 80mm). POBA of TPT (4 x 40mm) and entire ATA (3 x 80mm), followed by proximal PTA.
Complications	Post-angioplasty showed widely patent popliteal stent, two-vessel runoff, and distal ATA spasm.
Closure	Hemostasis achieved with 7fr Mynx closure.

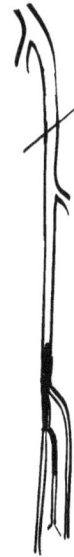

CONCISELY SUMMARIZE THE PROCEDURE USING KEY TERMS (ANSWER BELOW).

CHECK YOUR KNOWLEDGE

Qs ON STRATEGY

Why was the 5mm Nav6 filter used before the atherectomy with Jetstream?

The Nav6 filter captures potential embolic debris during atherectomy, reducing the risk of downstream complications.

Qs ON BALLOONING

How might the use of a drug-eluting balloon (DEB) angioplasty, as mentioned in the procedure (6 x 80mm), offer advantages or challenges over a plain old balloon angioplasty (POBA) in the context of a recanalized stent?

DEB angioplasty releases drugs that inhibit restenosis by reducing smooth muscle proliferation. This could be advantageous in preventing re-occlusion of a previously occluded stent. However, DEB might also pose challenges, including potential allergic reactions to the drug, cost implications, or concerns about uneven drug delivery in certain lesion morphologies. In comparison, POBA is a straightforward mechanical dilatation without drug involvement.

IN-DEPTH ANALYSIS

PROCEDURE : ATHERECTOMY AND RE-ALIGNMENT OF STENT.

COMMENTS:

- Atherectomy involves the mechanical removal of plaque from blood vessels, and in this case, the Jetstream rotational atherectomy device was used. This device is beneficial in treating complex peripheral arterial disease (PAD) due to its ability to modify both soft and calcified plaque, and also its potential to treat total occlusions.

- In the biomechanical aspect, the Jetstream consists of a catheter with rotating blades at the tip. The high-speed rotation (up to 70,000 RPM) is designed to cut the plaque into tiny particles that are then aspirated into the catheter and removed from the patient's body. This helps restore the lumen's diameter and improves blood flow. The device also has infusion ports distal to the cutting blades to continuously infuse saline and prevent heat build-up, which could injure the vessel.

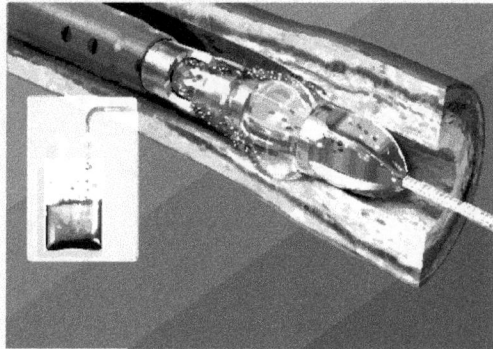

- In this scenario, however, a complication arose when the atherectomy device became entangled on the guidewire of the Nav6 filter, leading to the en bloc removal of the Nav6 filter and Jetstream catheter. This could have led to potential hemodynamic implications, such as abrupt vessel closure or dissection due to mechanical stress on the vessel wall. It also could lead to a period of compromised blood flow, depending on how long it took to manage the situation.

- The post-procedural observation of spasm in the distal ATA could have been a consequence of the mechanical trauma that occurred when the setting up the devices. Vessel spasm is a physiological response to injury and could potentially limit flow in the treated area until it resolves. Careful monitoring and pharmacological management (i.e., vasodilators) are usually required in such situations.

- After the complications were managed, there was successful recanalization, and hemostasis was achieved. The vessel showed satisfactory post-angioplasty appearances with widely patent popliteal stent and two-vessel runoff, suggesting that any potential negative hemodynamic effects were successfully managed.

MODEL CASE:
Right superficial femoral artery occlusion
with right popliteal artery stenosis

WATCH LIVE:
https://tinyurl.
com/4mdj3syb

NOTES, TIPS AND TRICKS:

STRATEGIC QUESTIONS- POPLITEAL ARTERY PROCEDURES

In a popliteal artery Chronic Total Occlusion (CTO), what would be your best strategy, and expected outcome, in relation to the following:

Point of discussion	Answer	Comment
What is the best Access point?	Antegrade femoral. Standard to achieve best pushability, manuerverability, and torque Retrograde using PT or AT. Can be considered in selected patients such as: - Previous fem-pop bypass where antegrade approach failed to 'engage' into the lesion.	
Which Guidewires and catheters to Consider?	CXI + Terumor (The 'horse' tools) NaviCross (more distal, 0.018 or 0.014 guidewire) Asahi for distal subintimal revascularisation	
What options for treatment are there?	• POBA • DCB • High chronic outward force (COF) stenting • Low chronic outward force (COF) stenting • Biomemitic stenting • Shockwave Lithotripsy • Atherectomy	

In POBA +/- Bail-out stenting:

What is the likelihood of performing a plain balloon procedure compared to a bail-out stenting procedure?	Estimated 70:30	The IPAD Multicenter Study (2018). 3 tertiary centres (Greece). 46 of 4717 PAD procedures.

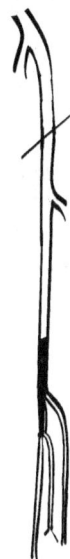

Restenosis rate at 1,2, and 3 years	Est. 15, 40, 45% @ 1,2&3 yr
TLR-free rate @ 1,2 and 3 years	Est. 90, 80, 75% @ 1,2&3 yrs
Limb salvage @ 5 years	Est. 75%
Survival @ 5 yrs	Est. 90%
Major Amputation Rate in claudicants vs . CLI	0% vs 10%

Is the treatment outcome for popliteal endovascular procedures different between patients with Chronic Total Occlusion (CTO) and those without CTO?

- In the non-CTO group, conventional balloon angioplasty was more common (33% vs. 21%, P<0.001), as was drug-coated balloon angioplasty (3% vs. 1%, P<0.001)

XLPAD registry (2023) on total of 3658 lesions

- In the CTO group, bare-metal stents were used more frequently (28% vs. 20%, P<0.001), as were covered stents (4% vs. 2%, P<0.001)

- Debulking procedures were performed more frequently in the non-CTO group (53% vs. 41%, P<0.001), despite similar levels of calcification between the two groups

- The non-CTO group had a higher procedural success rate (97% vs. 90%, P<0.001)

- The CTO group experienced more procedural complications (7% vs. 5%, P=0.002), primarily due to a higher rate of distal embolization (2% vs. 1%, P=0.015)

- One year after treatment, the CTO group had a higher rate of major adverse limb events (22% vs. 19%, P=0.019), which was mainly driven by a higher rate of target limb revascularization (19% vs. 15%, P=0.013)

What is the current estimated 5-yr clinical improvement, primary patency, secondary patency, freedom from TLR outcome and amputation-free survival for each of the following procedures:

The IPAD Multicenter Study (2018). 3 tertiary centres (Greece). 46 of 4717 PAD procedures.

POBA — Est. 65, 50, 65, 50 & 90%

DCB — Est. 70, 50, 70, 45 & 90%

LOW COF — Est. 70, 55, 80, 45 & 95%

HIGH COF — Est. 65, 55, 85, 50 & 95%

DAART — Est. 85, 60, 80, 60 & 95%

SIMPOD™ TRAINING CASES

https://www.vssmasterclass.co.uk

SIMPOD™ POP 1

LESION: Lt SFA+POP. 50, 70, & 67; 85%, 95%, & 81%. Sim diameter: 6.5, 6.5, & 6.6
YOUR TASK: Angioplasty +/- stenting via Lt femoral

Notes:

SIMPOD™ POP 2

LESION: Rt SFA+POP. 110mm long. 60% stenosis. Sim EIA diameter: 5mm
YOUR TASK: Angioplasty +/- stenting via Rt femoral

Notes:

SIMPOD™ POP 3

LESION: Lt SFA+POP. 90mm long. 90% stenosis. Sim EIA diameter: 6.5mm
YOUR TASK: Angioplasty +/- stenting via Lt femoral

Notes:

CHAPTER 5
TIBIAL
ENDOVASCULAR
THERAPIES Q&A

TIBIAL CASE: 1

A 48-year-old diabetic patient presented with tissue loss in the dorsum of the left foot. Duplex scan shows a likely distal tibial/microvascular disease. A decision was agreed to attempt a tibial angioplasty to establish circulation to the ulcer area.

READ CAREFULLY ...

Access	Pre Op checklist, supine, GA, cleaned and draped, Antegrade L CFA puncture via US with 4Fr sheath.
Equipments	Standard (Micro-access. J Wire. Glidewire+Cobra. Amplatz+Proglide. Pigtail. contrast+HepSaline)
Angiogram Findings	Femoropopliteal clear. ATA: proximal stenoses, ankle occlusion. PerA patent, limited arch supply. Proximal PTA occlusion.
Procedure	ATA stenoses dilated (2.5mm Ultrascore). ATA occlusion negotiated, dilated (2mm balloon). Pedal arch supply minimally improved. PTA recanalisation not attempted.
Complications	Hypotension, tachycardia during haemostasis. Prolonged compression, fluid resuscitation, 1 unit PRBC. Stable Hb on venous gas.
Closure	Retroperitoneal haematoma on US. CTA: no puncture-related haemorrhage. Noted: decreased L iliopsoas haematoma from 9/1/23.

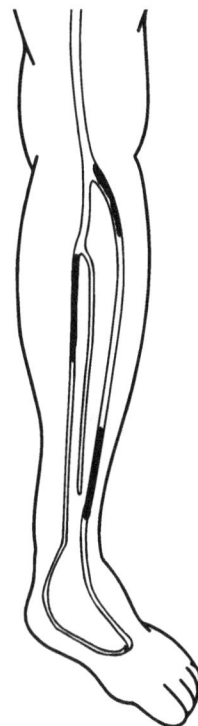

CONCISELY SUMMARIZE THE PROCEDURE USING KEY TERMS (ANSWER BELOW).

CHECK YOUR KNOWLEDGE

Qs ON RECANALISATION

Is the cannulation of the DP frequently correlated with a sustained positive arterial response?

Not usually.

Qs ON BALLOONING

Why is a scoring balloon suitable for AT angioplasty?

The PTA scoring balloon is a non-slip peripheral angioplasty catheter with three nylon scoring elements which produce controlled scoring of the vessel wall and work to reduce slipping during balloon inflation.

IN-DEPTH ANALYSIS

PROCEDURE : TIBIAL ANGIO. 2.5MM ULTRASCORE BALLOON. COMPLICATED. PARTIALLY SUCCESSFUL

COMMENTS:

- The angioplasty and scoring balloon dilation techniques utilized illustrate the delicate balance between vessel wall shear stress and radial force needed for successful recanalization. A scoring balloon is suitable for anterior tibial (AT) angioplasty because it provides controlled and focused dilation of the vessel, particularly in cases with calcified or resistant lesions.

- The scoring balloon features raised elements, or "scores," on its surface that create circumferential stress points within the arterial plaque during inflation. This action facilitates the fracturing of the plaque in a more predictable and uniform manner, reducing the risk of vessel injury, dissection, or excessive arterial wall stress. In AT angioplasty, where the vessels are smaller and often tortuous, the precise and controlled dilation offered by scoring balloons is advantageous for improving luminal gain while minimizing potential complications.

- The hypotension and tachycardia encountered during compression hemostasis necessitated immediate intervention, involving prolonged compression, fluid resuscitation, and transfusion of 1 unit PRBC. Given the stable hemoglobin level on venous gas, the response appears to have been effective. However, the finding of a retroperitoneal hematoma on ultrasound raises concern. Although the CTA did not show any haemorrhage related to the day's puncture, the patient's previous left iliopsoas haematoma warrants monitoring. This case accentuates the complex challenges of hemostasis and the potential for hidden complications in vascular procedures, necessitating an astute approach to patient monitoring and intervention in the post-procedural period.

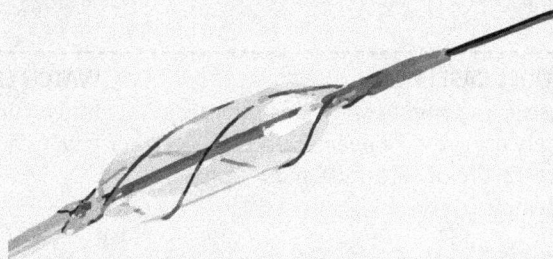

MODEL CASE:
diabetic foot triage

WATCH LIVE:
https://tinyurl.
com/37uu88d8

NOTES, TIPS AND TRICKS:

MODEL CASE:
Rescue angioplasty of the posterior tibial
artery using the Pioneer Re-entry device
after failure of antegrade and retrograde
attempts

WATCH LIVE:
https://tinyurl.com/
fpw5m9jn

NOTES, TIPS AND TRICKS:

MODEL CASE:
Optimal complex recanalization of BTK
arteries with drug-coated balloon angioplasty for re-occlusion

WATCH LIVE:
https://tinyurl.
com/4yf8ccsu

NOTES, TIPS AND TRICKS:

TIBIAL CASE: 2

A 42-year-old diabetic patient presented with right foot gangrene following a recent unsuccessful antegrade tibial angioplasty. A decision was agreed to re-attempt a tibial angioplasty to establish circulation to the foot.

READ CAREFULLY ...

Access	Pre Op checklist, supine, GA , cleaned and draped. Challenging antegrade access of CFA due to overlying soft tissue and haematoma from previous intervention. Proximal SFA puncture and 4Fr long sheath. Retrograde DP puncture, 4Fr pedal access sheath.
Equipments	Standard (Micro-access. J Wire. Glide-wire+0.014 wire+CXI. Amplatz+Proglide. Pigtail. contrast+HepSaline.
Angiogram Findings	Proximal occlusion of AT and PT. Patent per-oneal artery with a few focal stenoses in the distal calf, supplying the incomplete plantar arch and filling the DP.
Procedure	Unsuccessful attempts to cross mid-ATA oc-clusion from both antegrade and retrograde approaches. Distal peroneal artery disease dilated with 3mm x 15cm standard balloon, improving flow down the peroneal artery to the foot.
Complications	none
Closure	Manual compression applied to both punc-ture sites, achieving haemostasis. No imme-diate post-procedure complications.

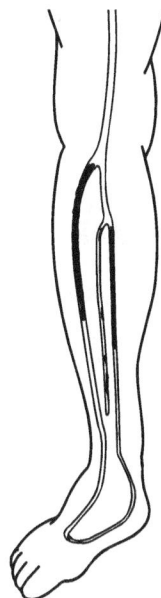

CONCISELY SUMMARIZE THE PROCEDURE USING KEY TERMS (ANSWER BELOW).

CHECK YOUR KNOWLEDGE

Qs ON STRATEGY

Qs ON ACCESS

What alternative is there if acquiring antegrade CFA access proves difficult (due to scarring or hematoma) but TPT or AT angioplasty is necessary?

Utilize antegrade SFA access, leveraging a 4Fr sheath, such as the Fortress sheath, for instance.

What characteristics of a Fortress sheath make it particularly beneficial?

A Fortress sheath is designed with a stainless steel coil which grants it both flexibility and stability. Additionally, it is equipped with a smooth taper tip that contains a radiopaque marker band, enhancing its visibility and aiding in accurate placement during procedures. Certain versions come with a hydrophobic coating, minimizing friction and facilitating smoother insertions. Reference: Fortress- Biotronik. https://www.biotronik.com/en-us/en-us/products/vi/peripheral/fortress. Accessed March 17, 2023.

Qs ON BALLOONING

Can the peroneal artery adequately supply blood to the foot in the presence of collaterals to the foot arteries?

The peroneal artery exhibits a flow velocity only marginally lower than that of the anterior tibial artery (AT). While it does branch out to nourish both the distal AT and posterior tibial (PT) arteries, the overall velocity and pressure it sustains seem to facilitate nearly equivalent perfusion to that offered by the AT, albeit to a slightly lesser extent in comparison to the PT. For further information, refer to the following article: https://www.jvascsurg.org/article/S0741-5214(18)30129-0/pdf

IN-DEPTH ANALYSIS

PROCEDURE : TIBIAL ANGIO. 2.5MM ULTRASCORE BALLOON. COMPLICATED. PARTIALLY SUCCESSFUL

COMMENTS:
• In this complex case, the patient presented with challenging vascular access due to previous intervention complications and anatomical constraints. Despite multiple attempts from both antegrade and retrograde approaches, the occlusion in the mid-ATA could not be successfully crossed. However, the treatment of distal peroneal artery disease with balloon angioplasty led to improved blood flow to the foot, which may have positive implications for the patient's limb perfusion and overall prognosis.

BIOMECHANICAL INSIGHT:
• The mid-ATA occlusion proved to be recalcitrant to both antegrade and retrograde approaches, suggesting the presence of a highly calcified or fibrotic lesion.
• The successful dilation of the distal peroneal artery disease with a 3mm x 15cm standard balloon angioplasty contributed to the augmentation of distal perfusion. This improvement in blood flow ameliorates tissue oxygenation and nutrient delivery, potentially mitigating the risk of critical limb ischemia and subsequent amputation..

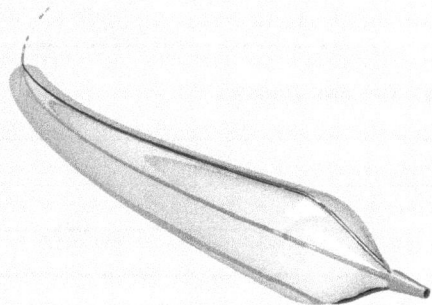

RESEARCH INSIGHT

• A study found that the success rate for tibial revascularisation was similar between the minimal calcification(MC (95.3%)) and the intermediate calcification (IC (91.7%)) groups but significantly lower in the extensive calcification (EC group (71.1%)). The causes of technical failure were inability to cross the lesion in 16/124 patients and arterial rupture in 2/124 patients. (1)
• (1) Semiquantitative assessment of tibial artery calcification by computed .... https://www.sciencedirect.com/science/article/pii/S0741521416302889.

MODEL CASE:
Big small vessels: the new scenario of PAD

WATCH LIVE:
https://tinyurl.
com/3czu6urk

NOTES, TIPS AND TRICKS:

MODEL CASE:
Angioplasty of the anterior tibial artery
and dorsalis pedis artery in a desert foot

WATCH LIVE:
https://tinyurl.com/
s37d5psc

NOTES, TIPS AND TRICKS:

MODEL CASE:
Subintimal angioplasty of full length
occlusion of the anterior tibial artery. The
Bolia technic

WATCH LIVE:
https://tinyurl.
com/2ak4ur4y

NOTES, TIPS AND TRICKS:

TIBIAL CASE: 3

A 69-year-old patient with a Left hallux gangrene. Duplex shows occluded AT . A decision was agreed to proceed to left AT angioplasty +/- stenting.

READ CAREFULLY ...

Access	Pre Op checklist, supine, GA , cleaned and draped. Antegrade approach via left Common Femoral Artery (CFA) under ultrasound guidance and retrograde access to left Anterior Tibial (AT) at the ankle using a micropuncture technique
Equipments	Standard (Micro-access. J Wire. Glidewire+0.014 wire+CXI. Amplatz+Proglide. Pigtail. contrast+HepSaline.
Angiogram Findings	Initial angiography revealed patent Superficial Femoral Artery (SFA), popliteal and peroneal arteries extending to the ankle, with AT occlusion post-origin and reconstitution proximal to the ankle. Following Percutaneous Transluminal Angioplasty (PTA), AT demonstrated patency extending to the Dorsalis Pedis (DP) into the foot
Procedure	Procedure initiated under General Anesthesia (GA). AT occlusion traversed in a retrograde manner using V18 guidewire and CXI support catheter. Administration of Heparin (5000 units). AT occlusion was also crossed from an antegrade direction, achieving rendezvous with the retrograde equipment within the lower extremity. AT dilated using 2x10 cm and 3x10 cm angioplasty balloons. Subsequently, a selective 100 microliter infusion of Glyceryl Trinitrate (GTN) was performed into the AT
Complications	none
Closure	Mynx Vascular Closure Device

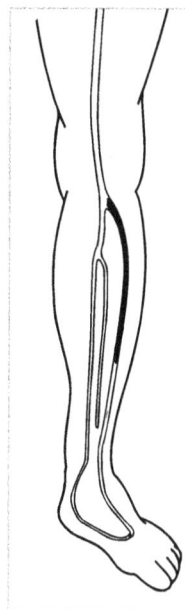

CONCISELY SUMMARIZE THE PROCEDURE USING KEY TERMS (ANSWER BELOW).

CHECK YOUR KNOWLEDGE

Qs ON STRATEGY

Given the use of both retrograde and antegrade approaches to traverse the AT occlusion, what might be the potential benefits of achieving a rendezvous within the lower extremity, compared to solely using one approach?

Achieving a rendezvous combines the advantages of both approaches. The retrograde provides a means to navigate challenging distal occlusions, while the antegrade offers a more conventional and direct approach to treat the lesion. This combined method can increase the success rate and decrease procedural time by leveraging the strengths of both techniques.

Qs ON COMPLICATIONS

What is the rationale behind the selective infusion of Glyceryl Trinitrate (GTN) into the AT post-dilatation, and how does it impact the vascular environment?

GTN acts as a vasodilator. After angioplasty, infusing GTN can help in preventing vasospasm, enhancing blood flow, and ensuring the treated vessel remains patent. Its administration aids in optimizing the post-angioplasty vessel diameter and ensuring smooth blood flow to the distal extremities.

IN-DEPTH ANALYSIS

PROCEDURE : LEFT AT ANGIOPLASTY.

COMMENTS:

- The Anterior Tibial (AT) artery, one of the major arteries supplying blood to the foot, plays a vital role in wound healing, especially when procedures like hallux gangrene management and amputation of hallux are planned. In such clinical contexts, it is important to restore and maintain the patency of the AT artery if it is the main runoff to ensure adequate tissue perfusion and oxygenation, both of which are fundamental for healing processes.
- From a biomechanical perspective, an occlusion in the AT artery disrupts the normal inline blood flow, causing a decrease in the shear stress experienced by the endothelial cells lining the arterial wall. This reduction in shear stress can lead to a state of endothelial dysfunction, contributing to further progression of the vascular disease. The percutaneous transluminal angioplasty (PTA) carried out in the procedure aims to mechanically dilate the occluded AT, re-establishing the blood flow, and therefore restoring the hemodynamic conditions necessary for healing post-procedure.
- Glyceryl trinitrate (GTN), also known as nitroglycerin, plays a crucial role in this context. GTN is a potent vasodilator that functions by releasing nitric oxide (NO), a molecule that promotes vasodilation. From a hemodynamic perspective, GTN aids in improving blood flow by reducing vascular resistance. In addition to its vasodilatory effects, NO has several other beneficial effects including inhibition of platelet aggregation, leukocyte adhesion, and smooth muscle cell proliferation, all of which can contribute to maintaining the patency of the dilated vessel post-angioplasty.
- Overall, maintaining adequate blood flow via the AT and employing agents like GTN is crucial to enhance the chances of successful healing post amputation and to potentially prevent further complications such as wound infection or need for higher level amputations.

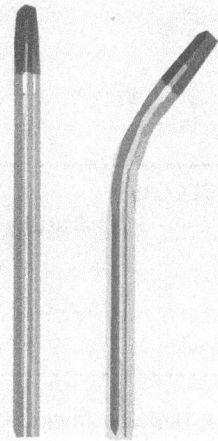

MODEL CASE:
foot arteries angioplasty

WATCH LIVE:
https://tinyurl.com/
yc2eutmn

NOTES, TIPS AND TRICKS:

MODEL CASE:
Left anterior tibial artery occlusion

WATCH LIVE:
https://tinyurl.com/
yn2fn89b

NOTES, TIPS AND TRICKS:

TIBIAL CASE: 4

A 65-year-old patient with a ulcers right foot. Duplex shows right runoff disease. A decision was agreed to proceed to right runoff angioplasty +/- stenting.

READ CAREFULLY ...

Access	Pre Op checklist, supine, GA , cleaned and draped. An antegrade approach to the right common femoral artery (CFA) was utilized, with an initial 4Fr dilator later escalated to a 6Fr.
Equipments	Standard (Micro-access. J Wire. Glidewire+0.014 wire+CXI. Amplatz+Proglide. Pigtail. contrast+HepSaline.
Angiogram Findings	non-critical proximal SFA stenosis, complex 70% distal SFA stenosis to proximal popliteal artery- suggestive of chronic dissection. Noted focal stenosis at proximal TP trunk. Preserved run-off via common peroneal artery with retrograde distal anterior tibial artery filling.
Procedure	overlapping 6 x 40 mm balloon angioplasty on distal SFA stenosis. Despite prolonged 6 mm angioplasty, residual dissection persisted. 2.5 x 20mm angioplasty on proximal TP trunk executed successfully. Deployed 5.5 x 60 mm Supera stent.
Complications	Patient exhibited poor procedure tolerance; general anesthesia recommended for future procedures. Noted residual dissection distal to stent, non flow-limiting. Suggested recanalisation of distal anterior tibial artery in future session.
Closure	Applied 6-Fr Angio-Seal for hemostasis.

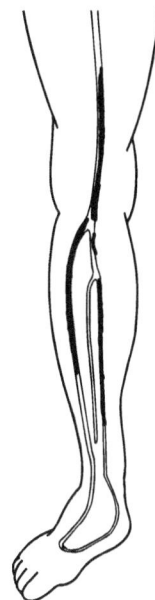

CONCISELY SUMMARIZE THE PROCEDURE USING KEY TERMS (ANSWER BELOW).

CHECK YOUR KNOWLEDGE

Qs ON STRATEGY

Given the presence of both non-critical proximal SFA stenosis and a complex 70% distal SFA stenosis with a chronic dissection, how might the decision to perform overlapping balloon angioplasty specifically on the distal SFA stenosis align with the observed hemodynamics and patient symptoms?

The decision likely prioritized addressing the complex distal SFA stenosis due to its severity and potential impact on blood flow, especially given its chronic dissection nature. The proximal non-critical stenosis might not have been the primary cause of significant hemodynamic compromise or the patient's symptoms.

Qs ON COMPLICATIONS

Despite successful angioplasty on the proximal TP trunk and the deployment of a 5.5 x 60 mm Supera stent, why might the presence of a non-flow-limiting residual dissection distal to the stent be a concern, and what could be potential implications for future interventions?

A non-flow-limiting residual dissection, though not immediately problematic, poses a potential risk for propagation or becoming flow-limiting in the future. It could lead to further stenosis or occlusion, warranting close monitoring and possibly necessitating future interventions, like the suggested recanalization of the distal anterior tibial artery.

IN-DEPTH ANALYSIS

PROCEDURE : LEFT AT ANGIOPLASTY.

COMMENTS:

- The complex approximately 70% stenosis in the distal superficial femoral artery (SFA), extending to the proximal popliteal artery, represents a significant alteration in the blood flow dynamics. Stenosis of this degree can potentially generate a turbulent flow distally, which may contribute to arterial wall damage, thrombus formation and further stenosis development. Moreover, it significantly impacts the ability to deliver oxygen-rich blood to the tissues distal to the stenosis, such as the lower leg and the foot.

- Furthermore, the presence of a chronic dissection, which was left unresolved despite the balloon angioplasty, may have biomechanical implications. The dissection alters the arterial wall's mechanical properties and might potentially compromise the artery's integrity. It can create a false lumen, thus affecting blood flow and leading to further complications like thrombosis or aneurysm formation.

- The angioplasty attempts, both initial and prolonged, could not significantly ameliorate the dissection, demonstrating the resilience of such chronic changes to conventional interventions.

- The deployment of the 5.5 x 60 mm Supera stent aimed to address these challenges.

  This stent, with its interwoven nitinol design, offers superior radial strength, flexibility, and fracture resistance. It adapts well to the biomechanical forces exerted by the distal SFA and proximal popliteal artery, which undergo significant bending, twisting, and compressive forces during limb movement.

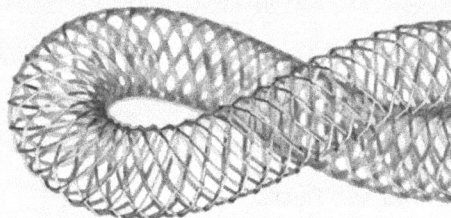

MODEL CASE:
Foot salvage very distal right posterior tibial artery balloon angioplasty with below-the-knee angioplasty

WATCH LIVE:
https://tinyurl.com/3p3pkpnd

NOTES, TIPS AND TRICKS:

MODEL CASE:
Right anterior tibial artery occlusion recanalization

WATCH LIVE:
https://tinyurl.com/jxm72my2

NOTES, TIPS AND TRICKS:

SIMPOD™ TRAINING CASES

https://www.vssmasterclass.co.uk

SIMPOD™ TIBIAL 1

LESION: Lt AT+PT. 50&80mm
long. 90%&80% stenosis. Sim
EIA diameter: 4.4&3.8mm
YOUR TASK: Angioplasty +/-
stenting via Lt femoral

Notes:

SIMPOD™ TIBIAL 2

LESION: Lt AT. 90mm long. 90%
stenosis. Sim EIA diameter:
3mm
YOUR TASK: Angioplasty +/-
stenting via Lt femoral

Notes:

SIMPOD™ TIBIAL 3

LESION: Lt PT&PN. 115mm
long. 85% stenosis. Sim EIA
diameter: 3.2mm
YOUR TASK: Angioplasty +/-
stenting via Lt femoral

Notes:

SIMPOD™ TIBIAL 4

LESION: Rt PT. 110mm long.
85% stenosis. Sim EIA diameter: 5mm
YOUR TASK: Angioplasty +/-
stenting via Rt femoral

Notes:

SIMPOD™ TIBIAL 5

LESION: Rt AT+PT. 80&100mm
long. 90% stenosis. Sim EIA
diameter: 4.2-4.4mm
YOUR TASK: Angioplasty +/-
stenting via Rt femoral

Notes:

SIMPOD™ TIBIAL 6

LESION: Lt AT. 90mm long. 90%
stenosis. Sim EIA diameter:
3.7mm
YOUR TASK: Angioplasty +/-
stenting via Lt femoral

Notes:

SIMPOD™ TIBIAL 7

LESION: Lt TPT. 70mm long. 90% stenosis. Sim EIA diameter: 4.1mm
YOUR TASK: Angioplasty +/- stenting via Rt femoral

Notes:

SIMPOD™ TIBIAL 8

LESION: Rt AT. 100mm long. 95% stenosis. Sim EIA diameter: 3mm
YOUR TASK: Angioplasty +/- stenting via Lt femoral

Notes:

SIMPOD™ TIBIAL 9

LESION: Lt AT+PN. 80&40mm long. 90%&85% stenosis. Sim EIA diameter: 3.4&2.6mm
YOUR TASK: Angioplasty +/- stenting via Lt femoral

Notes:

SIMPOD™ TIBIAL 10

LESION: RT PN. 90mm long. 90% stenosis.
YOUR TASK: Angioplasty +/- stenting via Rt femoral

Notes:

SIMPOD™ TIBIAL 11

LESION: Rt PT&PN&AT. 115mm long. 85% stenosis. Sim EIA diameter: 3.2mm
YOUR TASK: Angioplasty +/- stenting via Lt femoral

Notes:

CHAPTER 6
RUPTURED AAA
ENDOVASCULAR
THERAPIES Q&A

RUPTURED AAA (ʀAAA) CASES Q&Aꜱ

Qs ON STRATEGY

In rAAA, should surgery proceed if the patient becomes severely unstable?

If the initial decision was to proceed, then yes.

During an aneurysm repair, if the patient loses BP upon placing the 6Fr femoral sheath in, what should be the next step?

Rule out iliac rupture during entry; using contrast through the sheath might be sufficient to identify this.

How can an iliac rupture be stabilized?

Insert an immediate angioplasty balloon; potential size: 8x10 cm.

Is CPR allowed/effective if the patient is peri-arrested?

No, CPR is considered futile in this scenario.

What is the optimal approach for a ruptured juxtarenal AAA?

Considering a chimney procedure is often the best option.

Is there scientific backing that LA is superior to GA in rAAA situations?

Yes.

What is the detailed protocol for C/L limb cannulation attempts in various scenarios?

Attempt to cannulate the C/L limb from contralateral side initially, then try ipsilateral to contralateral sharply; if unsuccessful, opt for brachial. If that fails, complete ipsilateral, plug contralateral from brachial, and proceed with fem-fem crossover.

What is the preferred access point for treating endoleak type Ia?

Brachial or axillary access is usually preferred.

What is a common risk associated with axillary access?

There is a risk of developing a large hematoma.

What is the standard management strategy for endoleak type Ia?

Common strategies include balloon dilation of the proximal sealing zone, using EndoAnchors (Medtronic), or a cuff insertion.

In cases of symptomatic AAA, is LA preferred over GA?

No, GA provides better control and possibly uses less contrast if equipped with enhanced 3D modules on the C-Arm.

For patients with a transplanted kidney, where should the main graft deployment aim to be?

The target is just below the superior mesenteric artery (SMA) (i.e. cover the unused renal arteries).

In cases with a transplanted kidney, where should the main graft be introduced from?

It should be introduced from the contralateral iliac.

Is it viable to use Local Anesthesia (LA) for EVARs utilizing a Chimney approach?

Not usually but possible.

Are there variations in the treatment methods for substantial inflammatory aneurysms?

No. The standard approach is used, which includes administering two more doses of antibiotics, then stopping, followed by prophylactic LMWH.

Can you explain what a bovine arch is and its impact on stent deployment?

A bovine arch is a normal variant of the aortic arch in which the right brachiocephalic artery and left common carotid artery arise from a common trunk, also known as the brachiocephalic trunk. This variant is named after the bovine anatomy, in which the aortic arch has a similar branching pattern.

Bovine arches can make stent deployment more challenging, particularly when the transfemoral approach is used. This is because the brachiocephalic trunk is typically more tortuous and difficult to navigate with a guiding catheter. Additionally, the common trunk may be shorter and have a smaller diameter than a normal aortic arch, which can make it more difficult to deploy the stent accurately.

Qs ON SECURING ACCESS & SETUP WIRES AND CATHETERS

Should Proglide be placed before or after finishing EVAR for rAAA?

Before

What is the common access for inserting a renal stent during ChimneyEVAR repair?

Left brachial 6Fr

What should be done if the iliacs are heavily diseased and there is a suspicion of narrowing?

Place supporting kissing iliac stents.

What is the usual brachial sheath size needed for ChEVAR?

7Fr long sheath

Where should the sheath be positioned?

In the suprarenal aorta

How to re-enter the true aortic lumen from the false lumen?

Multiple manipulations until penetrating the separating wall via natural/artificial fenestration, then confirming with contrast and expanding with a 10x4 balloon.

What is the solution to regain flow from the true lumen to the graft?

Insert an additional stable graft, such as an AUI.

Qs ON USING CODA BALLOON

Following the stabilization of the patient using an aortic occlusion balloon, what should be the subsequent step in the event of a blood pressure drop?

Proceed if it seems reasonable to complete the procedure.

Should consideration be given to relocating the occlusion balloon lower, within the main graft, as opposed to maintaining its position in the thoracic aorta?

Yes, it might be beneficial

In situations where the patient becomes unstable, where is the recommended placement for the CODA balloon?

Position it in the visceral region rather than the thoracic area.

Is it advisable to hold the balloon stationary at one location (like the suprarenal visceral region) or to systematically lower its position?

The standard procedure is to progressively lower it

Qs ON INSERTING MAIN BODY

| What type of graft is suitable for addressing an infrarenal aortic dissection?

Valiant Navion Captive.

| Under what circumstances would an AUI be deemed appropriate in the remediation of a ruptured or inflammatory AAA?

In situations where cannulation of the contralateral limb is impracticable, or the contralateral iliac is too diseased to allow for standard EVAR.

| When is the employment of a bifurcated EVAR stent advised or discouraged for mending a CIA aneurysm?

Advisable when the CIA aneurysm protrudes into the aortic bifurcation, making sealing with a straightforward iliac stent unviable, given that the aortic diameter permits the contralateral limb to unfurl and be accessible for cannulation.

| What is regarded as the minimum aortic dimension that facilitates a satisfactory deployment of the contralateral limb?

A measurement between 16 and 18 mm is typically sufficient for specific grafts.

| Should an extension be utilized even when no endoleak is evident in the angiogram? |

Yes, particularly when a CT scan substantiates the presence of an endoleak.

| Is it permissible to obstruct a single renal artery during a rupture scenario?

Yes, as exemplified in this instance where three left renal arteries were enveloped while the right one retained an atrium and necessitated a chimney approach to remain open.

| When there is an anticipation of a renal artery being occluded, what should be encapsulated in the documentation?

A transparent dialogue with the patient or their family regarding the potential long-term repercussions of probable renal failure, coupled with a notation accentuating the deliberate obstruction of the renal artery.

Qs ON DEPLOYING MAIN BODY

When using chimney EVAR, what condition should the renal stent maintain during the deployment of the EVAR main body?

It should have a balloon inflated within it during the deployment.

In the case of bilateral CIA aneurysms, is it necessary to seal both IIAs?

Yes

What risks are associated with covering both IIAs?

It can lead to a high occurrence of buttock pain, with a small but established risk of distal colon ischaemia

If the individual becomes restless while the graft is being deployed, is it acceptable to cover a renal artery?

Yes, it is allowed; however, it is essential to record the rationale behind this decision.

Is a chimney approach mandatory for every juxtarenal ruptured aneurysm?

No, there are successful cases managed without adopting the chimney approach.

What does the presence of a conical neck in a ruptured aneurysm necessitate?

Ensuring consistent coverage with a suitably sized diameter throughout the neck section.

In the context of a ruptured AAA, is it more advantageous to employ one or two chimneys when necessary?

Utilizing a single chimney is preferable, as it is faster and has a diminished propensity for leakage

What could potentially prevent the contralateral gate from unfolding correctly?

A narrow aortic bifurcation could be a hindrance.

s it permissible to position the AUI entirely within the existing graft

Yes, doing so is viewed as the optimal strategy to restore true lumen flow in certain scenarios.

Qs ON DEPLOYING EVAR LIMBS

What challenges may arise when opening the c/l limb in a narrow aorta?

Difficulty in cannulation can occur if the opening faces the aortic wall rather than the iliac.

Can you anticipate this difficulty?

In theory, yes, but it depends on knowing the orientations well. For instance, orienting to the front and side may lead to cannulation in the right iliac.

What is the best solution if patient movement affects the deployment of the main body and causes the c/l limb to become stuck?

Attempt cannulation from the c/l side, or attempt to cannulate from the i/l side sharply back into the c/l. If both fail, try the brachial approach. If that fails, complete the i/l, plug the c/l (from brachial), and perform fem-fem crossover.

How easy is it to cannulate a detached iliac limb (from a previous EVAR) from the i/l side in a ruptured setting?

Not easy, as observed in many cases.

What should be attempted if i/l cannulation from the i/l side fails?

Consider cannulation from the c/l side and use wire snaring if necessary.

How easy is it to cannulate a detached iliac limb (from a previous EVAR) from the c/l side and snare it in a ruptured setting?

Not easy and sometimes impossible.

If both cannulation attempts fail in this context, what is the 3rd step?

Attempt cannulation via a brachial access, using a large 7Fr sheath (Anseal sheath), then snare the wire down to the detached i/l limb.

Can snaring result in more complications?

Yes, the tip of the Cobra catheter can break and detach from the wire, requiring snaring from the top.

Is it always necessary to cover the IIA in the presence of iliac aneurysm?

No, it is not necessary if a good seal is achieved.

Should the i/l iliac be supported with Zilver routinely?

Possibly yes, as iliacs tend to be tortuous due to previous surgery or kidney implantation

When it is not possible to cannulate the c/l gate, what should be the next step in a ruptured aneurysm setting?

Consider a brachial approach if the gate is reasonably open. If not, plug the gate and proceed to a fem-fem crossover. A third option is to place another stent (AUI) through the i/l limb and deploy it.

Qs ON MOULDING & CLOSING

What is the procedure for closing a 6Fr brachial access?

Utilize Proglide after completing the procedure and apply manual pressure.

After deploying stents, where should the balloon be applied?

Apply the balloon in overlapping and sealing zones.

Qs ON COMPLICATIONS

What should be done if there is suspicion of an IVC injury?

Puncture the femoral vein and perform an IVC evaluation with a pigtail catheter.

Is treatment required for a tight area identified in completion angiography during a rAAA procedure?

Yes, utilize a Zilver Stent to address it.

Is treatment of endoleak Type Ia typically successful?

No, addressing persistent Type Ia endoleak is challenging and occurs in 2.9% to 6.9% of all EVAR procedures.

What should you do if there is suspicion of kinking or incomplete apposition in the iliac limb?

Use a balloon and consider deploying a Zilver stent.

In a straightforward EVAR for a rAAA, is ITU admission necessary?

Yes, it is necessary.

What can occur when deploying a kissing stent over calcified tight iliac arteries within an EVAR graft?

Possible fabric tear, resulting in a blush on completion angiography.

How should you handle a fabric tear?

If the endoleak is mild and not Type I, it may be left alone.

What happens if the proximal graft is deployed lower than planned?

It may deploy within the aneurysmal area, causing a Type I endoleak.

How should this be treated?

Consider using a cuff.

Does the aortic cuff have supra renal fixation?

Yes, it can.

If a persistent slow Type I leak is discovered after this, what should be done?

Perform more ballooning and assessment, then decide if it's acceptable within the context of rCIA or chimney procedures.

If there is bleeding in the brachial access after sealing, what action should be taken?

If bleeding is controlled with pressure and has no impact on distal pulses, then no further action is necessary.

What effect can a tight, tortuous C/L iliac have on completing the EVAR procedure?

It can hinder gate cannulation by affecting catheter manipulation, including pushability and torquability.

What risks are associated with applying a clamp on the proximal femoral during the X-Over procedure?

There's a risk of occluding one limb of the EVAR graft.

What should be done if the EVAR limb is occluded due to clamp application?

Prophylactic measures, such as using a shunt, should have been taken to maintain graft flow. If not, attempt to pass a fogarty catheter up. If unsuccessful, consider puncturing the SFA more distally and trying to advance a wire.

What should be done if there is no remnant flow in the EVAR limb and unblocking is not possible?

Consider an ax bifemoral bypass procedure.

MODEL CASE:
Percutaneous endovascular abdominal aortic aneurysm repair

WATCH LIVE:
https://tinyurl.com/36wdrhj5

NOTES, TIPS AND TRICKS:

MODEL CASE:
evar-tevar co2

WATCH LIVE:
https://tinyurl.com/xts4ttkw

NOTES, TIPS AND TRICKS:

MODEL CASE:
Nexus aortic arch stent graft in a patient with prior TEVAR type 1A endoleak

WATCH LIVE:
https://tinyurl.com/ycydtw6w

NOTES, TIPS AND TRICKS:

MODEL CASE:
Evar and anchors chimney

WATCH LIVE:
https://tinyurl.com/ynaaxh68

NOTES, TIPS AND TRICKS:

SIMPOD™ TRAINING CASES

https://www.vssmasterclass.co.uk

SIMPOD™ EVAR 1

LESION: AAA. NECK: 18- Sim
Sac: 36; bifurcation: 18; length: 80
YOUR TASK: EVAR via right femoral

Notes:

SIMPOD™ EVAR 2

LESION: AAA. NECK: 27- Sim
Sac: 46; bifurcation: 25; length: 50
YOUR TASK: EVAR via right femoral

Notes:

SIMPOD™ EVAR 3

LESION: Aortic Dissection.
NECK: 22- length: 90

YOUR TASK: STENT via right femoral

Notes:

SIMPOD™ EVAR 4

LESION: AAA. NECK: 20- Sim
Sac: 36; bifurcation: 20; length: 50
YOUR TASK: EVAR via right femoral

Notes:

SIMPOD™ EVAR 5

LESION: AAA. NECK: 20- Sim
Sac: 36; bifurcation: 18; length: 75
YOUR TASK: EVAR via right femoral

Notes:

SIMPOD™ EVAR 6

LESION: AAA. NECK: 20- Sim
Sac: 45; length: 90
YOUR TASK: EVAR via right femoral

Notes:

CHAPTER 7
AORTO-ILIAC ENDOVASCULAR THERAPIES Q&A

AORTOILIAC CASE: 1

A 62-year-old patient with a history of bilateral IC. Duplex showed occluded distal aortic and iliac occlusion. A decision was agreed to proceed to CERAB.

READ CAREFULLY ...

Access	Pre Op checklist, supine, GA , cleaned and draped. 7 Fr ansell sheath in left brachial and left mid SFA; Standard 7 Fr sheath in right mid SFA.
Equipments	Standard (Micro-access. J Wire. Glidewire+0.014 wire+CXI. Amplatz+Proglide. Pigtail. contrast+HepSaline.
Angiogram Findings	occlusions in distal aorta, bilateral iliacs, and femorals; Identified heavy calcification in bilateral common femorals
Procedure	After securement of access, performed recanalisation on the left side with a through-and-through wire; Multiple attempts to advance the wire into the right SFA were made, but all were unsuccessful, even with distal attempts using an outback catheter; Successfully advanced the wire into the PFA, resulting in good SFA filling; Bilateral CFA underwent angioplasty with a plain balloon, followed by shockwave lithoplasty utilizing an 8 mm balloon, extending the procedure to include EIA and CIAs; Placement of bilateral iliac kissing stents extending to the distal aorta below the renals, using 8x59, 7x79, and 7x39 VBX stents; Insertion of a Zilver stent (7x60 mm) in the left EIA; Placement of bilateral CFA supera stents, each 6x100 mm
Complications	none
Closure	Femoseal closure in left brachial and both groins.

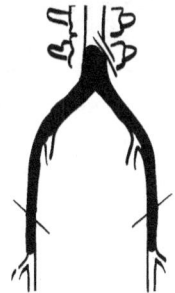

CONCISELY SUMMARIZE THE PROCEDURE USING KEY TERMS (ANSWER BELOW).

CHECK YOUR KNOWLEDGE

Qs ON STRATEGY

What is the ideal level of arterial wall calcification for shockwave?

Brachial and distal regions are generally more suitable.

Qs ON RECANALISATION

What is the technique for securing the wire in aortoiliac reconstruction (CERAB)?

Pass the wire through and through for stabilization.

Can the PFA (Profunda Femoris Artery) be utilized as the primary exit artery in aortoiliac recanalization?

Yes, it can be used as the primary exit artery.

Qs ON STENTING

If the CFA entry point is not suitable, which stent is recommended for use in the CFA?

The Supera stent is the preferred choice.

IN-DEPTH ANALYSIS

PROCEDURE : CERAB. CONVERTED TO CFA STENT +KISSING STENTS. SHOCKWAVE AND SUPER IN CFA.

COMMENTS:
- This case presents a highly complex vascular scenario marked by considerable occlusion and calcification across multiple areas. The difficulties in achieving right SFA cannulation underline the technical challenges encountered in such heavily diseased vessels. The inability to effectively advance the wire, despite using advanced techniques such as distal approach with an outback catheter, testifies to the severity of the occlusion.
- The switch from the initial plan of Covered Endovascular Reconstruction of the Aortic Bifurcation (CERAB) to the placement of iliac kissing stents is noteworthy. CERAB is typically favored in extensive aortoiliac occlusive disease for its potential benefits including superior patency rates and fewer reinterventions. However, in this case, the challenges related to vascular

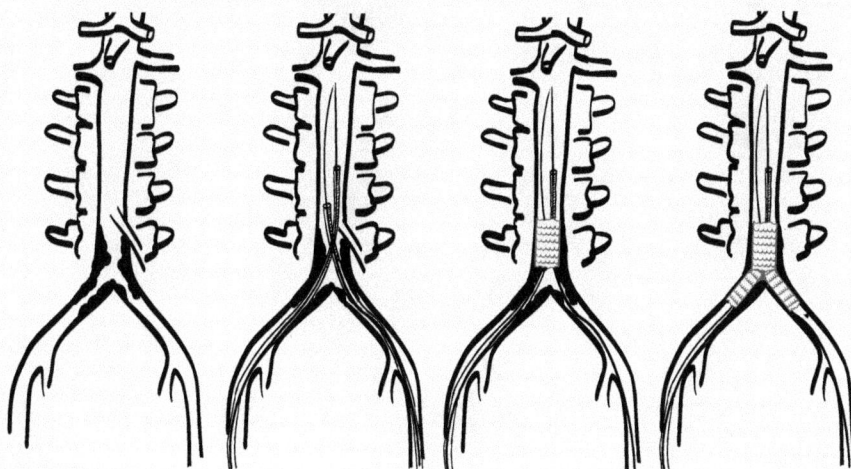

access, the patient's overall condition, and the complexity of the lesions may have prompted the shift towards the simpler and less invasive strategy of iliac kissing stents.
- While both CERAB and kissing stents can restore unobstructed blood flow, the choice between them is dictated by factors such as anatomical constraints, severity and extent of disease, risk of complications, and technical expertise. The main difference in hemodynamic effects lies in the pattern of blood flow, where CERAB seeks to replicate physiological flow across the aortic bifurcation while iliac kissing stents can lead to flow disturbances due to stent overlapping and guttering effect across the heavily diseased aortic wall. However, in real-world scenarios, these theoretical differences may not translate into substantial variations in clinical outcomes, and the primary goal remains the successful restoration of blood flow with minimal complications.

MODEL CASE:
How to treat symptomatic abdominal
aortic calcified occlusion

WATCH LIVE:
https://tinyurl.
com/3mbt4uye

NOTES, TIPS AND TRICKS:

AORTOILIAC CASE: 2

A 69-year-old patient with a left sfa stent occlusion, occluded fem-pop bypass and recent iliac stenting with residual rest pain on left. CTA showed 75% stenosis at right CIA. A decision was agreed to proceed to CIA stent for a stenotic CIA following CERAB.

READ CAREFULLY ...

Access	Pre Op checklist, supine, GA , cleaned and draped. Bilateral CFAs percutaneously accessed under general anesthesia with ultrasound assistance.
Equipments	Standard (Micro-access. J Wire. Glidewire+0.014 wire+CXI. Amplatz+Proglide. Pigtail. contrast+HepSaline.
Angiogram Findings	Angiogram revealed slow opacification of IMA.
Procedure	1. Left CFA preclose with Proglides. 2. 7 Fr sheath on right, 10 Fr on left. 3. Iliac arteries crossed. 4. Aortic graft (12x29 mm) deployed at IMA level. 5. Graft proximal end flared using 16x20 Atlas balloon. 6. VBX stents (right 8x59, left 9x59) placed.
Complications	No immediate adverse events post-procedure.
Closure	Hemostasis achieved with left CFA Proglide and right CFA Femseal.

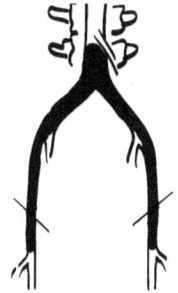

CONCISELY SUMMARIZE THE PROCEDURE USING KEY TERMS (ANSWER BELOW).

CHECK YOUR KNOWLEDGE

Qs ON STRATEGY

How do you determine the appropriate size and type of aortic graft and VBX stents to use in an endovascular procedure, and what are the implications of improper sizing?

The appropriate size of an aortic graft and VBX stents is determined based on pre-operative imaging, such as a CT angiogram, which provides detailed measurements of the vessel's diameter and length.

It's crucial to select a graft and stents that are slightly larger than the native vessel to ensure a secure fit and to prevent migration or endoleaks.

Improper sizing can lead to complications such as graft/stent migration, endoleaks, or occlusion of the vessel.

IN-DEPTH ANALYSIS

PROCEDURE : STANDARD CERAB

COMMENTS:

- This case illustrates the use of endovascular techniques in a complex aortic intervention. The Bentley stent's usage demonstrates its flexibility and conformability, essential for securing a seal in difficult anatomies.
- The Bentley graft, with its specific dimensions, was used effectively at the level of the IMA, which is critical for maintaining the patency and flow in visceral vessels. This aligns well with the philosophy of the CERAB technique, which aims to maintain perfusion to all critical vessels while managing aortic pathology.
- The Atlas Balloon's utilization stands out due to its unique features - it offers high-pressure non-compliant dilation, which is crucial for creating a precise, controlled flare of the graft's proximal end. This step ensures an optimal seal at the graft-arterial wall interface, reducing the risk of guttering.
- Finally, the deployment of VBX stents indicates the need for adjunctive procedures to ensure patency of the parallel stents. These balloon-expandable stents offer flexibility, accuracy, and improved radial force. Their use here reinforces the need for vigilant planning and technique to ensure the optimal outcome in these complex aortic interventions.

CHAPTER 8
BYPASS
ENDOVASCULAR
THERAPIES Q&A

BYPASS CASE: 1

A 42-year-old diabetic patient presented with right foot Gangrene. The patient has had a right fem pop bypass with critical stenosis on a follow up duplex despite a recent angioplasty attempt. A decision was agreed to perform a bypass angioplasty to establish circulation to the foot.

READ CAREFULLY ...

Access	Pre Op checklist, supine, GA , cleaned and draped, Successful puncture of right CFA (below injection sinus area) under ultrasound guidance. 6Fr Brite-tip sheath.
Equipments	Standard (Micro-access. J Wire. Glidewire+Cobra. Amplatz+Proglide. Pigtail. contrast+HepSaline) + 5mm x 4cm Mustang balloon. 5mm x 4cm DCB. (no 6mm DCB available for this case).
Angiogram Findings	CFA, PFA, and proximal SFA show normal opacification. Right femoral-popliteal bypass is patent with improved proximal and patent distal anastomoses ends (compared to the recent angiogram). Three-vessel run-off reaches ankle, while a stable, short focal occlusion is still present in the right PT at the ankle.
Procedure	Catheter and wire navigated through proximal anastomosis into bypass; POBA performed using 5mm x 4cm Mustang balloon, followed by 5mm x 4cm DCB.
Complications	None observed.
Closure	6Fr Mynx- successful hemostasis.

CONCISELY SUMMARIZE THE PROCEDURE USING KEY TERMS (ANSWER BELOW).

CHECK YOUR KNOWLEDGE

Qs ON ACCESS

What is the recommended access point for treating a fem-pop bypass?

Any access point that offers sufficient working space to visualize and address the anastomotic lesion.

What are the characteristics of a Brite Tip sheath that make it particularly useful in this context?

Some of the properties that make Brite Tip sheath specially useful are:

- It has a **tungsten-filled radiopaque tip** that allows excellent visualization and accurate positioning of the sheath's distal tip under fluoroscopy[12].
- It has a **co-extruded kink resistant cannula** that provides flexibility and support for easy tracking through tortuous vessels[1].
- It has a **unique SLIX valve** that ensures minimal hemostasis and prevents blood loss or air embolism[1].
(1) BRITE TIP™ Interventional Sheath. https://cordis.com/emea/products/peripheral-interventions/evar/catheter-sheath-introducers/brite-tip-interventional-sheath.

Qs ON BALLOONING

What are the characteristics of a Mustang balloon?

- It is a high-pressure and non-compliant balloon, making it resistant to deformation and suitable for treating highly calcified lesions.
- It has a rated burst pressure of up to 24 ATM (2431 kPa), allowing it to handle high inflation pressures without rupturing.
- It offers superior cross and track performance, enabling easy navigation through tight lesions and tortuous vessels.
- It comes in longer lengths (up to 300 mm) and smaller sheath sizes (compatible with 4 Fr), providing coverage for longer lesion segments and reducing access site complications.

Is it acceptable to use a smaller diameter DCB if the right size is unavailable?

Yes, using a smaller diameter DCB is acceptable when the ideal size is not available.

IN-DEPTH ANALYSIS

PROCEDURE : FEM POP BYPASS PLASTY. MUSTANG BALLOON (DIFFICULT MANIPULATION TO POSITION). DCB. SUCCESSFUL.

COMMENTS:

- In this case, the patient underwent a successful endovascular intervention to treat a previously treated femoral-popliteal bypass. The use of angioplasty and drug-coated balloons demonstrated good post-procedure angiographic appearances and preserved run-off, highlighting the effectiveness of minimally invasive techniques in managing anastomotic stenosis.

BIOMECHANICAL INSIGHT:

- The Mustang balloon, utilized in this femoral-popliteal bypass angioplasty, exemplifies the integration of advanced biomechanical principles and material science in the field of endovascular interventions. This semi-compliant, high-pressure balloon is designed to offer controlled, targeted dilatation of the stenosed vessel segment, while minimizing the risk of vessel wall injury and minimizing barotrauma. The balloon's material composition, often consisting of durable polymers like polyethylene terephthalate (PET), ensures optimal radial expansion force and retraction capabilities, resulting in precise vessel dilation and rapid deflation times.

- Biomechanically, the Mustang balloon's design allows for even distribution of pressure across the balloon surface during inflation, preventing uneven or excessive stress on the vessel wall. This is particularly important in femoral-popliteal bypass angioplasty, as it minimizes the risk of intimal dissection, plaque disruption, or vessel perforation, which could lead to acute closure, embolization, or subsequent restenosis.

- Moreover, the Mustang balloon's low-profile design and hydrophilic coating enhance its deliverability and crossability, enabling smooth navigation through tortuous vascular anatomy and tight lesions. The advanced tracking and pushability of the balloon catheter further contribute to its biomechanical efficiency in complex endovascular interventions.

HAEMODYNAMIC INSIGHT:

- Stenosis in the fem-pop anastomosis can result in turbulent flow patterns, characterized by a high Reynolds number and localized vortices, which exacerbate endothelial dysfunction, activate platelets, and promote a pro-thrombotic environment. This hemodynamic environment contributes to the development of further atherosclerosis, intimal hyperplasia, and restenosis.

- Following a successful balloon angioplasty, the stenotic lesion is dilated, leading to a marked improvement in the vessel's luminal diameter and cross-sectional area. This mechanical intervention ameliorates the adverse hemodynamic effects by reducing the resistance to blood flow, increasing flow velocities, and decreasing the pressure gradients across the treated segment. Consequently, the blood flow becomes more laminar, characterized by a lower Reynolds number, which mitigates endothelial stress and reduces

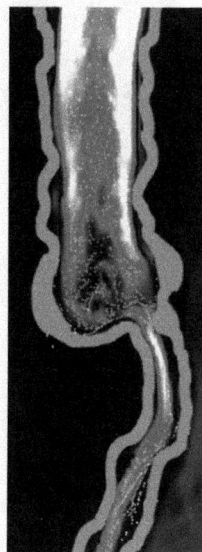

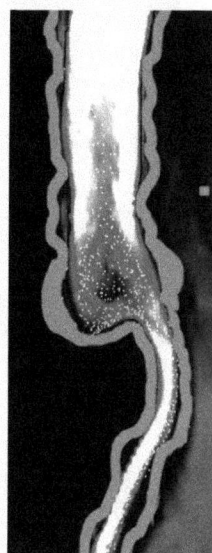

the likelihood of thrombus formation and subsequent complications.

RESEACH INSIGHT

- Cochrane Database of Systematic Reviews on Endoluminal interventions versus surgical interventions for stenosis in vein grafts following infrainguinal bypass (2021) found no RCTs that compared endoluminal interventions versus surgical intervention for stenosis in vein grafts following infrainguinal bypass. Currently, there is no high certainty evidence to support the use of one type of intervention over another. High quality studies are needed to provide evidence on managing vein graft stenosis following infrainguinal bypass.
- (1)https://www.cochranelibrary.com/cdsr/doi/10.1002/14651858.CD013702.pub2/full

BYPASS CASE: 2

A 72-year-old patient with a history of fem- BTK popliteal graft. Duplex showed a proximal, focal significant stenosis. A decision was agreed to proceed to left graft angioplasty +/- stenting.

READ CAREFULLY ...

Access	Pre Op checklist, supine, GA , cleaned and draped, Utilized 6Frs sheath across challenging aortic bifurcation.
Equipments	Standard (Micro-access. J Wire. Glidewire+Cobra. Amplatz+Proglide. Pigtail. contrast+HepSaline) + 5mm x 4cm Mustang balloon. 5mm x 4cm DCB. (no 6mm DCB available for this case).
Angiogram Findings	CFA and profunda patent. Graft patent with proximal, significant stenosis. P3 popliteal patent. Three-vessel runoff confirmed. Mid-peroneal exhibits significant stenosis.
Procedure	Treated proximal graft stenosis with 4x40mm standard and 5x40mm DCB, improving flow and vessel lumen diameter.
Complications	Mynx Control failure.
Closure	Left groin haemostasis achieved manually. No immediate complications.

CONCISELY SUMMARIZE THE PROCEDURE USING KEY TERMS (ANSWER BELOW).

CHECK YOUR KNOWLEDGE

Qs ON STRATEGY

Does accessing a fem-pop bypass present unique challenges?

Yes, as demonstrated in this case, it can pose challenges due to anatomical factors.

Qs ON BALLONING

Should incidental isolated tight run-off disease be treated simultaneously?

No, in this case, the tibial issue is diseased but left untreated.

Is a standard POBA adequate for bypass plasty?

Likely not. Consider using a DCB for better results.

IN-DEPTH ANALYSIS

PROCEDURE : FEM POP BYPASS PLASTY. MUSTANG BALLOON (DIFFICULT MANIPULATION TO POSITION). DCB. SUCCESSFUL.

COMMENTS:

- Balloon angioplasty, a conventional method, offers immediate relief by physically dilating the stenotic lesion, restoring blood flow. However, it carries a risk of vessel wall injury, dissection, or recoil, leading to restenosis. The technique's effectiveness might be transient, as it does not prevent neointimal hyperplasia, a significant cause of restenosis.
- Drug-coated balloons (DCBs) offer a more advanced solution. These are standard balloons coated with antiproliferative drugs that are delivered directly to the lesion during inflation. The pharmacological agent helps inhibit neointimal hyperplasia, reducing the chance of restenosis. Consequently, DCBs might offer a more durable solution for bypass graft stenosis, as indicated by the improved flow and lumen diameter in this case, potentially improving the graft's longevity and the patient's overall clinical outcome.

CHAPTER 9
ENDOVASCULAR
VISUAL QUIZ

GENERAL APPROACH

Describe the following topics in three sentences?

BEST POSITION FOR ENDO OPERATOR?

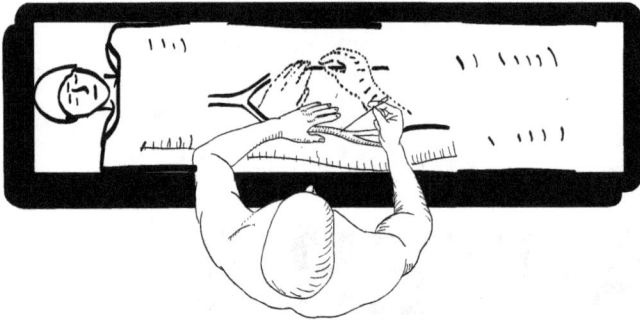

- Forehand operation preferred.
- Right-handed surgeon stands on patient's right for femoral artery puncture.
- Forehand used for brachial puncture.

ANATOMY LANDMARKS FOR FEMORAL PUNCTURE?

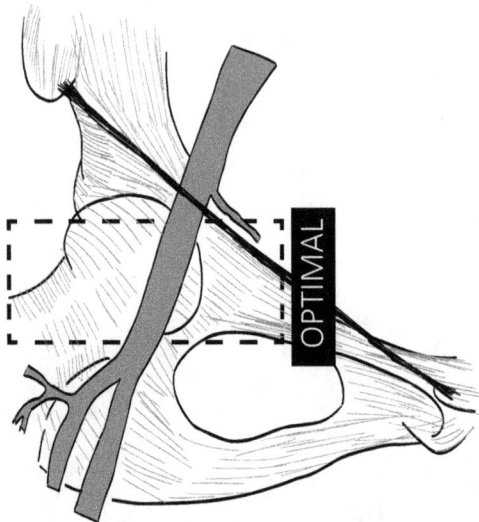

OPTIMAL

- The inguinal ligament delineates the upper border for femoral access.
- Palpate the femoral pulse below the midpoint of the inguinal ligament for puncture guidance.
- Within the femoral triangle, the artery lies medial to the vein and lateral to the nerve.

GENERAL APPROACH

COMPONENTS FOR PUNCTURE SET?

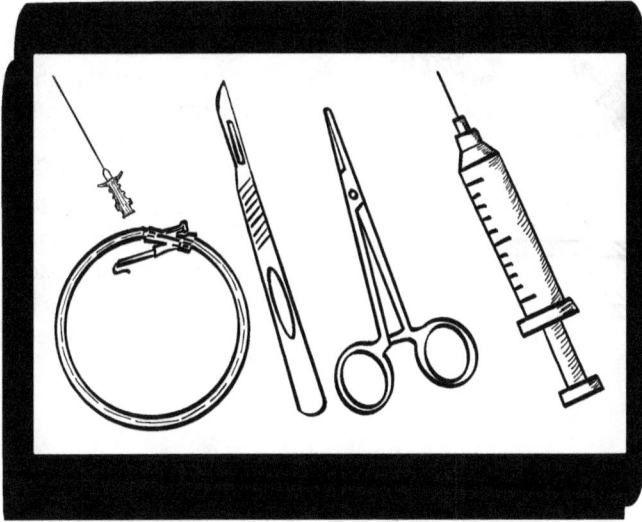

- Sterile tools for percutaneous arterial entry include a scalpel, hemostat, needle, anesthetic syringe, and guidewire.

WHERE TO ACCESS FEMORAL ARTERY?

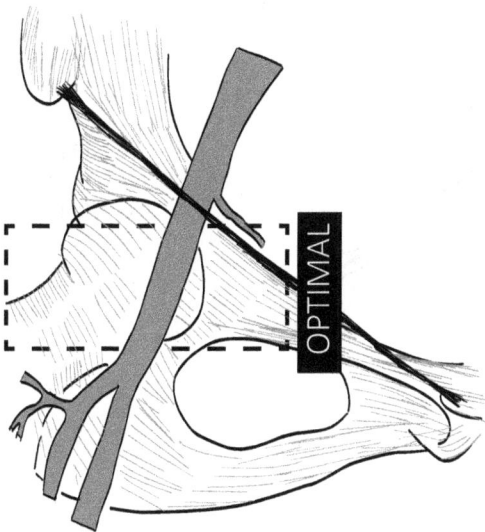

OPTIMAL

- Operator uses nondominant hand to hold tissue while injecting anesthetic, making femoral pulse pronounced.
- Needle enters the artery at 45-degrees; arteriotomy is safest in the proximal to middle femoral artery.
- Upon successful needle insertion, nondominant hand steadies it and dominant hand inserts a guidewire.

GENERAL APPROACH

TYPES OF ARTERIAL PUNCTURES?

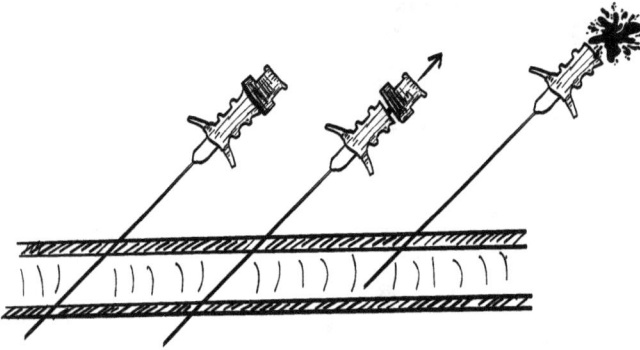

- Single-wall puncture uses a beveled-tip needle for the artery's anterior wall.
- Double-wall puncture utilizes a trochar with a sharp beveled tip through the artery.
- After needle removal, the blunt-tip casing is withdrawn until pulsatile backbleeding is seen in the arterial lumen.

How and what causes Retroperitoneal bleeding?

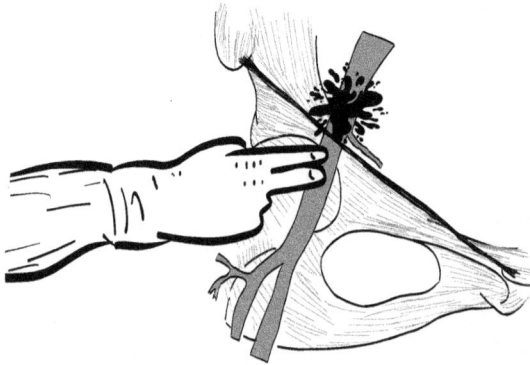

- Groin puncture too far proximal can cause retroperitoneal hemorrhage.
- Unrecognized pressure at the skin site might worsen the bleeding.
- Relaxing the abdominal wall and applying manual pressure can manage a distal external iliac artery puncture.

GENERAL APPROACH

HOW TO DEAL WITH OBESE PATIENT?

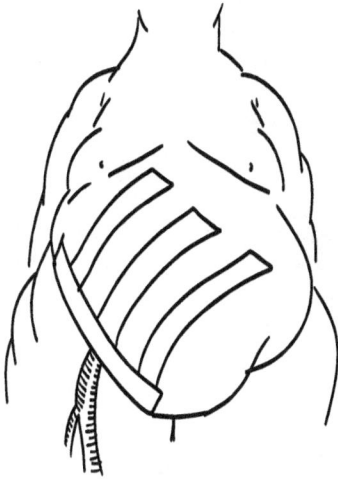

- Abdominal pannus taped up.
- Procedure enhances femoral exposure.
- Taping aids visibility during operation.

PULSELESS FEMORAL. WHAT NEXT?

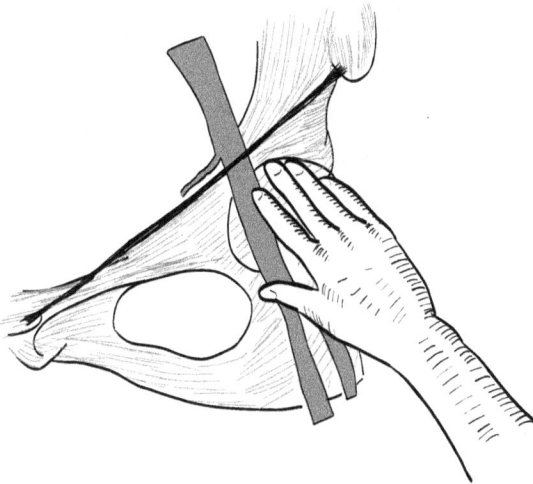

- Percutaneous puncture is used on pulseless femoral arteries, often palpable despite the lack of pulse.
- Arteriograms and fluoroscopy help determine the artery's location and guide puncture.
- Consider contralateral and proximal access.
- An arteriographic catheter can provide a contrasted road map for precise puncture.

GENERAL APPROACH

PERFORMING BRACHIAL ACCESS?

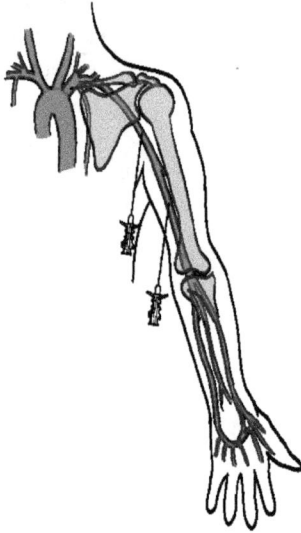

- Proximal access involves brachial or axillary artery entry, typically on the left side.
- Brachial artery interventions can be via cutdown or puncture near the antecubital crease.
- "Axillary artery puncture" is done just beside the axilla, essentially a high brachial artery puncture.

WHAT TO DO BEFORE YOU INSERT THE SHEATH?

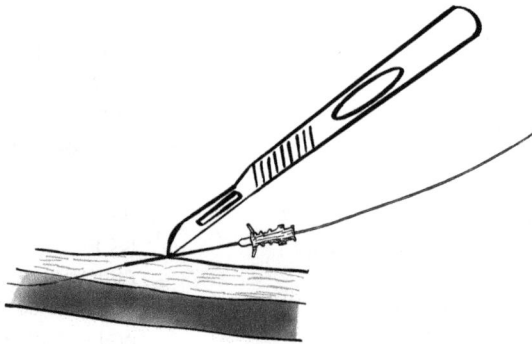

- Make a precise skin incision at the entry site.
- Place a 4 or 5 Fr dilator over the confirmed arterial guidewire.
- Use the scalpel on skin above the dilator; it's tougher than a regular sheath so can withstand the scalpel.

GUIDEWIRES AND CATHETERS

Describe the following topics in three sentences?

TYPES OF LESION-WIRE INTERACTIONS?

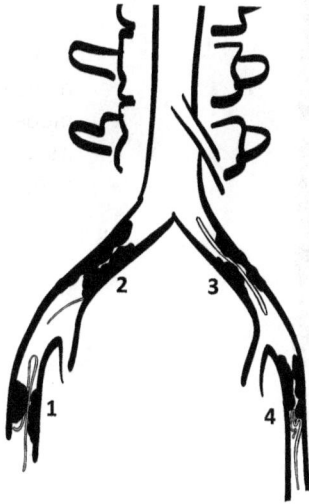

- Guidewire interacts with occlusive lesions in various ways.
- Outcomes include successful traversal, catching on plaque, or causing plaque disruption.
- Specific scenarios include buckling, piling up, finding subintimal planes, and embolization.

STIFFENING FLOPPY TIP - HOW TO?

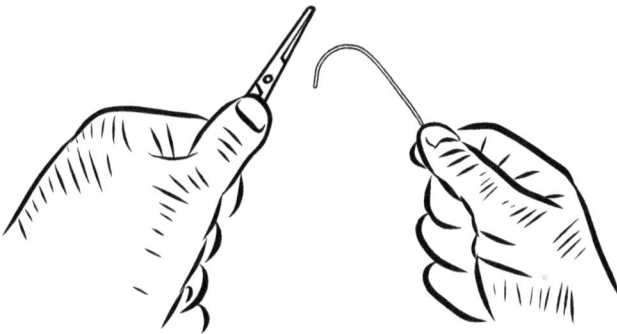

- Stiffen the guidewire's floppy tip for easier handling.
- Use one-handed traction to pass it through the needle's hub.
- Grasping and applying traction straightens the tip.

GUIDEWIRES AND CATHETERS

ROUTE GUIDEWIRE CAN TAKE?

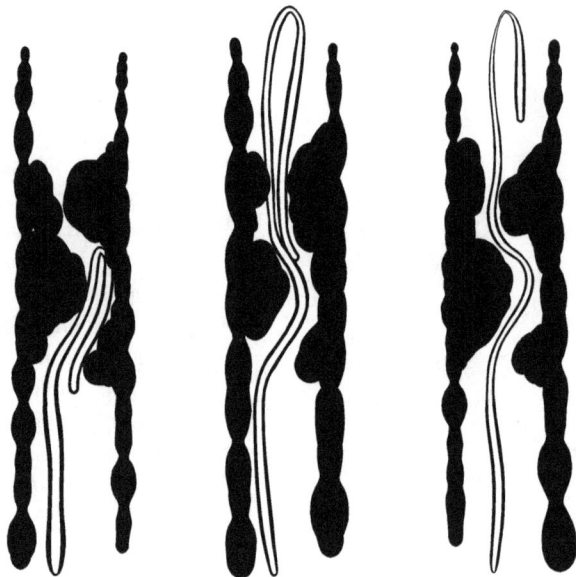

- Buckling the guidewire helps navigate eccentric lesions.
- If the tip buckles, use the created elbow as the leading edge for safer passage.
- The buckling technique is best for moderate arterial issues, not critical ones.

GUIDEWIRES AND CATHETERS

CATHETER INTERACTING WHEN INSERTING WIRE?

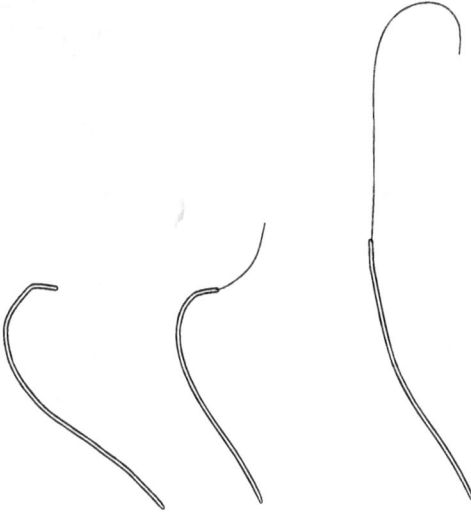

- Catheter head shape is influenced by guidewire position.
- Guidewire presence affects the curvature of the catheter.
- Specific guidewire sections can cause the catheter to splay or straighten.

PRIMARY AND SECONDARY CURVES?

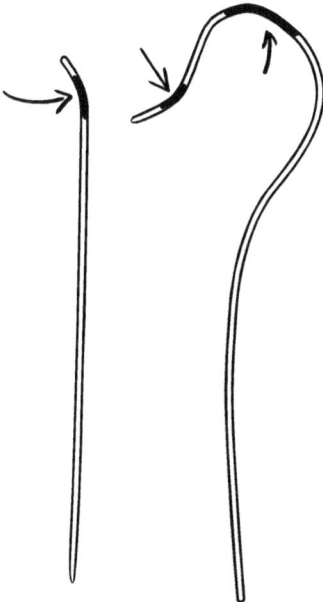

- Simple vs. complex curve.
- Simple curve catheters have just a primary curve.
- Complex curve catheters possess both primary and secondary curves, occasionally more.

GUIDEWIRES AND CATHETERS

KEEPING WIRE IN WHILE REMOVING CATHETER?

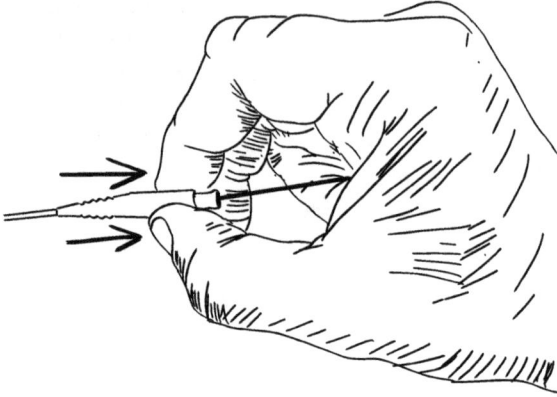

- "Walk along" the guidewire to remove the catheter.
- Grasp the catheter hub with thumb and forefinger; hold guidewire with fourth and fifth fingers.
- Withdraw catheter while maintaining guidewire position; repeat by moving hand further along guidewire.

COAXIAL VS. MONORAIL SYSTEMS?

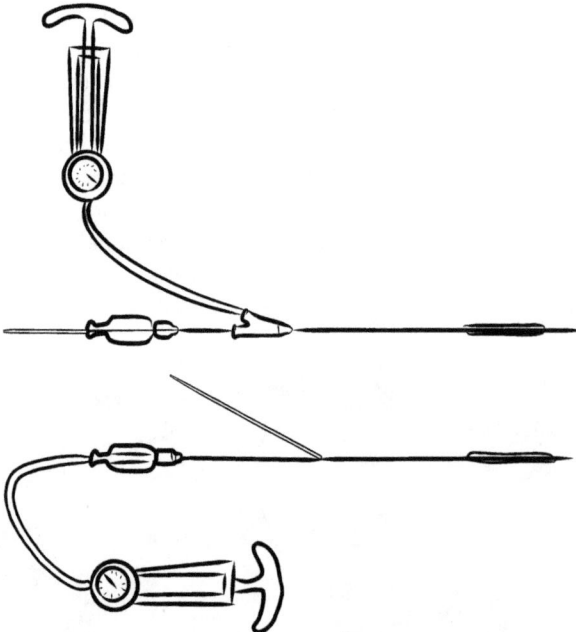

- Coaxial catheters have a guidewire lumen throughout their length, while monorail catheters have it only partially.
- The monorail catheter's guidewire starts at the tip and exits along the shaft, allowing for one-handed insertion.
- When using the monorail, operators can manage the guidewire and catheter separately, utilizing a two-handed technique for complete removal.

MARKING AND PASSING LESIONS

Describe the following topics in three sentences?

USING LANDMARKS FOR CATHETER POSITIONING

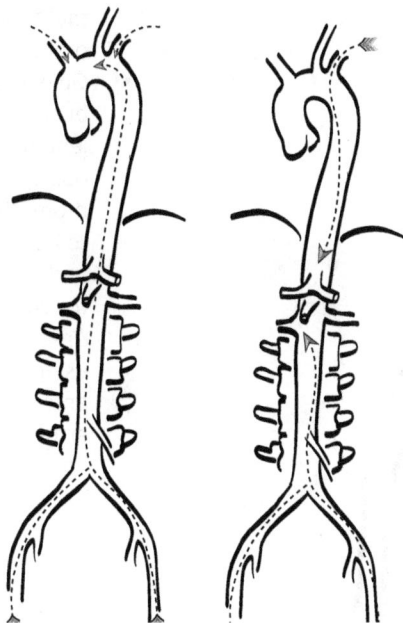

- Use landmarks for catheter positioning, especially bony ones.
- The renal arteries are near the L1-L2 vertebral junction; identify T12 with attached ribs to count down.
- Position catheter head near L1-L2 for contrast injection; aortogram shows renal artery origins.

PASSING THROUGH LONG LESION?

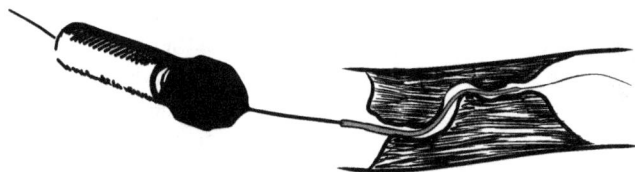

- Navigating through diseased arteries is tough.
- A steerable guidewire assists in making turns across long lesions.
- The guidewire tip probes the lesion.

MARKING AND PASSING LESIONS

BUCKLING GUIDEWIRE AND CATHETER

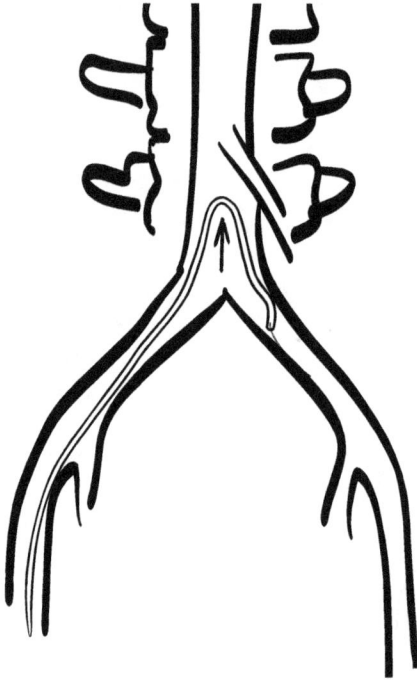

- In this case, a contralateral approach is chosen for proximal superficial femoral artery stenosis.
- Guidewire-catheter buckling occurs with lengthy or tortuous approaches, prompting a switch to a stiffer guidewire and curved sheath to reduce friction.
- An alternative is using an ipsilateral antegrade femoral artery puncture.

CROSSING AN ANEURYSM?

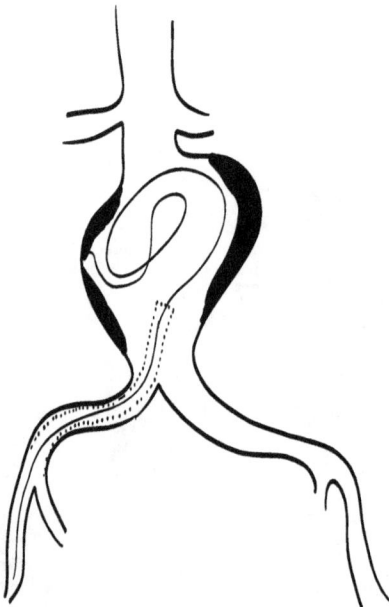

- Guidewire-catheter buckling highlighted.
- Guidewire accumulates in the aorta during passing an aneurysm.
- A simple-curve catheter directs the guidewire through twisted iliac and aortic segments.

MARKING AND PASSING LESIONS

C ARM VS IMAGE SIZE

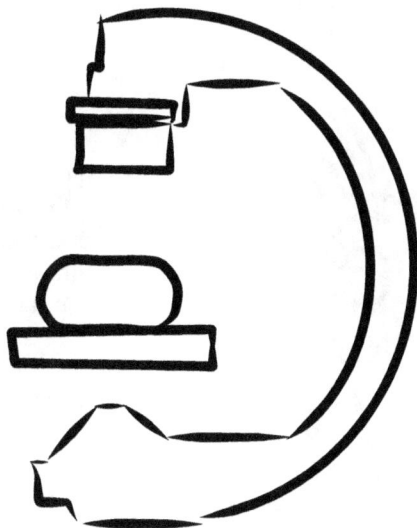

- X-ray tube emits energy, partially absorbed by patient.
- Remaining beam hits image intensifier, creating an X-ray image.
- Closer image intensifier reduces radiation scatter and broadens view.

SELECTIVE CATHETARIZATION

Describe the following topics in three sentences?

RIGHT SUBCLAVIAN ARTERY CATHETARIZATION?

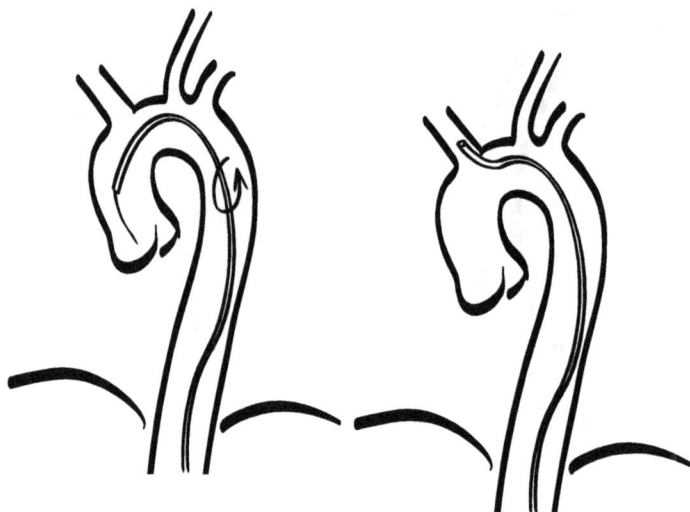

- A guidewire is placed in the ascending aorta with a simple-curve cerebral catheter over it.
- After removing the guidewire, the catheter head shapes as the catheter is withdrawn and rotated clockwise.
- The catheter tip enters the arch branch, and the guidewire secures access.

LEFT SUBCLAVIAN ARTERY CATHETARIZATION?

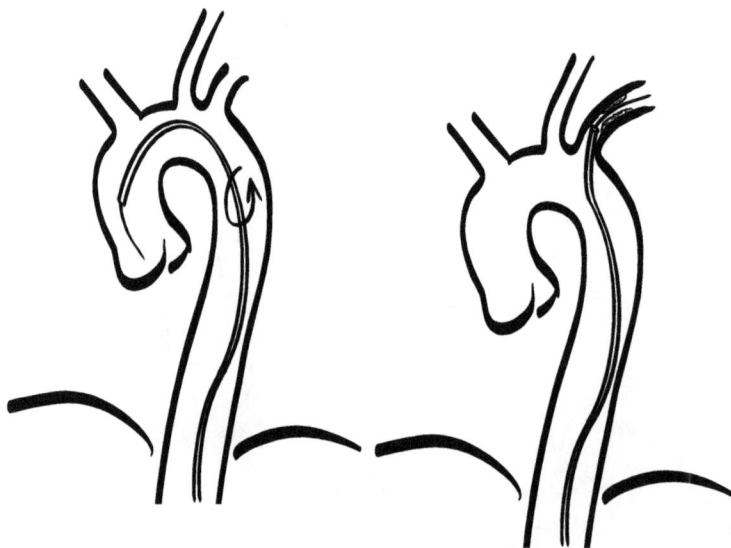

- A simple-curve catheter is exchanged for a complex-curve one in the subclavian artery.
- The catheter is adjusted, rotated, and advanced into the ascending aorta, engaging the arch branches.
- When the catheter tip reaches the desired arch branch, it is advanced further as its curve straightens.

SELECTIVE CATHETARIZATION

LEFT TRANSBRACHIAL SUBCLAVIAN ARTERY CATHETARIZATION?

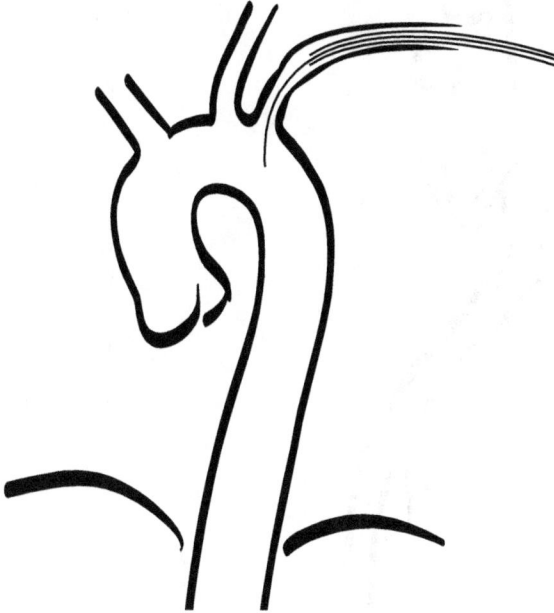

- Retrograde catheterization of the subclavian artery starts with a brachial puncture using a micropuncture set.
- The guidewire's natural progression is towards the ascending aorta, but a selective catheter can be advanced into the distal arch.
- The guidewire is adjusted, and the catheter is oriented posterolaterally before being redirected into the descending aorta.

RENAL ARTERIES CATHETARIZATION?

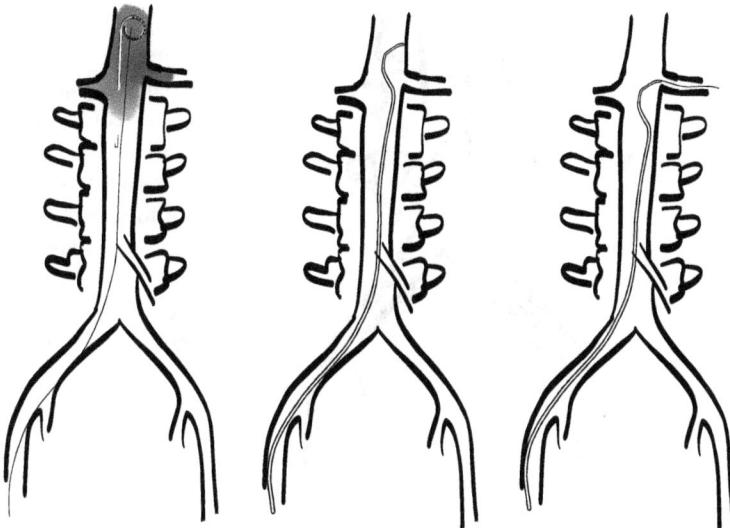

- A guidewire is placed in the aorta.
- An arteriographic catheter is used for an aortogram and renal arteriogram, then exchanged for a cobra catheter near the renal artery.
- The cobra catheter's tip enters the renal artery orifice, and the guidewire navigates through the renal artery lesion.

SELECTIVE CATHETARIZATION

POPPING OUT INTO THE AORTA?

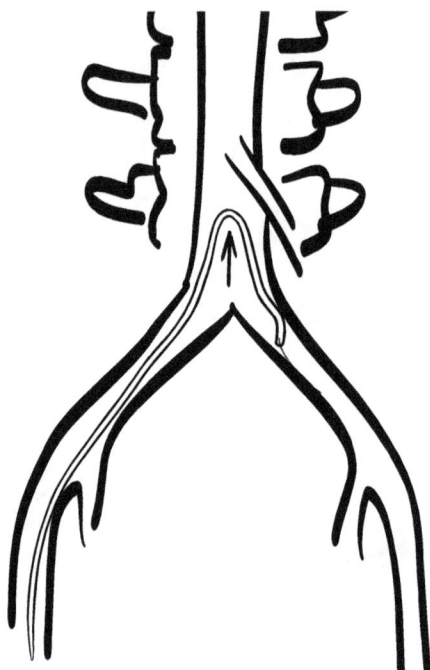

- Catheter may dislodge from contralateral iliac artery.
- Advancing the catheter without careful observation can lead to buckling in the infrarenal aorta.
- To prevent issues, extend the guidewire deep into the contralateral iliac system before advancing the catheter, especially in diseased arteries.

CATHETER ENTERS INTERNAL ILIAC?

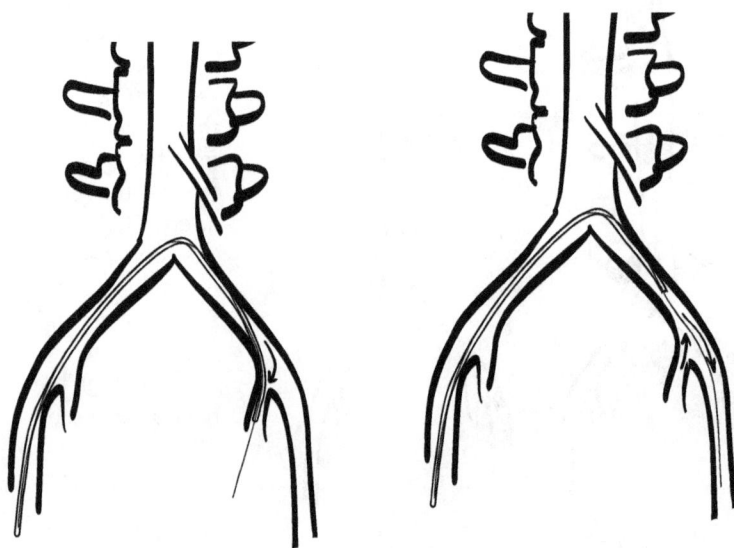

- The guidewire often enters the internal iliac artery, especially in a tortuous iliac system.
- The catheter and guidewire are withdrawn towards the common iliac artery.
- A torque device directs the guidewire anterolaterally, after which both guidewire and catheter move to the external iliac artery.

SELECTIVE CATHETARIZATION

GETTING CATHETER INTO AT?

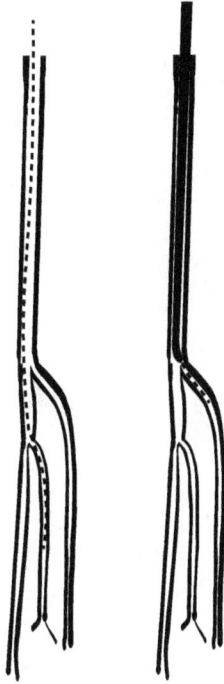

- Guidewire prefers peroneal artery after below-knee popliteal.
- Steerable guidewire with Berenstein catheter used for challenging anterior tibial artery angles.

ARTERIOGRAPHY

Describe the following topics in three sentences?

CEREBRAL ANGIOGRAPHY?

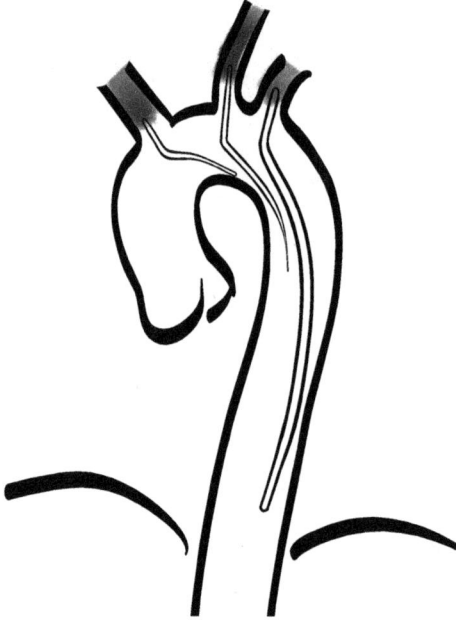

- Cerebral arteriography uses a simple-curve selective cerebral catheter in arch branches.
- The catheter tip should be positioned deep in the artery to prevent displacement.
- Recoil can occur during contrast administration.

RENAL AND VISCERAL ANGIOGRAPHY?

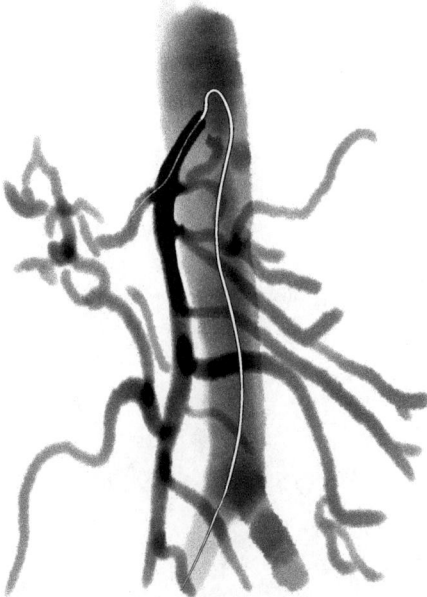

- Selective visceral and renal arteriography involves specific catheter techniques.
- A C2 cobra catheter is used for renal artery cannulation, requiring its tip to be inside the artery for detailed imaging.
- A hook-shaped catheter is utilized for arteriography of the celiac and superior mesenteric arteries.

ARTERIOGRAPHY

PROJECTION FOR RENAL ANGIOGRAPHY?

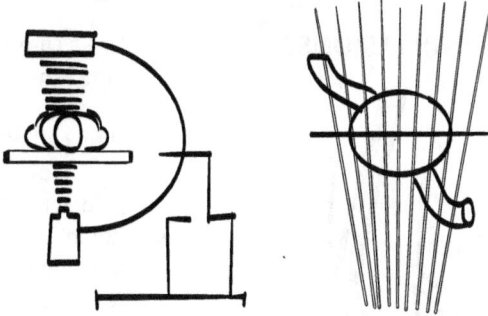

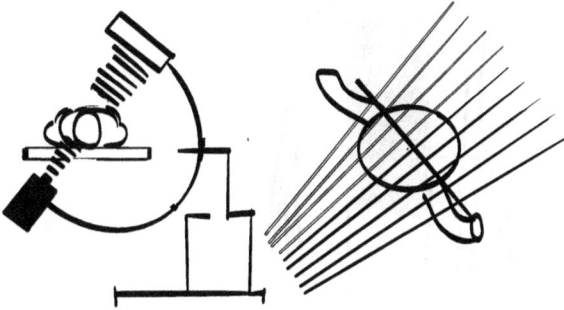

- Oblique projection improves renal arteriography.
- Renal artery starts postero-laterally.
- Anterior oblique view offers clearer view of renal artery origin, avoiding obstructions from aortic plaque or contrast.

ROJECTION FOR ILIACS AND FEMORAL ANGIOGRAPHY?

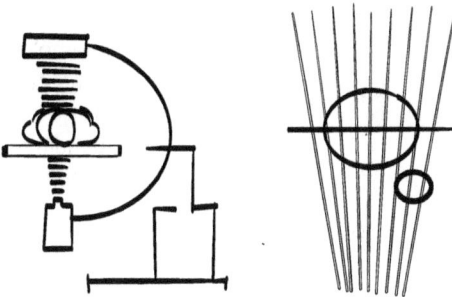

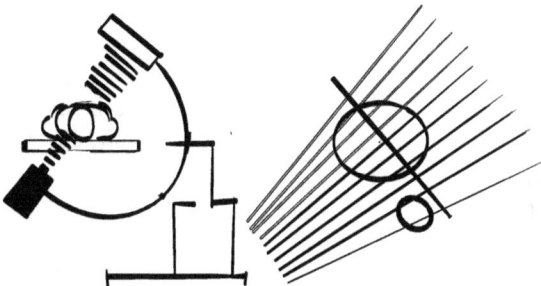

- Oblique projections show iliac and femoral bifurcations.
- Standard anteroposterior projection might not clearly show common iliac artery disease.
- Contralateral and ipsilateral oblique projections enhance visibility of bifurcations and reduce overlap.

CROSSING THE LESION

Describe the following topics in three sentences?

STEERING GUIDWIRTE TO PASS THROUGH LESIONS?

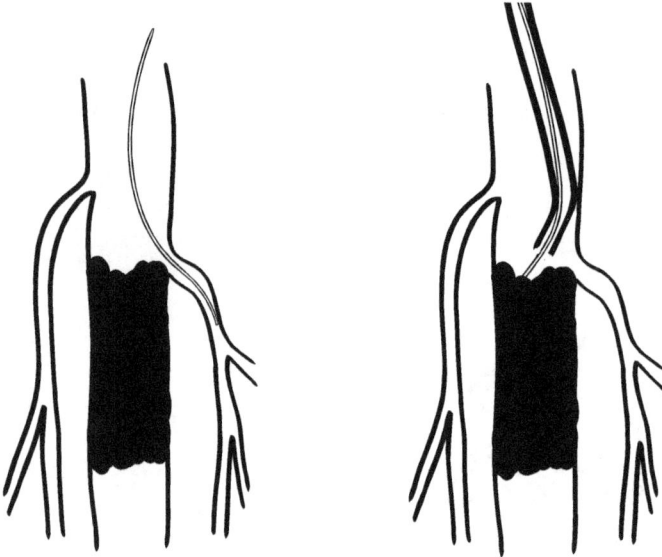

- Use a catheter to direct the guidewire.
- A bent-tip Berenstein catheter is placed over the guidewire.
- Rotate the catheter to guide the guidewire into the lesion.

FINDING THE WAY THROUGH USING PUFFS?

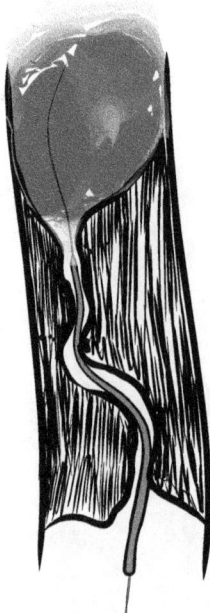

- 1. After a challenging guidewire passage, a multi-side-hole exchange catheter is placed over the guidewire to maintain position through the lesion.
- 2. Contrast is administered through the catheter, with side holes enabling the lesion to fill with contrast.
- 3. The guidewire can be removed, and contrast directly applied with the catheter tip, or a smaller guidewire and a Tuohy-Borst adapter can be used.

CROSSING THE LESION

IS THE GUIDEWIRE STILL IN THE LUMEN?

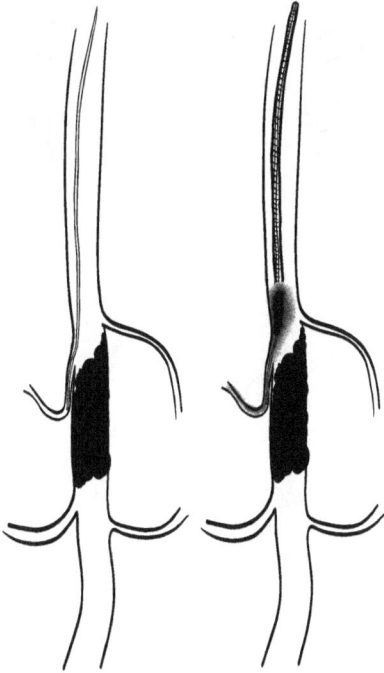

- Ensure the guide-wire is in the lumen.
- Under fluorosco-py, guidewire may falsely appear to cross the proximal popliteal artery.
- Arteriography shows the actual guidewire path and untra-versed lesion.

MAG AND OBLIQUE TO SEE BETTER?

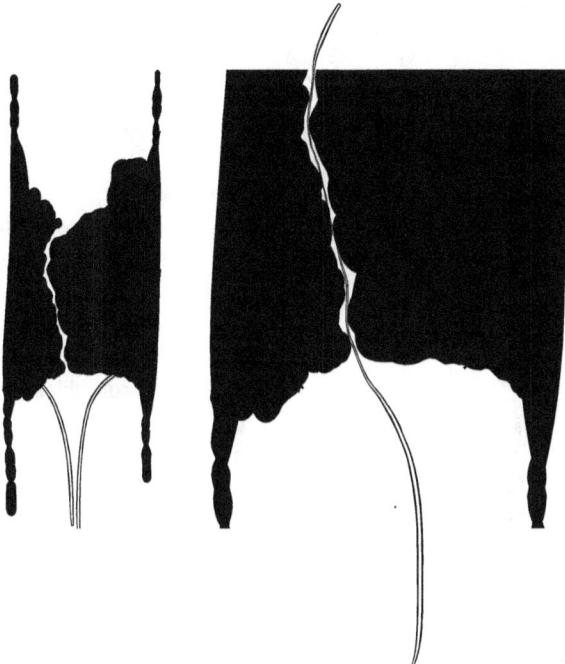

- Oblique view is magnified.
- Guidewire encoun-ters a complex lesion.
- Magnification and oblique projection reveal the lesion entrance.

CROSSING THE LESION

THE DOUBLE GUIDEWIRE APPROACH?

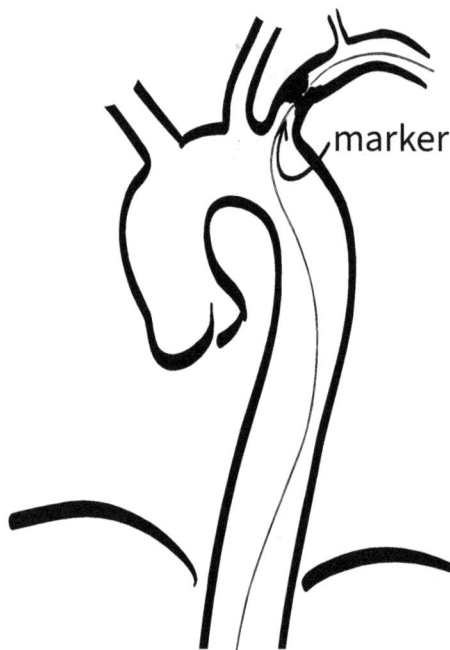

marker

- Subclavian artery occlusion has antegrade or retrograde approaches.
- If antegrade fails, use the first guidewire as a marker for a retrograde approach, assessing distance with fluoroscopic guidance.

SHEATH PLACEMENT?

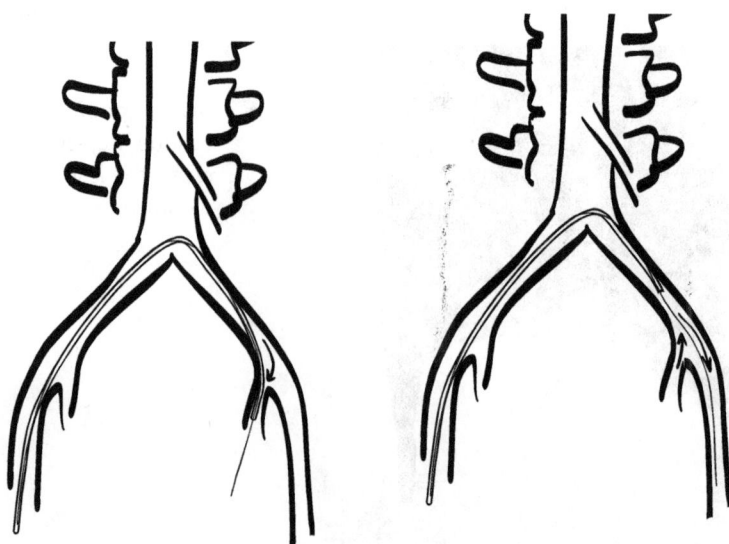

- The stiff exchange guidewire is directed from the lesion in the superficial femoral artery to the safer profunda femoris artery.
- The sheath's tip is positioned in the common femoral artery.
- After removing the exchange guidewire and dilator, the treatment guidewire crosses the superficial femoral artery lesion.

CROSSING THE LESION

SHEATH NEAR THE LESION?

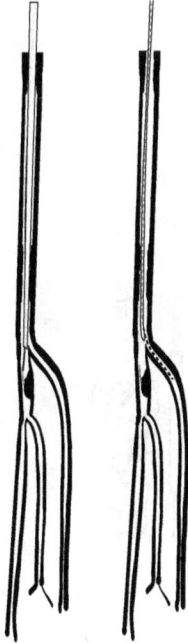

- Place the sheath tip close to the target lesion.
- Ensure adequate guidewire length for sheath advancement without adding risk.
- Redirect guidewire to a smaller branch, advance sheath, ensuring it's close to the lesion after removing exchange guidewire and dilator.

UP AND OVER SHEATH?

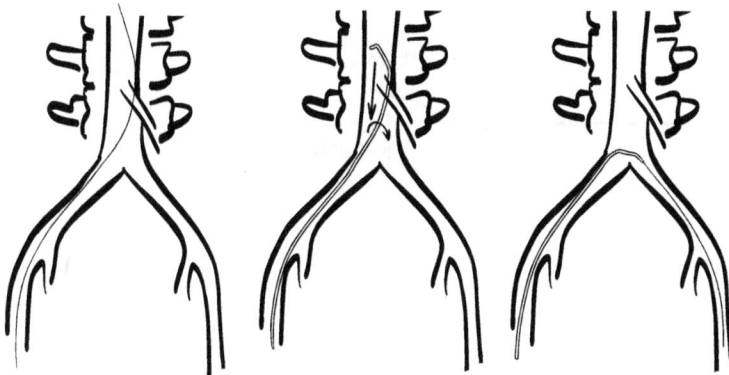

- Guidewire and catheter are positioned over the aortic bifurcation and then advanced to the contralateral femoral level.
- An exchange guidewire is placed, arteriotomy is dilated, and the up-and-over sheath is oriented and advanced over the guidewire with careful monitoring.
- If sheath faces resistance, ensure guidewire support; once in position, the dilator is removed, preparing the sheath for use.

BALLOON ANGIOPLASTY

Describe the following topics in three sentences?

BALLOON EFFECTS?

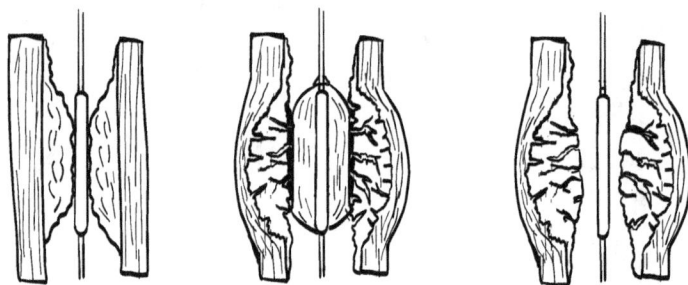

- A cross-sectional view displays an atherosclerotic lesion.
- A balloon catheter is positioned within the lesion and dilated.
- This dilatation generates radial force, leading to plaque fracture and observed dissection in completion studies.

BALLOON COMPONENTS?

- What are the balloon components in this schematic drawing?

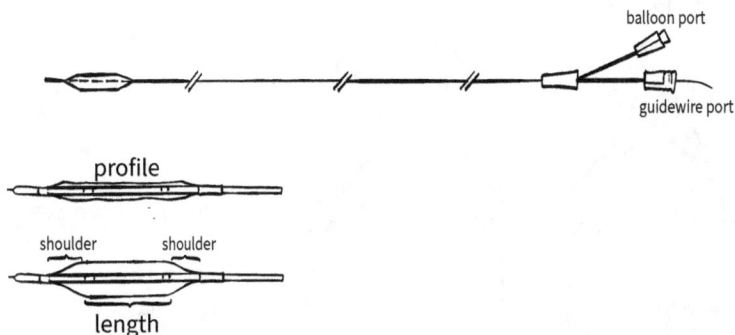

balloon port

guidewire port

profile

shoulder   shoulder

length

BALLOON ANGIOPLASTY

BALLOON PRESSURE?

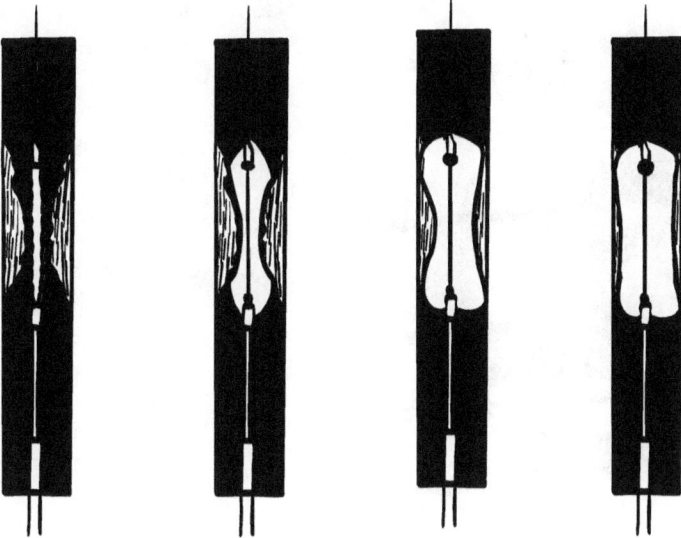

- Balloon catheter is placed to dilate atherosclerotic waist.
- At 4 atm pressure, residual stenosis is visible.
- At 8 atm pressure, atherosclerosis waist is fully dilated.

BALLOON RUPTURE?

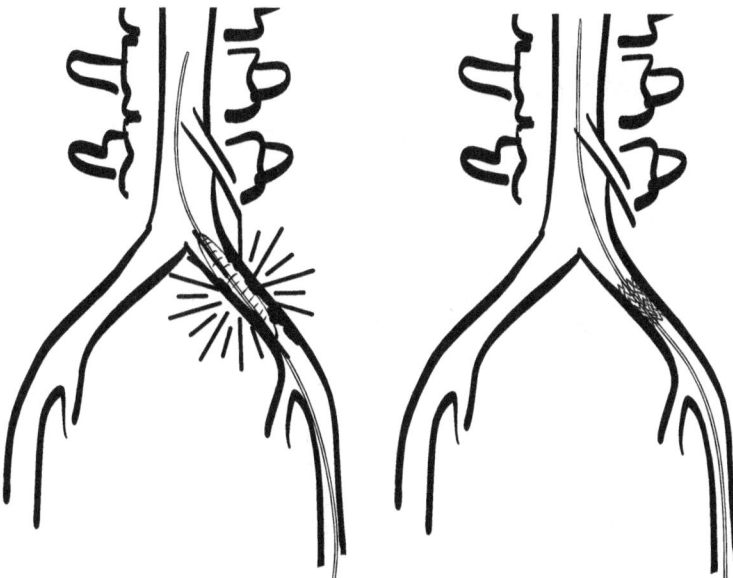

- Guidewire placed across iliac artery stenosis; balloon ruptures during inflation, showing contrast extravasation.
- Polymer balloon dilates lesion, possibly needing a larger sheath; lesion can be incrementally dilated using balloon's shoulder.
- Stent placement can also dilate calcified lesion; sharp lesions might perforate balloon during stent placement.

BALLOON ANGIOPLASTY

BALLOON HERNIATION?

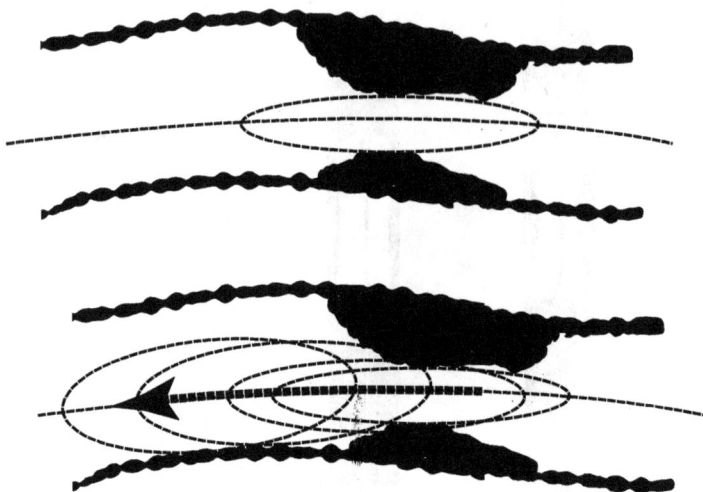

- A guidewire is passed through a stenosis.
- The balloon starts to migrate out of the lesion during inflation and might pop out of the angioplasty site.
- If this happens, deflate the balloon catheter, advance it, and reinflate while applying manual traction; or exchange for a longer balloon catheter.

ARTERIAL RUPTURE?

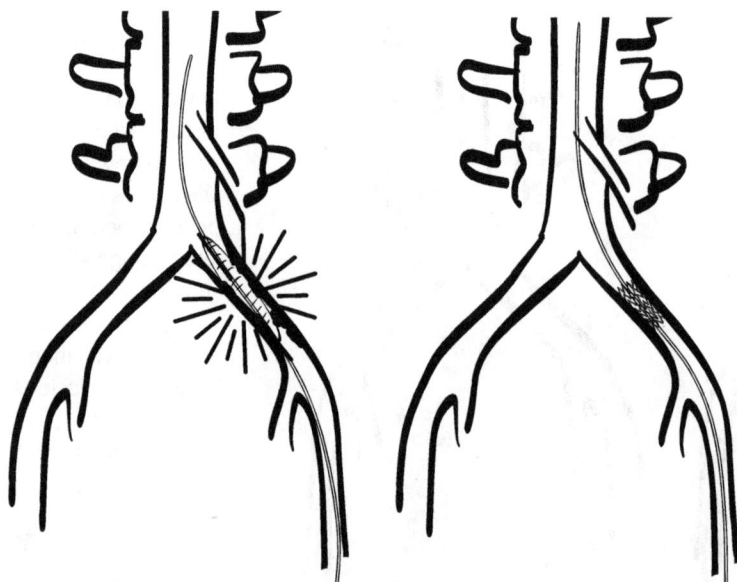

- Arterial rupture occurs at angioplasty site between hard plaque and soft artery.
- Rupture results from the contrast between calcified plaque and adjacent artery post-angioplasty.
- To control bleeding, the angioplasty balloon is reinserted and reinflated.

BALLOON ANGIOPLASTY

ACUTE OCCLUSION

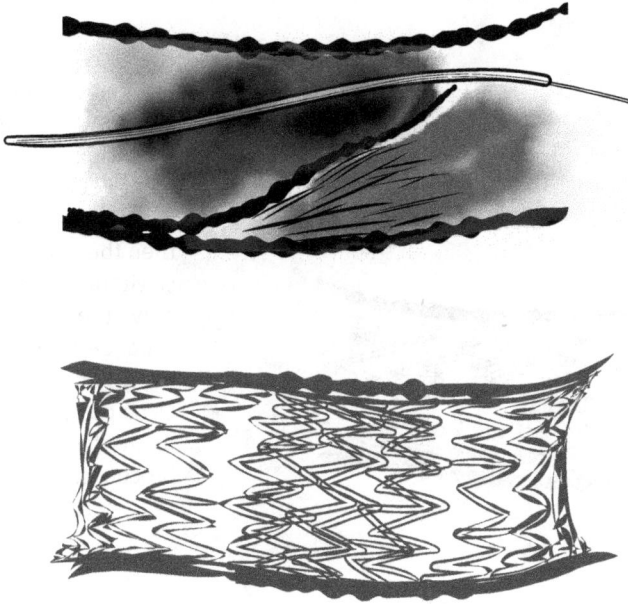

- Acute occlusion after angioplasty is often due to dissection.
- A dissection flap at the angioplasty site blocks flow.
- The issue is addressed by using a catheter, sheath, dilator, and stent to secure the dissection flap.

STENTING

Describe the following topics in three sentences?

MOVING SELF-EXPANDABLE STENT

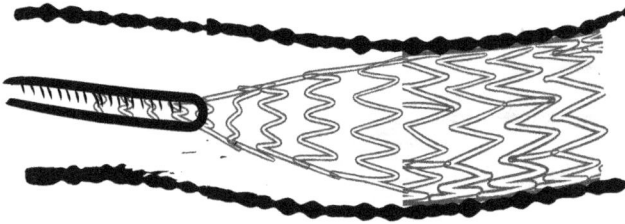

- The guidewire is positioned across the lesion.
- Stent deployment starts proximally, then the apparatus is withdrawn to move the stent's expanded end into the lesion.
- Once positioned correctly, deployment proceeds.

CROSSING A STENT?

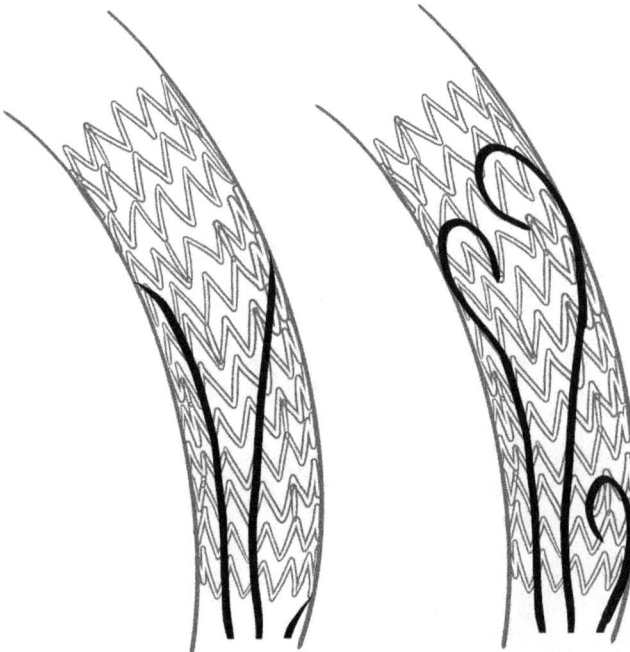

- Stent deployment has multiple false passage routes.
- Passage through stent struts is typically avoided.
- J-tip guidewires assist in preventing this passage.

STENTING

STENTING THE SUBCLAVIAN ARTERY

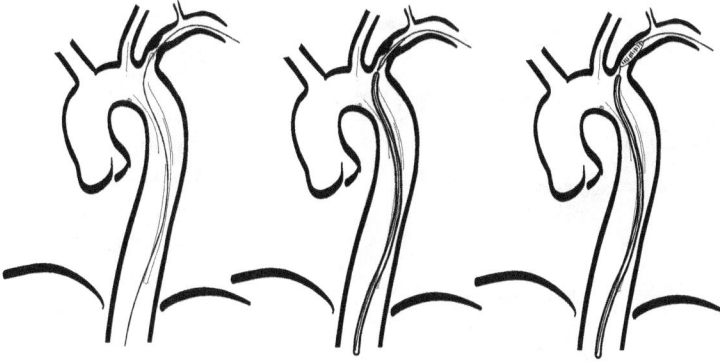

- Guidewire positioned at subclavian artery lesion origin.
- Transbrachial sheath inserted, but artery's tortuosity prevents safe sheath passage.
- Angioplasty balloon with stent navigated beyond sheath and through lesion; stent deployed.

KINKED SHEATH?

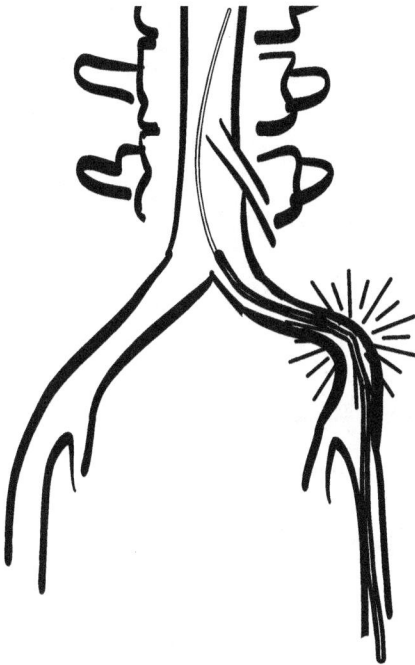

- Guidewire passes through lesion in tortuous iliac artery.
- Sheath and dilator advance for stent preparation; dilator removal causes sheath kinking.
- Kinked sheath prevents balloon-mounted stent passage.

STENTING

LOOSE STENT ON THE BALLOON

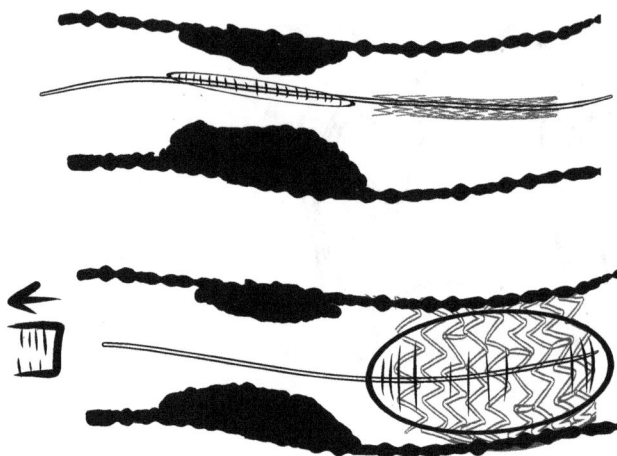

- Balloon-expandable stent becomes dislodged from the balloon catheter.
- Attempts are made to pull the stent back; if unsuccessful, it's pinned and the balloon is reloaded.
- The sheath is removed, and the remounted stent is deployed neutrally.

STENTED WRONGLY DISMOUNTED FROM BALLOON?

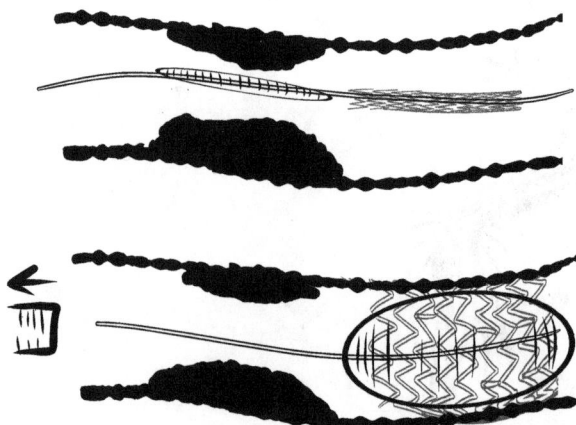

- Balloon-expandable stent is loose; risk of shooting forward if improperly mounted.
- Guidewire advanced for maneuvering; smaller balloon exchanged; one stent end flared.
- Appropriate balloon substituted; stent deployed neutrally.

STENTING

DISSECTION AT THE END OF THE BALLOON

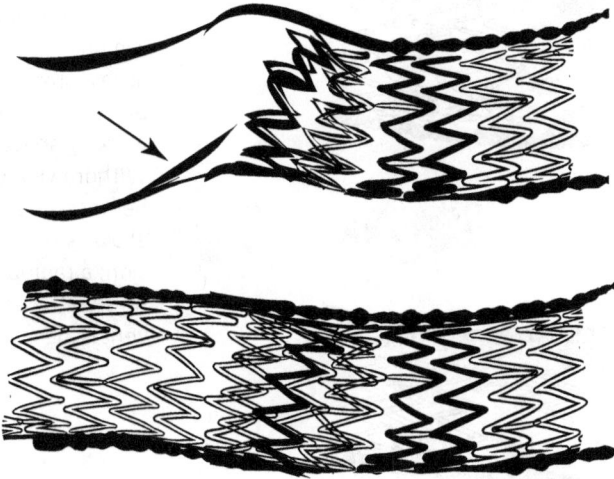

- A guidewire is positioned across the lesion.
- A stent is inserted, but a dissection occurs at the lesion's edge.
- A second stent is placed, overlapping the first, repairing the dissection.

SELF EXPANDING STENT INACCURATE?

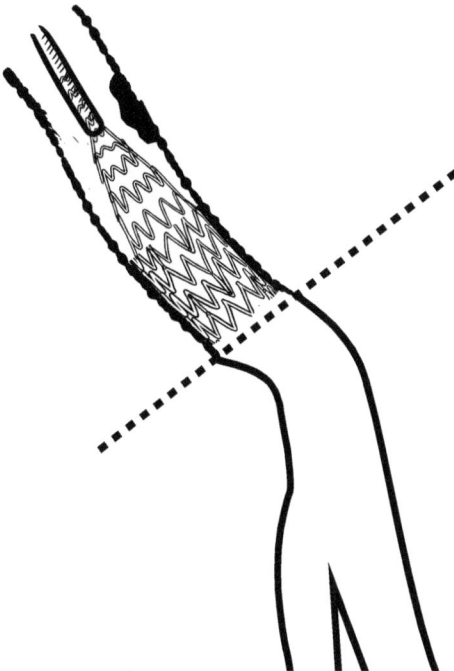

- Self-expanding stent placement is often imprecise.
- Retrograde Wallstent placement ensures accuracy at the stent's proximal end.
- Antegrade placement prioritizes the distal end due to limited working space near the inguinal ligament.

STENTING

SELF EXPANDING STENT PARTIALLY DEPLOYED?

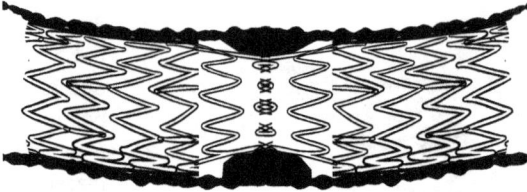

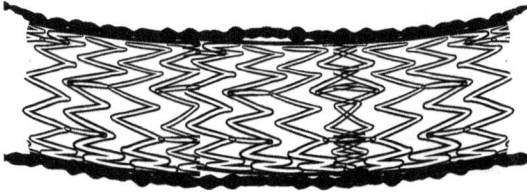

- Self-expanding stent partially deploys into hemostatic introducer sheath.
- Stent deployment is hindered due to access sheath impingement in limited working space.
- Withdrawing the hemostatic sheath allows stent expansion; a radiopaque tip sheath can prevent issues.

SELECTIVE PROCEDURES

Describe the following topics in three sentences?

AORTIC ANGIOPLASTY?

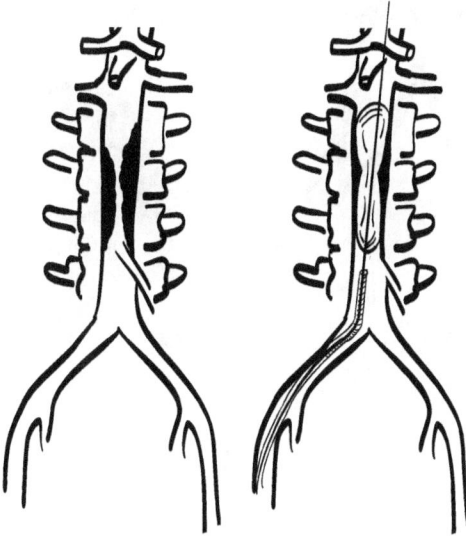

- Focal lesion found in infrarenal abdominal aorta.
- Balloon angioplasty treats aortic lesions.
- Complex lesion in infrarenal aorta addressed with retrograde guidewire and kissing balloons at bifurcation.

CERAB?

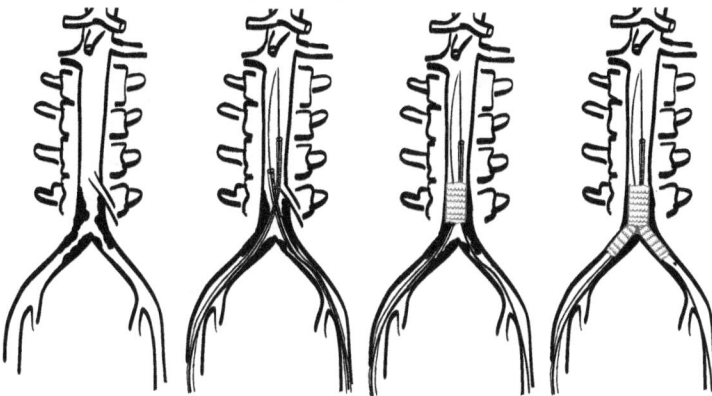

- A lesion in the infrarenal aorta and iliac arteries is treated with multistent reconstruction.
- Sheaths and guidewires are positioned; aortic stent delivered and contralateral guidewire adjusted.
- Kissing stents are inserted up to or inside the aortic stent.

SELECTIVE PROCEDURES

ILIAC KISSING STENTS?

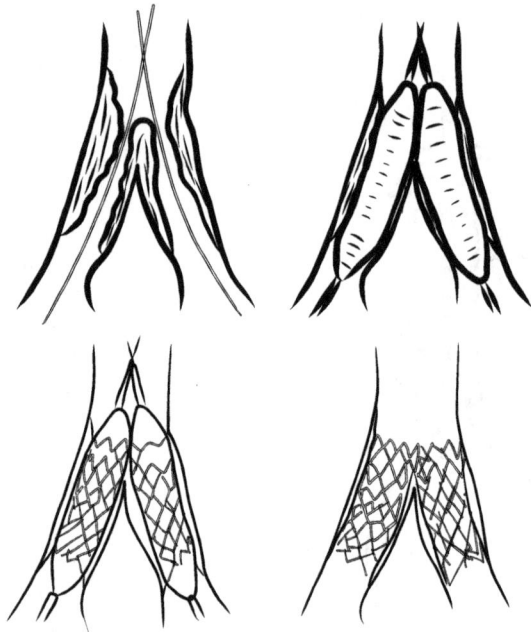

- Lesion in aortic bifurcation managed with kissing balloons.
- Bilateral guidewires placed across stenosis; balloon catheters inserted through femoral arteries with overlapping markers.
- Equal-sized balloons inflated simultaneously to dilate the bifurcation lesion.

SFA/POPLITEAL ANGIOPLASTY?

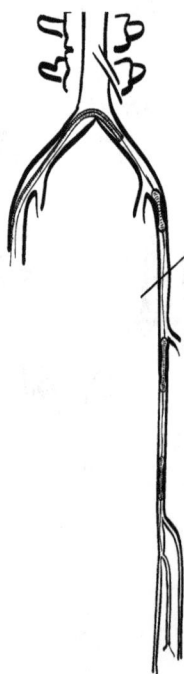

- Balloon angioplasty targets the SFA stenosis.
- The stenosis is approached antegrade, and the angioplasty balloon is passed through and dilated.
- Post-dilation, the balloon is removed, but the guidewire's position is maintained for completion arteriography.

SELECTIVE PROCEDURES

ANGIOPLASTY OF A BYPASS GRAFT —UP AND OVER APPROACH?

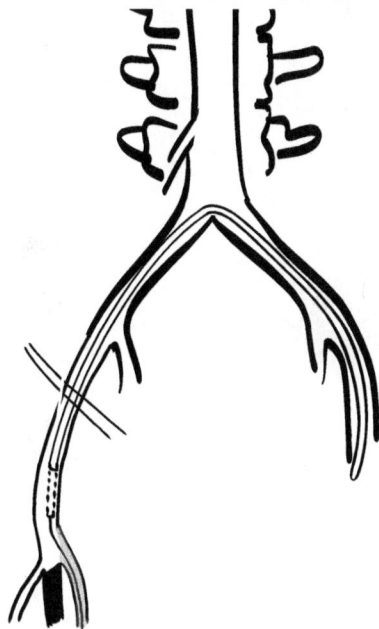

- Infrainguinal bypass graft originates from the common femoral artery and has a proximal graft lesion.
- An up-and-over sheath is used for arteriography and guiding the guide-wire through the lesion.
- Balloon angioplasty is executed, followed by completion arte-riography through the sheath.

SANGIOPLASTY OF A BYPASS GRAFT —ANTEGRADE APPROACH?

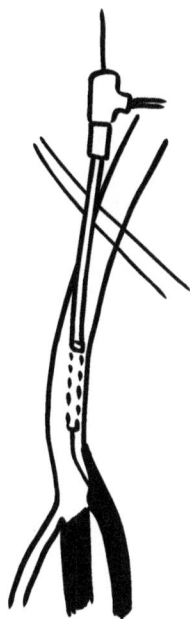

- Balloon angioplasty is done on infrain-guinal bypass grafts via an antegrade ipsilateral approach.
- An antegrade femo-ral sheath is used for arteriography, and a guidewire is directed into the vein graft with a selective catheter.
- After removing the catheter, balloon angioplasty is per-formed, followed by completion arteriog-raphy.

SELECTIVE PROCEDURES

ANGIOPLASTY OF AORTO-BIFEM GRAFT?

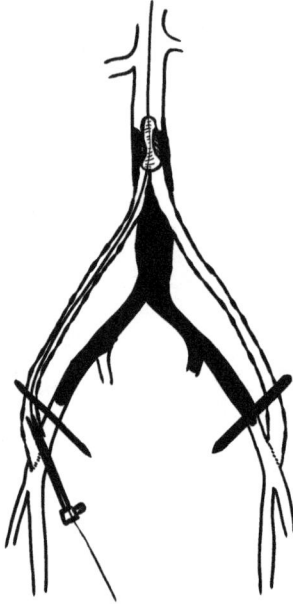

- Disease progresses in the aorta after aortofemoral graft.
- A femoral sheath is placed, followed by stent placement below renal arteries.
- Post-stent balloon angioplasty is done, concluded by completion arteriography.

CAROTID STENTING?

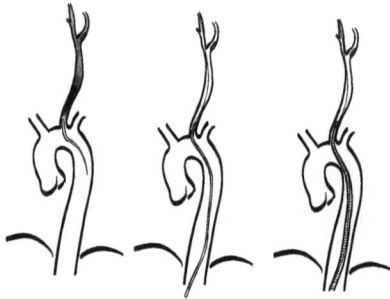

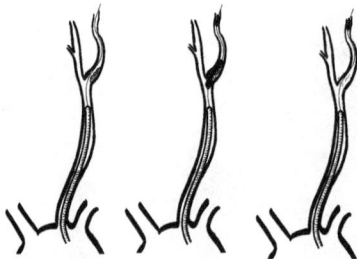

- Carotid bifurcation stent placement described.
- Normal aortic arch has distinct branch origins; elongated arch seen in elderly and hypertensive individuals.
- Left common carotid artery catheterized with a roadmap.

SELECTIVE PROCEDURES

SUBCLAVIAN ANGIOPLASTY?

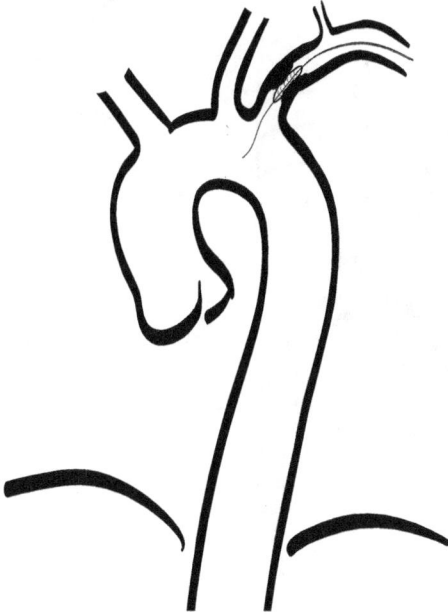

- Balloon angioplasty is done on the subclavian artery via a transfemoral approach.
- A guidewire and long sheath are positioned in the subclavian artery, followed by an angioplasty catheter.
- After the angioplasty, completion arteriography is executed through the sheath.

SUBCLAVIAN STENTING?

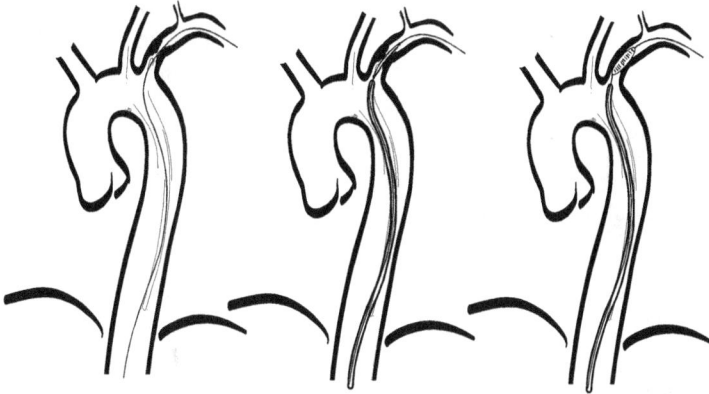

- The Glidewire, catheter, and guidewires are advanced and adjusted in the carotid arteries.
- Devices for embolic protection are placed, the lesion is pre-dilated, and a stent is deployed across the bifurcation.
- Post-stent dilation is done, and after angiography, the filter is removed.

MODEL CASE:
Left subclavian artery stenting and left internal carotid artery stenting in a single step

WATCH LIVE:
https://tinyurl.com/53kurzzn

SELECTIVE PROCEDURES

CELIAC AND MESENTERIC ARTERY CATHETERIZATION?

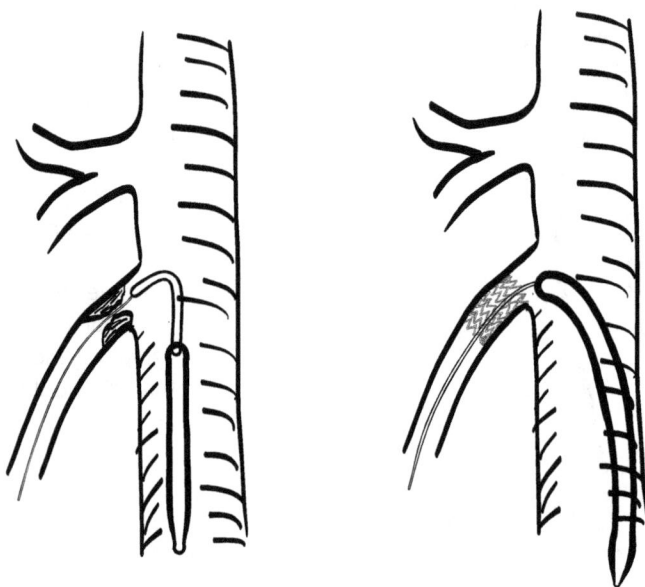

- Catheterization targets the celiac and superior mesenteric arteries.
- A hook-shaped catheter with an image intensifier in a lateral position is used.
- The celiac artery has a curving path, while the superior mesenteric artery has a straighter course with Glidewire.

CELIAC AND MESENTERIC STENTING?

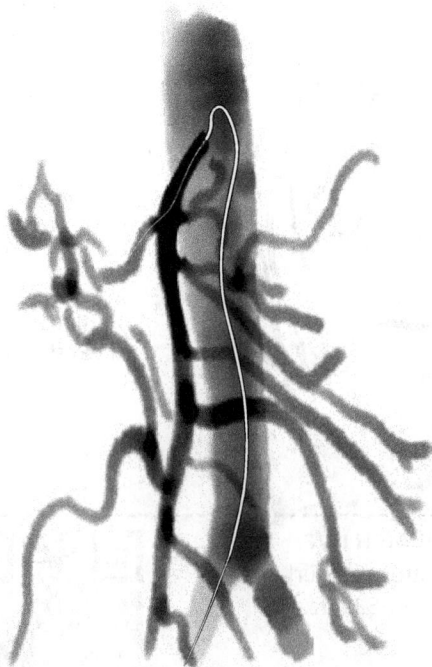

- Guiding sheath is placed near the SMA with a hook-shaped angiographic catheter.
- 0.014 in. guidewire is directed using the angiographic catheter and stabilized.
- A balloon-expandable stent is advanced into the lesion and positioned at the artery's orifice.

SELECTIVE PROCEDURES

SUBINTIMAL ANGIOPLASTY?

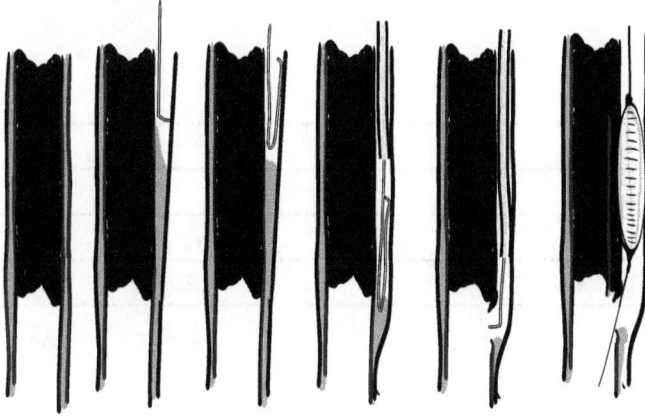

- A sheath is positioned near the occlusion, using the profunda femoris artery for guidewire insertion.
- An angled tip catheter directs the guidewire away from major branches, utilizing available stumps.
- The Glidewire tip buckles into the subintimal space, with the catheter advancing over it while maintaining the loop.

SUBINTIMAL ANGIOPLASTY?

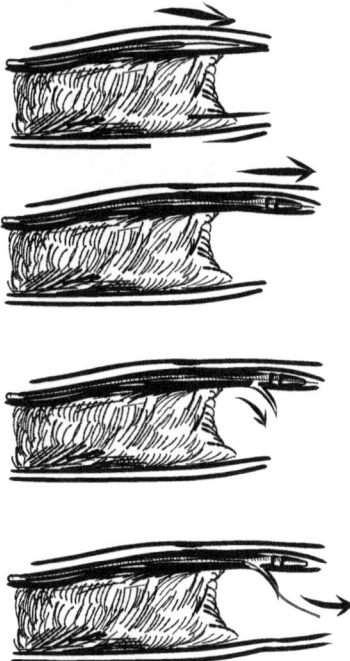

- Manage the guidewire loop by incrementally advancing the catheter for support.
- Ensure the guidewire advances easily, with the loop remaining narrow.
- Avoid allowing the loop to become too large to maintain its effectiveness as a re-entry tool.

MODEL CASE:
Multi Level Lower Limb Angioplasty
Through Contra-Lateral Access Outback
Re-Entry Device, Femoral Artery Stenting,
Popliteal Artery Stenting, Btk Angioplasty

WATCH LIVE:
https://tinyurl.
com/4fxb5wwx

NOTES, TIPS AND TRICKS:

CHAPTER 10
ENDOVASCULAR DECISION-MAKING QUIZ

WHAT IS THE BEST STRATEGIC ACTION PLAN

CASE 1:
Multilevel stenosis in the superficial femoral artery (SFA), significant in the proximal and distal SFA, with a patent popliteal artery, and calcification in the tibial arteries without significant disease.

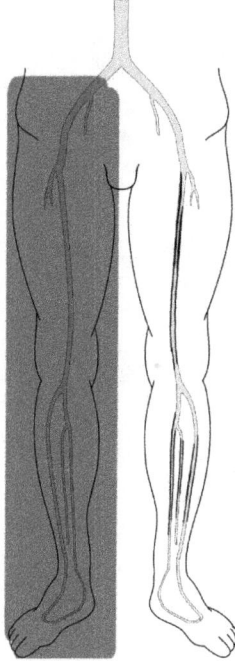

OUR SOLUTION:
The SFA lesions were crossed using a long terumo and CXI catheter intraluminally with ease, and two angioplasties were performed using 6mm x 14mm balloons on the entire length of the SFA.

CASE 2:
1- Proximal stenosis in the bypass graft.
2- Lesser stenosis at the distal graft near the popliteal artery.
3- Non-flow limiting stenosis in the popliteal artery (less than 30%).

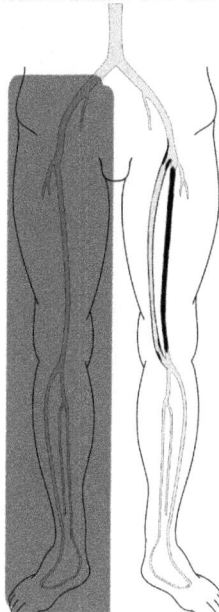

OUR SOLUTION:
Both the proximal and distal stenoses in the bypass graft were treated using a 6 mm balloon followed by a 6 mm drug-eluting balloon plasty.

CASE 3:

Patent SFA, with popliteal and peroneal arteries to the ankle, and an AT artery that occludes after its origin, reconstituting above the ankle.

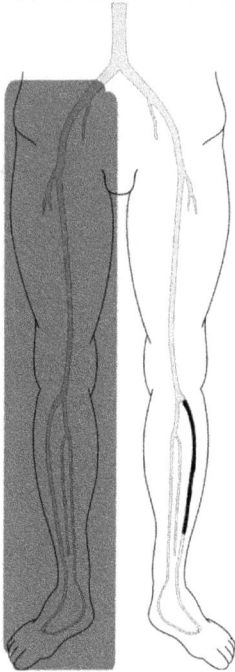

OUR SOLUTION:

AT was crossed with V18 and CXI, followed by a rendezvous with the bottom catheter in the lower leg, PTA of the AT using 2x10 cm and 3x10 cm, and an angiogram revealed that AT is patent to the DP into the foot. Selective injection of 100 mic GTN into the AT was used.

CASE 4:

The right distal popliteal artery and tibioperoneal trunk have a narrowing (stenosis) occurring distal to the femoral-popliteal bypass.

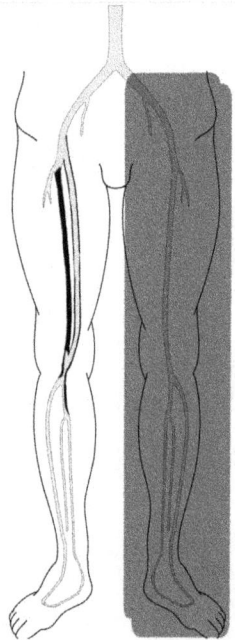

OUR SOLUTION:

A V18 wire was passed into ATA, with 3 x 10 POBA procedures to ATA and distal popliteal/TPT achieving good angiographic results, a Terumo wire was inserted into the peroneal artery, a small area of spasm was treated with 50 micrograms GTN, Proglide was avoided due to groin scarring, and manual pressure was applied to the puncture side.

CASE 5:

Multiple high-grade stenoses in the distal SFA, a short stenosis in the popliteal artery, and a single vessel runoff via the peroneal artery with two short high-grade stenoses proximally and at the mid-calf leve.

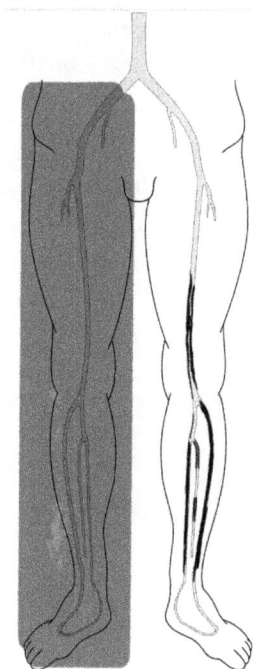

OUR SOLUTION:

A 4-French sheath was replaced with a 6-French sheath. Manipulation with wire and catheter to SFA and Pop, angioplasty with a 5 mm drug-eluting balloon, and treatment of distal and proximal PN lesions with 2.5 mm and 3 mm balloons, respectively.

CASE 6:

Nonsignificant stenosis in the proximal SFA, a 70% moderate-length stenosis in the distal SFA extending to the proximal popliteal artery, possibly due to chronic dissection, and a significant focal stenosis at the proximal TP trunk.

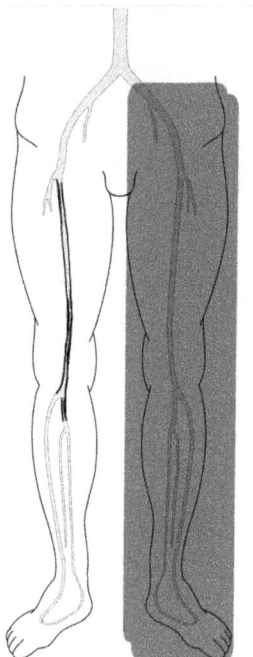

OUR SOLUTION:

Overlapping and prolonged balloon angioplasty were performed on distal SFA stenosis with significant residual dissection and no significant improvement, a 2.5 x 20mm angioplasty was conducted on the proximal TP trunk with good results, and a 5.5 x 60mm Supera stent was deployed in the SFA.

CASE 7:

SFA, popliteal, TPT, proximal AT, and peroneal, PT origin are unobstructed, but there is an occlusion beyond these areas with possible reconstitution in the distal segment, and the foot is mainly supplied by collateral vessels.

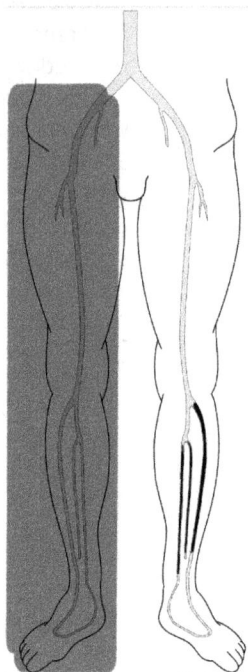

OUR SOLUTION:
The procedure to recanalize PT and AT was abandoned after multiple unsuccessful attempts, facing difficulties in tracking catheters and wires due to heavy calcification and other issues.

CASE 8:

SFA in-stent stenosis, with distal SFA stenoses, and good run-off mainly achieved through PT and Peroneal Artery.

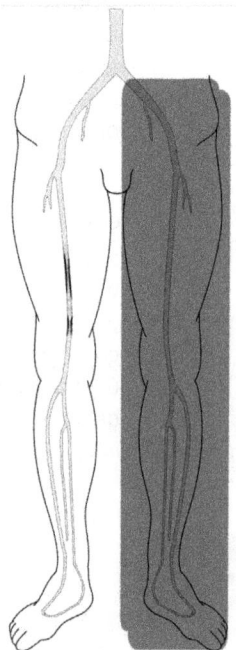

OUR SOLUTION:
The procedure involved crossing lesions with a command wire, performing several angioplasties (POBA) and using drug-coated balloons (DCB) in the distal SFA, followed by a stent placement (Zilver Flex 6x80mm) with subsequent angiographic checks showing good results and preserved brisk flow.

CASE 9:

Calcified arterial tree with bilateral iliac kissing stents in place, various levels of stenosis in different arteries including the right EIA and SFA, and occlusion of the peroneal artery and PT, with a patent AT supplying an incomplete plantar arch.

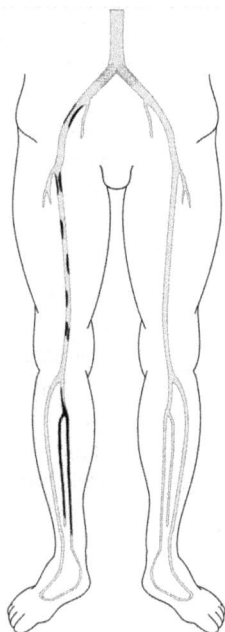

OUR SOLUTION:

Overlapping SFA angioplasties (using a 5mm x 15cm Mustang), followed by a 0.018 catheter and 0.014 to cross the PT occlusion.

Balloons were unable to pass a tight lesion in the mid-PT. Angioplasties were conducted up to this lesion with a 3mm x 25cm POBA, but further advancement was unsuccessful, leading to extravasation.

CASE 10:

50% blockage in the distal left SFA, possible mild stenosis in the proximal peroneal artery, an occlusion in the PT at its origin, and a proximal occlusion in the AT.

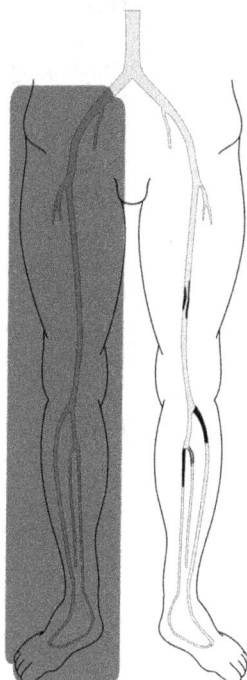

OUR SOLUTION:

Up and over access with a 6Fr 45cm destination sheath used. Wire and catheter (0.018 and 0.014) manipulated into the AT; poor pushability. Proximal AT angioplasty done with 2mm x 15cm POBA; unable to advance catheter/balloon distally. Overlapping angioplasty of distal SFA with 6mm x 8cm balloon.

Small extraluminal contrast foci noticed near SFA angioplasty site; prolonged angioplasty performed with the 6mm balloon (2 x 4 minute inflations).

CASE 11:

CTA left CIA
with calcified
arteries.

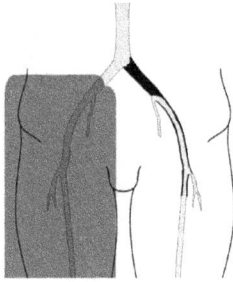

OUR SOLUTION:

Severe calcified CFA
(Common Femoral Artery)
disease identified. Access
secured using Hydophilic
wire/catheter, then
Standard wire, and a 6Fr
Sheath. Multiple failed
attempts to cross LEFT
CIA calcified lesion using
various wire/catheter;
limited dissection planes
created. Decision reached
that completing the pro-
cedure endovascularly is
likely hazardous.

CASE 12:

Left SFA is
occluded from
the origin.
The hood of
the previous
bypass is open.
Flow recon-
stitutes at the
adductor.
Diseased P1
segment iden-
tified.
Three vessels
run off..

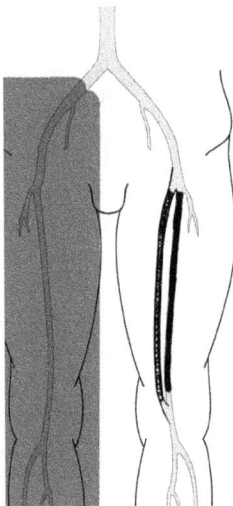

OUR SOLUTION:

SFA occlusion extremely
challenging to cross.
Various attempts with
different wires and catheters. Wire passed into the
SFA with no way back to
popliteal artery.
Using outback was unsuc-
cessful.
Attempts to cannulate the
popliteal artery above the
knee failed.
procedure abandoned

CASE 13:

Patent CFA and
PFA .
SFA flush
occlusion;
reconstitution
at P2 Popliteal
Artery. Patent
TPT with runoff
through PA
and moderate
stenosis at ATA
origin.
Incomplete
pedal arch.

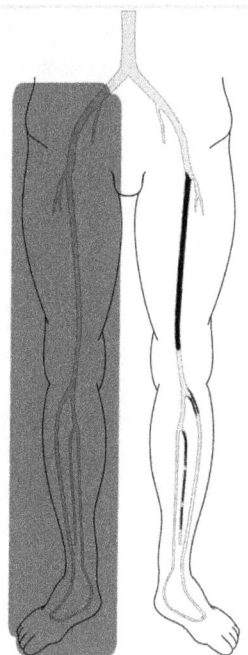

OUR SOLUTION:

subintimal SFA occlusion
crossing, with outback
re-entry device at P2
PopA. angioplasty with
3mm POBA to distal SFA
and P1 PopA, followed
by 5mm and 6mm POBA
throughout the SFA.

Post angiogram showed
long flow limiting dis-
section. SFA stenting
perforemd using A total
of four Supera stents.
Completion angiogram
demonstrates rapid flow
via the patent SFA and P1
PopA with improved fill-
ing of the crural vessels.

CASE 14:

Patent CFA and
profunda
Graft is patent;
proximal, focal
significant ste-
nosis
Patent P3
popliteal
Three vessel
run-off
Focal, signifi-
cant stenosis in
mid-peroneal.

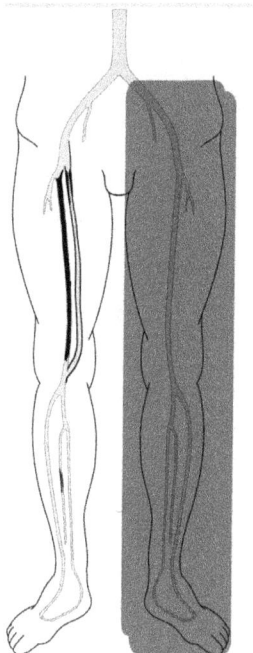

OUR SOLUTION:
A 4x40mm standard and a
5x40mm DCB were used
to treat the proximal graft
stenosis.

CASE 15:

Angiograms through the sheath reveal two short-segment blockages in the distal SFA and popliteal arteries. The anterior tibial artery is blocked at its origin, reopening approximately 3 cm further down. The AT artery is again obstructed for more than 10 cm at the ankle level. The dorsalis pedis artery receives blood flow from collateral vessels. There's no identifiable tibioperoneal trunk, or peroneal or posterior tibial arteries. Numerous collateral vessels are present over the knee and calf regions.

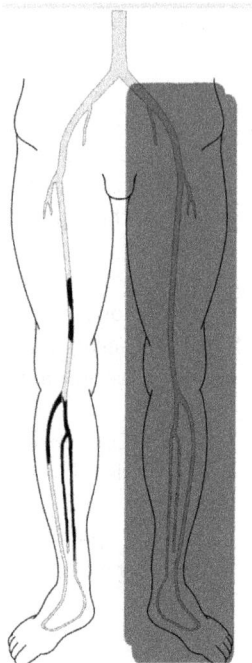

OUR SOLUTION:

The occlusion in the proximal anterior tibial artery was navigated and managed with a 3 mm balloon.

A distal occlusion was also crossed and addressed with a 2.5 mm balloon. Short segment distal SFA lesions were treated using a 6 mm balloon.

The angiographic appearance showed significant improvement.

CASE 16:

Constriction in the distal EIA above the patch, with stenosis at the patch itself. Complete blockage in the SFA from its origin, with flow resuming in the mid Pop. Closure in the proximal PT, accompanied by a large branch and collateral connections. Existence of a three-vessel runoff.

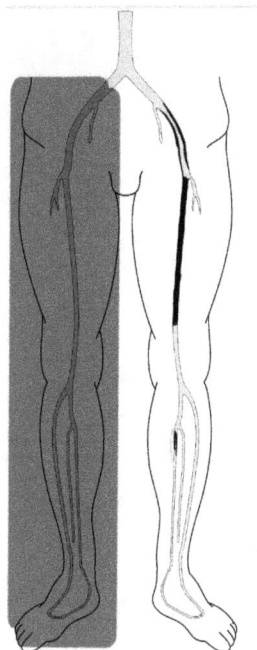

OUR SOLUTION:

Command, V18, and advantage wire and navi-cross used for subintimal crossing

PTA performed on the SFA and Pop using 4x15 cm and 5x17 cm balloons

Angiography shows dissection in the distal SFA and pop arteries, but very fast flow ensures run-off is maintained

PTA executed on the EIA and CFA utilizing a 6x4 cm balloon

Angiography reveals positive outcomes.

MODEL CASE:
Complex multi-vascular patient with occluded brachiocephalic trunk

WATCH LIVE:
https://tinyurl.com/mrxy46nc

NOTES, TIPS AND TRICKS:

SIMPOD™ TRAINING CASES

https://www.vssmasterclass.co.uk

SIMPOD™ MISC 1

LESION: Lt renal artery stenosis. 8mm long. 90% stenosis. Sim renal diameter: 5.2mm
YOUR TASK: Angioplasty +/- stenting via Rt femoral

Notes:

SIMPOD™ MISC 2

LESION: Lt renal artery stenosis. 8mm long. 85% stenosis.

YOUR TASK: Angioplasty +/- stenting via Rt femoral

Notes:

SIMPOD™ MISC 3

LESION: SMA. 16mm long. 90% stenosis. Sim renal diameter: 3.5mm
YOUR TASK: Angioplasty +/- stenting via Rt femorall

Notes:

SIMPOD™ MISC 4

LESION: Rt renal artery stenosis. 14mm long. 90% stenosis. Sim renal diameter: 3.7mm
YOUR TASK: Angioplasty +/- stenting via Rt femoral

Notes:

SIMPOD™ MISC 5

LESION: Lt IMA stenosis. 24mm long. 85% stenosis. Sim renal diameter: 2.5-4.2mm
YOUR TASK: Angioplasty +/- stenting via Rt femoral

Notes:

SIMPOD™ MISC 6

LESION: Lt IIA bleeding.
YOUR TASK: Coiling via Rt femoral

Notes:

SIMPOD™ MISC 7

LESION: SMA bleeding.
YOUR TASK: Coiling via Rt femoral

Notes:

SIMPOD™ MISC 8

LESION: Lt renal artery bleeding.
YOUR TASK: Coiling via Rt femoral

Notes:

SIMPOD™ MISC 9

LESION: IMA bleeding.
YOUR TASK: Coiling via Rt femoral

Notes:

SIMPOD™ MISC 10

LESION: Rt IIA bleeding + stenotic EIA and CIA.
YOUR TASK: Coiling via Lt femoral

Notes:

SIMPOD™ MISC 11

LESION: Lt SMA bleeding.
YOUR TASK: Coiling via Rt femoral

Notes:

SIMPOD™ MISC 12

LESION: Rt renal artery stenosis. 20mm long. 95% stenosis. Sim renal diameter: 4.4mm
YOUR TASK: Angioplasty +/- stenting via Rt femoral

Notes:

CHAPTER 11
ENDOVASCULAR
EVIDENCE REVIEW

AORTIC ANEURYSMS

Qs ON SCREENING AND PREVENTION

For which age group should AAA screening programme be established?

A screening programme for AAA should be setup for all men aged 65.

Which patients should be included in AAA surveillance programme?

Patients with AAA > 3 cm should be enrolled into a surveillance programme: every 3 yrs for 3-3.9cm; annually for 4-4.9cm; and every 3-6 months for >5cm.

When should men with an initial aorta diameter of 2.5-2.9 cm be rescreened?

Consider men with an aorta 2.5-2.9 cm in diameter at initial screening for rescreening after 5-10 years.

How should a family history of AAA affect screening recommendations?

Patients with a first degree relative with AAA should be considered for a screening ultrasound scan, at interval of 10 years, begining at age 50.

When is it recommended to consider AAA surveillance for patients with a true peripheral aneurysm?

Patients with a true peripheral aneurysm should be considered for AAA surveillance at 5-10 yr intervals.

When should elderly women with additional risk factors be considered for AAA screening?

Females aged 70 yrs or older should be considered for a scan (if AAA not excluded before) if they have another risk factor such as COPD, hypertension, or family history of AAA.

How should incidental AAA findings be managed in patients with a limited life expectancy?

No need to keep reviewing a patient with incidental AAA findings if they have very limited life expectancy.

What advice should be given to all patients regarding smoking, especially if a repair is being considered?

Advise all patients to stop smoking, for at least 2 weeks if a repair is considered. Ensure they receive appropriate help to support this. Ensure blood pressure is well controlled.

Are any medical therapies recommended to reduce the expansion of AAA?

There are currently no approved medical therapies that can be used to reduce the expansion of AAA, and none should be advised to patients. Alternatively, encourage a healthy life style (improved diet and ample excercise).

What should be the approach when a patient's AAA reaches 5.5cm but they aren't suitable for surgery?

Where the patient is not a good candidate for surgery when their AAA reaches 5.5cm, consider continuing the surveillance and aim to optimise their medical condition. Consider whether a procedure has become more suitable (risk:benefit ratio) if they reach a higher threshold (for example 7cm).

Qs ON DIAGNOSIS

What should be offered if AAA is suspected on a physical exam?

Offer an USS if AAA is suspected on physical exam.

Which modality should be used as a first line for diagnosis and surveillance of small AAA?

Use ultrasound scan as a first line modality for diagnosis and surveillance of small AAA.

How should the ultrasound scan be performed and where should the caliper be placed consistently?

Use anterio-posterior plane and be consistent in calipre placement.

What part of the aorta should be reported in an ultrasound scan?

Report the inner-to-inner maximum anterior-posterior aortic diameter.

What is recommended once a decision to consider AAA repair is made?

Once a decision to consider AAA repair is made, a CTA scan is recommended.

What should be used for measurements in a CTA scan and how to maintain consistency?

Use a dedicated softeware to make your measurements and uphold consistency.

Qs ON INDICATIONS FOR TREATMENT

For which group of men should an elective repair be considered if they have AAA?

Consider elective repair for all fairly fit men with AAA ≥ 5.5 cm.

When should an elective repair be considered for women with AAA and what should be taken into account in these cases?

Consider elective repair for all suitable women with AAA ≥ 5 cm. Be aware that AAAs are more likely to rupture in women than men.

Should the repair option be considered for patients with small aneurysms who require chemotherapy, radiotherapy, or solid organ transplantation, and how should the decision-making process be approached?

Consider the repair option (and not observation only) in patients with small (4-5.4cm) aneurysms who require chemotherapy, radiotherapy, or solid organ transplantation. A shared decision-making approach regarding treatment options is required.

What is the goal for the timeline to repair a threshold AAA from the time of diagnosis?

Aim to repair a threshold AAA within 8 weeks from diagnosis.

When should patients with AAA be considered for fast-tracking?

Consider fast tracking patients with AAA expanding ≥ 1cm/yr.

Should screening for unknown carotid artery disease be performed prior to AAA repair, and what about performing a prophylactic carotid endarterectomy for asymptomatic patients?

Do not screen for unknown carotid artery disease prior to AAA repair. Only treat the carotid prior to AAA repair if the patient has been symptomatic in the last 6 months.

When should the carotid be treated prior to AAA repair?

Do not routinely perform a prophylactic carotid endarterectomy for asymptomatic patients prior to AAA.

Should AAA repair be offered for patients with limited life expectancy?

Do NOT offer AAA repair for patients with limited (2-3 yrs) life expectancy.

Should the decision to proceed or not be based solely on any one risk assessment tool?

Do NOT base your decision to proceed (or not) on any one risk assessment tool.

What should be used in place of a single risk assessment tool for making decisions about AAA repair, and when can the Vascular Quality Initiative (VQI) perioperative mortality risk score be considered?

Use objective testing and specialist opinion instead. The Vascular Quality Initiative (VQI) perioperative mortality risk score can be considered to inform the patient where appropriate.

Qs ON OPTIMISATION FOR TREATMENT

When is it recommended to refer patients with poor functional capacity or significant risk factors for cardiac workup?

Once the repair is indicated, refer patients with poor functional capacity or significant risk factors for cardiac workup and optimisation.

Do patients with stable coronary artery disease require routine revascularisation?

No. Patients with stable coronary artery disease do not need routine revascularisation.

When should coronary disease be considered for prophylactic preoperative coronary revascularisation?

Unstable coronary disease should be considered for prophylactic preoperative coronary revascularisation.

Should dual antiplatelets be stopped after interventional coronary revascularisation to perform AAA repair?

Do NOT stop dual antiplatelets after interventional coronary revascularisation to perform AAA repair. Either wait for patients to move onto monotherapy, or consider EVAR under dual antiplatelets.

What tests and assessments should be considered prior to surgery?

Consider checking pulmonary function tests (excluding chest X-ray), renal function tests, nutritional assessment (via serum albumin measurements) prior to surgery.

Should patients be started on β blockers prior to AAA repair, and if they are of high importance, when should they be commenced?

Do NOT commence patients on β blockers (if not already been on) prior to AAA repair. If β blockers are considered of high importance (for example, to treat multiple comorbidites), commence well in advance.

When is it advised to start statins, and should monotherapy antiplatelets be stopped prior to surgery?

Commence statins where possible (ideally at least 4 weeks prior). Do NOT stop monotherapy antiplatelets prior to surgery.

Should remote ischaemic preconditioning be offered to people having AAA repair?

Do NOT offer remote ischaemic preconditioning to people having AAA repair.

What should be the hydration procedure if EVAR is performed, and how should Metformin usage be managed if eGFR is <60 mL/min?

Commence overnight hydration for non-dialysis patients with renal insufficiency. Maintain hydration (with normal saline or 5% dextrose/sodium bicarbonate) in the perioperative period if EVAR is performed.
Hold Metformin before using the contrast if eGFR is <60 mL/min (up to 48h if eGFR <45). Restart Metformin 48h postprocedure if renal functions remain relatively stable.

What alternatives should be considered for patients with a history of heparin-induced thrombocytopenia?

Consider using alternative thrombin inhibitor such as bivalirudin or argatroban.

Qs ON ELECTIVE ENDOVASCULAR REPAIR

What should be ensured in all EVAR cases?

Ensure radiation safety all the time.

When should the preservation of a large accessory renal artery be considered?

Consider preserving large accessory renal artery (>3mm) or accessory arteries feeding large proportion of kidney.

Should angioplasty and stenting of symptomatic renal artery stenosis or SMA stenosis be considered on doing EVAR?

Yes. Consider angioplasty and stenting of symptomatic renal artery stenosis or SMA stenosis BEFORE doing EVAR or open repair.

What should be preserved in terms of blood flow to intenral iliac artery during the EVAR or open repair procedure? And how?

Preserve blood flow to at least one internal iliac artey. A branched endograft should be considered to achieve this if need be.

If occlusion of both internal iliacs is necessary, what should be considered in terms of timing?

Consider staging this by at least 1-2 weeks

In which cases should EVAR be considered as the preferred treatment modality, and what factors might render open surgery a less suitable option?

This applies specifically for patients who have abdominal co-pathology (hostile abdomen, horseshoe kidney or a stoma), anaesthetic risks and/or medical comorbidities, or other considerations, specific to and discussed with the person, that may render open surgery a less suitable option.

In most patients with suitable anatomy and reasonable life expectancy, EVAR should be considered as the PREFERRED treatment modality with full patient informed consent.

Qs ON EMERGENCY ENDO-VASCULAR REPAIR

What is the recommended timeframe from arrival to intervention in ruptured AAA?

90min of door-to-intervention.

In what situations should a thoracoabdominal CTA be obtained for patients with suspected ruptured AAA?

Obtain thoracoabdominal CTA for stable and even relatively unstable patients with suspected ruptured AAA.

How should symptomatic non-ruptured AAA be managed in terms of repair timing and patient monitoring?

Do NOT repair symptomatic non-ruptured AAA urgently. If possible, repair under more elective conditions. Consider monitoring those patients in an intensive care unit (ICU) setting with blood products available.

What is the recommended first option for repair in patients with a ruptured abdominal aortic aneurysm and suitable anatomy, and who does this recommendation particularly apply to?

In patients with ruptured abdominal aortic aneurysm and suitable anatomy, endovascular repair is recommended as a first option. This is especially for men over 70 and women of any age. Highly consider open repair for men under 70.

In which patients should permissive hypotension be used?

Use permissive hypotension preferably in conscious patients.

Should a palliative decision be based on age or a scoring system?

Do NOT base a palliative decision on age or a scoring system.

What should be the first choice of anaesthetic for access in EVAR for ruptured AAA?

Where possible, use local anaesthetic as a first choice for access to stabilise the patient (with a balloon) or for performing EVAR.

What should always be considered for stabilising unstable patients undergoing open or EVAR repairs?

Always consider using aortic balloon to stabilise unstable patients undergoing open or EVAR repairs.

In EVAR for ruptured AAA, what type of graft should be considered as a first choice when suitable?

IN EVAR for ruptured AAA , Consider bifurcated graft as a first choice whenever suitable over aorto-uniiliac devices.

How much oversizing might be required in EVAR for ruptured AAA?

An over sizing of around 30% may be required.

When is the use of intraoperative Heparin perhaps optimal, and what kind of VTE prophylaxis should be used?

Use of intraoperative Heparin remains controversial. Heparin use is perhaps optimal when administered after controlling the aneurysm. Similarly, use mechanical VTE prophylaxis untill risk of bleeding reduces.

When should the use of NGT be considered intraoperatively?

Consider using NGT intraoperatively, and only if nausea and distension present postoperatively.

What should be monitored post open and EVAR repair and how should high pressures be acted upon?

Monitor intra-abdominal pressure post open and EVAR repair and act quickly where needed.

What actions should be taken when medical treatment fails and pressure remains high post-surgery, and what should be considered to manage the wound?

Perform decompressive laparotomy where medical treatment fails and pressure remains high (>20mmHg), in case of organ failure or if the pressure is very high (>30mmHg). Consider using vacuum-assisted closure to manage the wound.

What should be done for all AAA-repaired candidates postoperatively regarding atherosclerosis risk factors?

Optimise patient atherosclerosis risk factors for all AAA-repaired candidates.

What is the current average survival post-operation?

The current estimated average survival is 9 years.

How should para-anastomotic aneurysm be treated?

Treat para-anastomotic aneurysm with endovascular (proximal) or open approach.

What immediate action should be taken if there's any kink or occlusion of graft limb?

Check and treat any kink or occlusion of graft limb immediately.

What potential side effect should patients be informed about following open and EVAR surgeries?

Inform patients of possible sexual dysfunction following EVAR (17% when covering one internal iliac artery, and 24% when covering both).

What should be considered for patients following successful deployment of EVAR regarding surveillance?

Consider surveillance programme for patients following successful deployment of EVAR, based on their individual risk for EVAR-related complications.

What should be used for surveillance, and what kind of leaks should not be excluded based solely on duplex?

Consider using CTA or colour duplex ultrasound scan for surveillance, but do not exclude endoleaks based on duplex only.

When should imaging with CTA be considered postoperatively?

Consider imaging (with CTA) in 30 days postoperatively.

What kind of follow-up should be considered for a low risk group, and how are these groups defined?

Low risk group (no endoleak, anatomy within IFU, adequate overlap and seal of ≥10 mm proximal and distal stent graft apposition to arterial wall): consider limited follow up with repeated CT scan in 1 yr or 5 years.

What is the recommended surveillance schedule for an intermediate risk group, and how are these groups defined?

Intermediate risk group (adequate overlap and seal, but presence of Type II endoleak: Consider DUS at 6 or 12 months intervals for 24 months then annually thereafter. Patients with sac shrinkage ≥1 cm (even in the presence of a Type II endoleak) can be regarded as low risk.

How should patients be managed if sac size increases?

If sac increases in size, continue annual surveillance, or (if sac increasing ≥ 1cm per yr) treat as high risk.

What further investigations should be considered for type 5 endoleak?

Consider further investigations for type 5 endoleak, i.e. continued AAA expansion without radiographic evidence of a leak site.

How should high risk groups be managed, particularly regarding types I, III, and kinking?

High risk group (presence of Type I or III endoleak, inadequate overlap or seal < 10 mm).Always consider reintervention for type I, III and kinking. Consider using open repair if endovascular intervention fails (→2).

When should intervention for type II be considered, and what steps should be taken afterwards?

Consider intervention for type II if sac is expanding. Repeat scans as required and re-evaluate.

Qs ON JUXSTARENAL AAA

When should repair be considered in justarenal aneurysms?

Consider repair when the 5.5cm threashold is reached.

What repair methods should be considered?

Consider using open repair or complex endovascular repair based on patient's features and large centre team experience.

What is currently the preferred first method for repair, and what should the patient be aware of regarding this method?

Fenestrated EVAR are currently the prefered first method, where feasible. Ensure the patient is fully aware of the lack of clarity regarding perioperative survival or long-term outcomes, as compared with open surgical repair.

What alternative repair technique could be considered, especially in an emergency setting, and should the same principles be applied for ruptured cases?

Alternatively (especially in emergency setting), consider using parallel graft technique (Chimneys). Apply same principles for ruptured cases.

How extensively should patients be followed up, and what method could be used for this?

Follow up patients more extensively, with annual CTA for example.

Qs ON ILIAC ANEURYSMS

When should common, external, or internal iliac aneurysms be considered for repair?

Consider repairing common, external or internal iliac aneurysms when reaching 3.5cm or above.

What information is known about the risk of rupture for iliac aneurysms based on their size?

They rarely ruptured when <4 cm and most ruptured cases are usually present from size >5cm.

How should patients with iliac aneurysm be entered into a surveillance program based on the diameter of the aneurysm?

Enter patients with iliac aneurysm into surveillance programme. For example, every three years for a diameter 2.0-2.9 cm, and annually for 3.0-3.4 cm.

What repair method should be considered as a first option for iliac aneurysms?

Consider endovascular repair as a first option, where possible.

What is the recommendation regarding the preservation of at least one internal iliac artery in open or endovascular repair?

Always strive to keep at least one internal iliac artery in open or endovascular repair, or at least preserve the distal collateral circulation to pelvis.

How should patients be followed up after repair of iliac aneurysms?

Follow up patients using the same AAA follow up principles

Qs ON MYCOTIC ANEU-RYSMS

What causes the formation of mycotic aneurysms?

By definition, mycotic aneurysms (or primary infected aortic aneurysms) result from septic emboli to the aortic vasa vasorum, by haematogenous spread or by direct extension, leading to an infectious degeneration of the arterial wall and aneurysm formation.

How should the diagnosis of mycotic aneurysms be approached?

Diagnosis should combine clinical, laboratory, and imaging parameters.

What antibiotics should be started for the treatment of mycotic aneurysms, and for how long should they be continued?

Start IV antibiotics against Staph aureous and G-ve rods. Consider continuing antibiotics for 6-12 months.

Should the repair of mycotic aneurysms be considered regardless of the size of the aneurysm?

Repair of the aneurysm should be considered regardless of the size.

What methods of repair are acceptable for mycotic aneurysms?

Use EVAR or open surgery as appropriate, both are acceptable.

Qs ON INFLAMMATORY ANEURYSMS

How is an inflammatory Abdominal Aortic Aneurysm (AAA) defined?

By definition, inflammatory AAA is the unusually thickened aneurysm wall, associated with shiny white peri-aneurysmal and retroperitoneal fibrosis, and dense adhesions of adjacent intra-abdominal structures.

What is the suspected aetiology of inflammatory AAA?

Aetiology remains widely unknown. Autoimmunity is likely to be involved.

What can be the implications for adjacent organs and other parts of the aorta in the context of an inflammatory AAA?

Adjacent organs might be entrapped. Other parts of the aorta may also be involved.

Are acute phase reactants such as ESR and CRP reliable for managing and monitoring an inflammatory AAA?

Acute phase reactants (ESR, CRP) alone are not reliable for management and follow up.

What anti-inflammatory medications should be considered in the treatment of an inflammatory AAA?

Consider using anti-inflammatory medications. These include corticosteroids, immunosuppressive agents (azathioprine and methotrexate), and tamoxifen.

When should surgical repair be considered for an inflammatory AAA and what method should be used?

Consider surgical repair using same criteria as elective AAA: 5.5cm diameter, with suitable anatomy, use EVAR where possible.

When should a retroperitoneal approach be considered for the repair of an inflammatory aneurysm?

Consider using a retroperitoneal approach for open inflammatory aneurysm repair, a horseshoe kidney, or an aortic aneurysm in the presence of a hostile abdomen.

Qs ON ACUTE AORTIC SYNDROME

What conditions are included in the acute aortic syndrome?

Acute aortic syndrome includes aortic ulcer, pseudoaneurysm, intramural haematoma, local dissection, and saccular aneurysm.

What should be optimized in all cases of acute aortic syndrome?

Optimise medical management, including blood pressure, in all acute aortic syndrome cases.

What should be done for uncomplicated aortic ulcers, intramural haematoma, and local dissection within acute aortic syndrome?

Apply serial imaging surveillance for uncomplicated aortic ulcers, intramural haematoma, and local dissection.

When is a repair indicated in the case of acute aortic syndrome?

Once symptomatic or complicated, a repair is indicated.

What approach should be considered for the repair in cases of acute aortic syndrome?

Consider endovascular approaches where possible.

What should be considered for saccular Abdominal Aortic Aneurysm (AAA)?

Consider early intervention for saccular AAA.

Qs ON MANAGING CONCOMITTENT MALIGNANCY

What should be the approach towards managing an Abdominal Aortic Aneurysm (AAA) when it is below the threshold in patients with concomitant malignancy?

Do not repair AAA prophylactically when below threshold.

What is the recommended approach in managing a large or symptomatic AAA with concomitant malignancy?

A staged repair, starting with EVAR (where possible) to the large or symptomatic AAA, is recommended.

How long should the prophylactic Low Molecular Weight Heparin (LMWH) be considered postoperatively in managing an AAA with concomitant malignancy?

Consider prolonged (up to 4 weeks) prophylactic LMWH postoperatively (IIa).

CHRONIC LIMB ISCHAEMIA

Qs ON PREVENTION

Who should be screened routinely for Peripheral Artery Disease (PAD)?

Do NOT screen routinely for PAD in the absence of risk factors or symptoms. However, certain patients such as those >70, diabetics, or smokers can be considered for screening for PAD.

When is single antiplatelet therapy (SAPT) recommended?

Consider single antiplatelet therapy (SAPT) for:
All symptomatic PADs
All patients who have had revascularisation

Which antiplatelet is preferred for SAPT?

Preferably use clopidogrel rather than Aspirin

When should dual antiplatelet therapy (DAPT) be considered?

Consider dual antiplatelet therapy (DAPT) for:
Infra-inguinal stenting- use for min of 1 month
Below knee bypasses using prosthetic graft

Should antiplatelet therapy be used routinely for asymptomatic, incidental, isolated disease without any other clinical cardiovascular condition requiring antiplatelet therapy?

Do NOT routinely use antiplatelet therapy for asymptomatic, incidental, isolated disease (without any other clinical cardiovascular condition requiring antiplatelet therapy).

When should oral anticoagulation (OAC) be considered in addition to SAPT?

Consider oral anticoagulation (OAC) :
In addition to SAPT (for at least 1 month)- in endovascular revascularisation cases, where the risk of thrombosis is considered high, and the risk of bleeding is considered acceptable. Do not add SAPT if the bleeding risk is high.

In patients with PAD and AF, under what circumstances should OACs be used?

In patients with PAD and AF- where other risk factors indicate the use of OACs (such as congestive heart failure, Diabetes mellitus, Stroke or TIA, etc.).

In patients already on OAC for another indication, should antiplatelets be added?

In patients already on OAC for another indication (AF, etc.), do NOT add antiplatelets.

In patients already on OAC for another indication, but with a clear indication for SAPT, what is the recommendation for long-term use?

In patients already on OAC for another indication (AF, etc.), but with clear indication for SAPT, use both for long term

Qs ON MEDICAL TREAT-MENT

What is the recommendation on exercise for patients with peripheral artery disease (PAD)?

Exercise- supervised exercise training is highly recommended. Non-supervised training is also recommended where supervision is not possible.

What are the observed benefits of exercise on PAD patients?

Exercise can improve maximal walking distance by 5 min, and pain-free and maximal walking distance by 82 and 109 m, respectively. Improvements have been observed for up to 2 years. Exercise also improves QOL as well.

How long should exercise programs typically last for PAD patients?

Most studies use programmes of at least 3 months, with a minimum of 3 h/week, with walking to the maximal or submaximal distance.

What is the role of statins in the treatment of PAD?

On top of general prevention, statins are indicated to improve walking distance.

What are the effects of most studied drugs such as cilostazol, naftidrofuryl, pentoxifylline, buflomedil, carnitine and propionyl-L-carnitine in treating PAD?

The beneficial effects of most studied drugs (cilostazol, naftidrofuryl, pentoxifylline, buflomedil, carnitine and propionyl-L-carnitine), if any, are generally mild to moderate, with large variability.

What could be the recommended course of treatment with drugs like Cilastozol or pentoxifylline?

A 3-months trial with Cilastozol (100 mg twice daily) or pentoxifylline (400 mg thrice daily) can be recommended.

Qs ON REVASCULARSA-TION

Under what conditions should revascularisation be considered in patients suffering from peripheral artery disease (PAD)?

When daily life activities and quality of life are compromised despite exercise therapy, revascularisation should be considered when there is a reasonable likelihood of symptomatic improvement with treatment.

What are the considerations before opting for revascularisation?

Revascularisation options have limited durability and may be associated with mortality and morbidity. Hence restricting them to debilitating symptoms that substantially alter daily life activities is advisable.

What is the recommendation on the patient's general condition before considering revascularisation?

The general condition of the patient should be evaluated. Revascularisation should only be considerd for reasonably fit patients.

Under what circumstances should short (<5cm) lesions or long occlusive lesions in high-risk patients be considered for treatment?

In aorto-iliac occlusive disease: Short (<5cm) lesions, or long occlusive lesions in high risk patients, should be considered for `endovascular-first` strategy.

When should primary stenting be considered in the treatment of occlusive lesions?

Primary (or selective) stenting should be always considered in treating occlusive (but not stenotic lesions.

What type of stents should be considered for occlusive disease and for severely calcified or aneurysmal disease?

Consider bare metal stents for occlusive disease, and covered stents for severely calcified or aneurysmal disease.

When should long occlusive aorto-iliac lesions in fit and young patients be considered for an 'open surgery first' strategy?

Long occlusive aorto-iliac lesions in fit and young patients should be considered for `open surgery first` strategy. A full discussion and shared decision with the patient are recommended.

What is recommended when dealing with occlusive aorto-iliac lesions extending to the common femoral artery (CFA) in fit patients?

Occlusive aorto-iliac lesions extending to CFA, in fit patients, should be considered for a hybrid approach first.

Under what circumstances should an extra-anatomical bypass be considered?

Consider extra-anatomical bypass where no other alternatives exist.

When can an endovascular approach be considered for occlusive aorto-iliac disease?

Where experience exists, and the procedure does not compromise future options, an endovascular approach can be considered for occlusive aorti-iliac disease.

When should short (<25cm) lesions or long occlusive lesions in high-risk patients or those lacking veins, not involving the origin of the superficial femoral artery (SAF), be considered for an 'endovascular-first' strategy in femoro-popliteal occlusive disease?

Femoro-popliteal occlusive disease: Short (<25cm) lesions, or long occlusive lesions in high risk patients or lack of veins, not involving the origin of SAF should be considered for `endovascular-first` strategy.

When should primary (selective) stenting be considered for short lesions in femoro-popliteal occlusive disease?

Consider primary (selective) stenting for short lesions with unsatisfactory technical results. Drug eluting balloons or stents may be considered.

Under what conditions may drug-eluting balloons or stents be considered?

Consider drug-eluting balloons for the treatment of in-stent restenosis

When should long occlusive lesions in fit patients with a life expectancy of more than 2 years be considered for an 'open/bypass surgery first' strategy?

Long occlusive lesions in fit patients with life expectancy >2yrs, should be considered for `open/bypass surgery first` strategy , where an autologous vein is available.

What should be considered if a suitable vein is not available for open/bypass surgery?

Consider prosthetic conduit where a suitable vein is not available.

When using an endovascular approach, what should be considered to improve patency?

Where endovascular approach is used, consider using self-expanding nitinol stents to improve patency.

When should a hybrid approach be considered first for common femoral artery (CFA) disease?

CFA disease should be considered for a hybrid approach first (open endarterectomy and angioplasty of SFA/POP)

Qs ON FOLLOW UP

What is the 5-year cumulative cardio-vascular-related morbidity of patients with intermittent claudication (IC) compared to a reference-control population?

Most patients with IC present increased 5-year cumulative CV-related morbidity of 13% vs. 5% in reference to control population.

What is the limb risk for patients with IC at 5 years, and what percentage of these patients have amputations?

Regarding the limb risk, at 5 years, 21% progress to CLTI, of whom 4-27% have amputations.

How often should patients with IC be followed up?

Consider following up patients with IC on annual basis, althogh most centres stopped doing so.

Why is annual follow up important for patients with IC?

This allows for proper assessment of compliance with lifestyle measures (e.g. smoking cessation, exercise) and medical therapies. This also aids in determining whether there is evidence of progression in symptoms or signs of PAD.

What should a follow-up program for patients with IC consist of?

A follow up programme should consist of clinical history and examination (including ABI), checking compliance with medical therapy, and record of subjective functional improvements.

When is duplex scan surveillance recommended in patients with IC?

Duplex scan surveillance is recommended where a vein bypass was used. Lesions detected in duplex should be treated with an endovascular or open approach.

CRITICAL LIMB ISCHAEMIA

Qs ON DEFINITIONS

How is Critical Limb Ischaemia (CLI) defined?

CLI (outdated)- The presence of: Ischaemic rest pain with an ankle pressure (AP) <40 mm Hg; or tissue necrosis (ulcer or gangrene) with an AP <60 mm Hg

How is Chronic Limb-Threatening Ischaemia (CLTI) defined?

CLTI (Preferable)- the presence of: ischaemic rest pain, ulcers, gangrene, or infection requiring amputation.

What qualifies as ischaemic rest pain in the context of CLTI?

Ischaemic rest pain with inadequate perfusion (measured using haemodynamic tests) sufficient enough to cause pain, to impair wound healing, and to increase amputation risk.

How is an ischaemic ulcer graded?

Ischaemic ulcer, graded 0-3, based on depth, location, size and magnitude of ablative/wound coverage procedure required to achieve healing.

How is ischaemic gangrene graded?

Ischaemic gangrene- graded 0-3, based on depth, location, size and magnitude of ablative/wound coverage procedure required to achieve healing.

What does the term "regional ischaemia" refer to?

Regional ischaemia- of any type (grade 0-3). Relatively normal hemodynamics when the limb or foot is considered as a whole but, nevertheless, suffers ulceration (or gangrene) as a result of diminished local perfusion (i.e. angiosomal or regional ischemia without adequate collateral flow), which can threaten the limb.

When does an infection require amputation in spite of adequate perfusion?

Infection- which is severe enough (grade 0-3) to require amputation despite apparent adequate perfusion.

What does the term "EBR" stand for and how should it be implemented for optimal management?

EBR- Evidence-based revascularisation. For optimal management, all plans should include three independent axes: Patient risk, Limb severity, and ANatomic complexity (PLAN).

How are average-risk and high-risk patients defined?

Average-risk and high-risk patients are defined by the estimated procedural and 2-year all-cause mortality.

How is limb severity defined?

Limb severity- as defined by WiFI classification system (see below)

What is the ANatomic complexity and how is it defined?

ANatomic complexity- as defined by the GLASS system and the preferred target artery path (TAP), which would then allow for estimating limb-based patency (LBP).

Qs ON PREVENTION

What are the recommended medications for all CLTI patients unless clearly contra-indicated?

All CLTI patients should be on antiplatelets (unless clearly contra-indicated). Clopidogrel, or Aspirin with low dose Rivaroxaban (2.5 mg bd) is recommended. Do not use warfarin for treating CLTI.
All CLTI patients should be on moderate- or high-intensity statin therapy (unless clearly contra-indicated)

What is the recommended systolic and diastolic blood pressure control for all CLTI patients?

All CLTI patients should have their systolic (<140) and diastolic (<90) blood pressure controlled.

What is the recommended diabetes control level for all CLTI patients?

All CLTI patients should have their diabetes well controlled, with HbA1c <7%.

What lifestyle improvements should be implemented for all CLTI patients?

All CLTI patients should have their life style improved, including stopping smoking cessation, implementing a healthy diet (low-fat or Mediterranean type), weight control and exercise.

How should pain be managed in preparation for revascularisation in all CLTI patients? What types of pain relievers are suitable?

All CLTI patients should have their pain managed well in preparation for revascularisation. Paracetamol +- Opioid are suitable.

Qs ON ASSESSMENT AND DIAGNOSIS

What assessment is essential to perform in all patients with CLTI, in addition to the peripheral arterial disease assessment?

A complete cardiovascular physical assessment is essential in all patients with CLTI

What are the recommended clinical tests for all patients with CLTI?

Perform neuropathy test and a probe-to-bone test on all CLTI pts

What measurements should be taken in all patients with suspected CLTI, and what should be the next steps if these measurements are abnormal?

Measure ABI, AP and doppler wave form in all patients with suspected CLTI; If abnormal, proceed to TP and TBI especially in patients with tissue loss

When should DUS be considered as a first-line diagnostic approach in CLTI patients?

Consider obtaining DUS as a first line if the patient is a candidate for revascularisation

When should CTA/MRA be used in patients with CLTI?

Use CTA/MRA if invasive angiography become required

What are the recommended clinical severity and anatomical staging methods for all patients with CLTI?

Perform appropriate clinical severity staging in all CLTI patients:
Use a suitable lower extremity threatened limb classification staging system (e.g. SVS's WIfI classification system- Wound, Ischemia, and foot Infection (WIfI)) in all CLTI patients.

Can you explain the WIfI classification system used in CLTI patients?

Wound (W)-
0: No ulcer. No gangrene
1: Small shallow ulcer. No bone exposed. No gangrene
2: Deeper ulcer with exposed bone or tendon or shallow heel ulcer. Digital gangrene
3: Extensive ulcer involving forefoot or midfoot or full thickness heel. Extensive gangrene
Ischaemia (I)-
0: ABI ≥0.80. AP ≥100. TP/TcPO2 ≥60
1: ABI ≥0.60. AP ≥70. TP/TcPO2 ≥40
2: ABI ≥0.40. AP ≥50. TP/TcPO2 ≥30
3: ABI <0.40. AP <50. TP/TcPO2 <30
Foot Infection (fI)-
0: No clinical infection
1: Localised infection. Localised signs. erythema <2cm around ulcer.
2: Regional infection. Erythema > 2cm. Infection involving deep structures such as bone or fasciitis.
3: Systematic infection.

How is the Global Limb Anatomic Staging System (GLASS) used for anatomical staging in CLTI patients?

Aorto-iliac (inflow) disease staging:
AI 1: Any of: stenosis in infrarenal aorta; occlusion of CIA only; occlusion of EIA only; or stenosis of CIA and/or EIA.
AI 2: Aortic chronic occlusion; CIA+EIA total occlusion; severe diffuse disease/small-caliber (<6 mm) in CIA+EIA; severe diffuse in-stent restenosis in aorto and iliac system; concomitant aneurysm disease.
A: no significant CFA disease.
B: significant (>50% stenosis) CFA disease.

Femoropopliteal (FP) disease grading:
FP 0: Mild or no significant disease.
FP 1: SFA disease < 1/3 of total length (<10cm); or focal single occlusion (<5cm)- POPLITEAL: normal or mildly diseased.
FP 2: SFA disease < 2/3 of total length (<20cm); or SFA occlusion <1/3 (<10cm- not flush occlusion); POPLITEAL: focal stenosis (<2cm- not in trifurcation).
FP 3: SFA disease > 2/3 of total length (>20cm); or non-flush occlusion (<20cm- or flush occlusion 10-20cm); POPLITEAL: short occlusion (<5cm- not in trifurcation).
FP 4: SFA occlusion - total length (>20cm); POPLITEAL: any occlusion; or disease > 5cm or involving trifurcation

Infrapopliteal (IP) disease grade:
IP 0: Mild or no significant disease in the primary target tibial artery (TTA) path.
IP 1: Focal stenosis of TTA < 3cm.
IP 2: TTA stenosis <1/3 of total length; or TTA occlusion <3 cm. Not including TTA origin or TP trunk .
IP 3: TTA stenosis <2/3 of total length; or TTA occlusion up to 1/3. May include TTA origin but not TP trunk.
IP 4: TTA stenosis >2/3 of total length; or TTA occlusion >1/3. May include TTA origin. any occlusion of TP trunk (unless AT is the TTA).

Pedal (infra-malleolar) disease grade:
P 0: TTA crosses ankle into foot, with intact pedal arch.
P 1: TAA crosses ankle into foot; absent or severely diseased pedal arch
P 2: No TTA crossing ankle into foot

What is the definition of severe calcification and how does it affect the segment grade?

Severe calcification is defined as calcification >50% of circumference; diffuse, bulky, or coral reef plaques likely within the FP and IP segments of the target artery path (TAP).
If present, increase the segment grade by one.

How is the Global Limb Anatomic Staging System (GLASS) stage estimated?

Estimate the Global Limb Anatomic Staging System (GLASS) stage:
Stage 0: FP: 0 & IP: 0
Stage 1: FP: 0 & IP <3 or IP: 0 & FP <3 or IP:1 & FP:1
Stage 2: everything else
Stage 3: FP or IP of grade 4; or FP 3 & IP 3

Qs ON DECISION MAKING

What is necessary to do to all CLTI patients prior to making treatment decisions?

Ensure all CLTI patients are discussed by a vascular multidisciplinary team

How are 'average' and 'high' surgical risks defined in terms of anticipated mortality and estimated 2-year survival?

An anticipated mortality of < 5% and an estimated 2-year survival of >50% defines an `average` surgical risk. Any higher mortality or lower 2-yr survival defines a `high` surgical risk .

What should be combined to obtain an estimated patient's risk?

Combine patient's risk, clinical severity (WIfI), and anatomic complexity (GLASS) to formulate an intergrated PLAN (Patient risk estimation, Limb staging, ANatomic pattern of disease)

What treatment options should be offered to patients with limited life expectancy, poor functional status, or an unsalvageable limb?

Patients with limited life expectancy, poor functional status, or an unsalvageable limb should be offered a palliation or primary amputation after joint discussion and decision making.

What should the treatment approach be for a patient presenting with a deep space foot infection or wet gangrene?

Perform urgent surgical drainage, debridement, and/or minor amputation. Commence antibiotic. Consider correcting inflow disease (if likely to be urgently essential).

When should the staging be repeated?

Repeat staging before next major treatment decision.

What should be the treatment approach for a patient presenting with mild limb critical disease (WIfI stage 1) and mild ischaemic grade (WIfI ischaemia grade 0 or 1)?

Mild limb disease (WIfI stage 1) + mild ischaemic grade (WIfI ischaemia grade 0 or 1): do NOT offer revascularisation. Optimise BMT first. If the wound fails to reduce in size by ≥50% within 4 weeks despite appropriate care, consider revascularisation. Consider improving circulation to an isolated ischaemic area if required.

What is the recommended treatment for intermediate or advanced limb disease (WIfl stage ≥1) coupled with moderate ischaemic grade (WIfl ischaemia grade 1-2)?

Intermediate or advanced limb disease (WIfl stage ≥1) + moderate ischaemic grade (WIfl ischaemia grade 1-2): Consider revascularisation where possible.

What should be the treatment approach for advanced limb disease (WIfl stage ≥2) and moderate or severe ischaemic grade (WIfl ischaemia grade ≥1)?

Advanced limb disease (WIfl stage ≥2) + moderate or severe ischaemic grade (WIfl ischaemia grade ≥1): Consider revascularisation where possible

What is the suggested treatment for advanced limb disease (WIfl stage ≥2) and severe ischaemic grade (WIfl ischaemia grade ≥1)?

Advanced limb disease (WIfl stage ≥2) + severe ischaemic grade (WIfl ischaemia grade ≥1): Consider revascularisation where possible

Qs ON TREATMENT

What is the recommendation regarding inflow treatment?

Always correct the inflow first

In which patient cases should the inflow be corrected only without outflow correction?

Correct inflow ONLY without outflow correction (where both exist) for patients with:
Low-grade ischemia grade.
Limited tissue loss.
Risk-benefit of additional outflow reconstruction is high or initially unclear
Re-stage the level of ischaemia AFTER correcting the inflow

What is the recommended approach for treating moderate to severe Aortoiliac (AI) disease?

use endovascular-first approach

When should open surgical reconstruction be used for AI disease?

Use open surgical reconstruction for failed endovascular, extensive AI disease in an average risk patient

What is the suggested approach for treating hemodynamically significant (>50% stenosis) disease of the common and deep femoral arteries?

Use open CFA endarterectomy with patch, with or without extension into the PFA, in patients with hemodynamically significant (>50% stenosis) disease of the common and deep femoral arteries.

How should AI disease be treated along with open CFA endarterectomy?

Use open CFA endarterectomy and endovascular treatment to AI disease where needed.

What is the recommendation regarding the correction of hemodynamically significant (>50% stenosis) PFA proximal disease?

Correct hemodynamically significant (>50% stenosis) PFA proximal disease where possible.

What treatment is considered for very high-risk patients/hostile groin?	consider angioplasty of CFA (but not stent)
What is the recommended treatment for average-risk patients with mild disease severity (WIfI stage 1)?	In average-risk patients with suitable autologous vein: revascularisation (endo or open) is rarely required regardless of anatomical complexity.
What treatment options should be considered for average-risk patients with advanced disease severity (WIfI 2,3,4)?	Advanced disease severity (WIfI 2,3,4)- preferably offer endovascular for low anatomical complexity cases (Stage 1 +- 2), and open surgery preferably for high anatomical complexity cases (stage 3).
What are the considerations for high-risk patients with intermediate disease severity (WIfI stage 2 or 3) and mild ischaemic derangement (WIfI ischaemic grade 1)?	consider endovascular revascularisation if wound fails to reduce in size within 4 weeks despite appropriate infection control, wound care, and offloading
How should high-risk patients with intermediate disease severity (WIfI stage 2) and significant ischaemic derangement (WIfI ischaemic grade 2 & 3) be treated?	consider endovascular revascularisation if at all possible
What is the recommended treatment for high-risk patients with advanced disease severity (WIfI stage 3 or 4) and moderate ischaemic derangement (WIfI ischaemic grade 1)?	consider endovascular revascularisation if wound fails to reduce in size within 4 weeks despite appropriate infection control, wound care, and offloading
How should high-risk patients with advanced disease severity (WIfI stage 3 or 4) and significant ischaemic derangement (WIfI ischaemic grade 2 & 3) be treated?	consider endovascular revascularisation if at all possible
What treatment is considered for high-risk patients with advanced disease severity (WIfI stage 3 or 4), significant ischaemic derangement (WIfI ischaemic grade 2 & 3), and advanced complex anatomy (Glass III)?	consider open surgery revascularisation primarily or after failed endovascular procedure
When should adjuncts to balloon angioplasty (e.g. stents, covered stents, or drug-eluting technologies) be considered?	Consider adjuncts to balloon angioplasty (e.g. stents, covered stents, or drug-eluting technologies) when there is a technically inadequate result (residual stenosis or flow limiting dissection) or in the setting of advanced lesion complexity (e.g., GLASS FP grade 2-4)

Is the durability and hemodynamic and clinical effectiveness of endovascular interventions in the pedal arch known?

Endovascular interventions in the pedal arch have been used. However, their durability and hemodynamic and clinical effectiveness remain unknown.

Has open bypass surgery been used for treating infra-malleolar disease?

Open bypass surgery has also been successfully employed to tarsal and plantar arteries. However, techniques and outcomes are not established. The impact of IM disease on the success of proximal revascularization, whether open or endovascular, is also unknown.

When should angiosome-guided revascularisation be considered for patients?

Consider angiosome-guided revascularisation in patients with significant wounds (e.g. WIfI wound grades 3 and 4), particularly those involving the midfoot or hindfoot, and when the appropriate TAP is available.

When should spinal cord stimulation be considered for reducing the risk of amputation and decreasing pain?

Consider spinal cord stimulation (see page <?>) to reduce risk of amputation and to decrease pain in carefully selected patients where revascularisation is not suitable.

Should lumbar sympathectomy be used for limb salvage in patients for whom revascularisation is not suitable?

Do not use lumbar sympathectomy (page <?>) for limb salvage in patients for whom revascularisation is not suitable.

When should Intermittent pneumatic compression therapy be considered for patients?

Consider Intermittent pneumatic compression therapy in carefully selected patients for whom revascularisation is not suitable.

Qs ON FOLLOW UP

What should be emphasized for all patients in terms of follow-up and outcome?

Emphasise the importance of best medical therapy for all patients

In the case of infra-inguinal vein bypass, should single antiplatelet therapy, which is standard for long-term PAD management, be continued?

Single antiplatelet therapy, recommended as standard for long-term PAD management, should be continued in these patients.

Under what circumstances can treatment with warfarin be considered for patients with infra-inguinal vein bypasses?

Treatment with warfarin may be considered in patients with high-risk vein grafts (e.g. spliced vein conduit, or poor runoff) who are not at increased risk for bleeding.

For how long should regular follow-ups be considered for patients who have had infra-inguinal vein bypasses?

Consider regular follow up for at least 2 years with a clinical surveillance program consisting of interval history, pulse examination, and measurement of resting APs and TPs. Consider DUS scanning where available.

In which situations should intervention for DUS-detected vein graft lesions be considered?

Consider intervention for DUS-detected vein graft lesions with PSV of >300 cm/s, PSV ratio >3.5 or grafts with significant low velocity (midgraft PSV <45 cm/s).

Why should long-term surveillance be maintained for patients with infra-inguinal vein bypasses?

Maintain long term surveillance to detect any recurrent in new lesions.

For infra-inguinal prosthetic bypasses, when should DAPT be considered?

Consider DAPT (aspirin plus clopidogrel) for 6-24 months.

How often should regular follow-ups occur for patients with infra-inguinal prosthetic bypasses, and what should these follow-ups involve?

Consider regular follow up for at least 2 years with interval history, pulse examination, and measurement of resting APs and TPs.

After infrainguinal endovascular interventions, when should DAPT be considered?

Consider DAPT for 12 months

What should follow-up in a surveillance program include for patients who have had infrainguinal endovascular interventions?

Consider follow up in a surveillance program that includes clinical visits, pulse examination, and noninvasive testing (resting APs and TPs).

After repeated catheter-based interventions, for how long should DAPT be considered?

For repeated catheter-based interventions-consider DAPT for 1-6 months.

When should reintervention be considered for patients with DUS-detected restenosis lesions after infrainguinal endovascular interventions?

Consider reintervention for patients with DUS-detected restenosis lesions >70% (PSV ratio >3.5, PSV >300 cm/s) especially where symptoms are unresolved.

ACUTE LIMB ISCHAEMIA

Qs ON ASSESSMENT

Should active revascularisation be considered in selected patients with cancer, and how does the immediate outcome compare to non-cancer patients?

Consider active revascularisation in selected patients with cancer; the immediate outcome is comparable to non-cancer patients.

What classification should be used when evaluating Acute Limb Ischaemia (ALI)?

Use Rutherford classification (viable, marginally threatened, immediately threatened, non-viable) when evaluating ALI.

How essential is diagnostic imaging in the treatment of ALI and under what conditions should it be used?

Diagnostic imaging is always essential, providing this does not delay treatment significantly, and a primary amputation is not clearly indicated

What imaging method should be considered as a first line imaging for ALI?

Consider using CTA as a first line imaging.

Should myoglobin or CK assessment be used to decide on what surgical option is available for ALI patients?

Do NOT use myoglobin or CK assessment to decide on what surgical option is available (revascularisation, primary amputation, etc.).

When should the source of embolism be investigated if present?

Investigate the source of embolism, if present, after revascularisation has taken place.

Qs ON TREATMENT

When should Heparin be started for patients with Acute Limb Ischaemia (ALI), and under what conditions it should not be administered?

Start Heparin immediately (if not contraindicated and a spinal anaesthesia is not planned) and administer oxygen.

What should be administered along with oxygen for patients with ALI?

Control the pain adequately.

When should prostacyclin analogues be considered for administration?

Consider starting prostacyclin analogues perioperatively if an open surgery is decided.

Where should patients with ALI be treated?

Treat patients with ALI in appropriate fully equipped hybrid theatre.

If open thrombo-embolectomy is chosen, under what conditions should local or regional anaesthesia be considered?

If open thrombo-embolectomy is chosen: Consider local or regional anaesthesia, but ONLY with anaesthetist involvement.

What is the recommended device for performing an embolectomy under fluoroscopy guidance?

Always consider using over the wire embolectomy catheter under fluoroscopy guidance.

What material is preferred for a bypass graft when indicated?

Use vein graft for a bypass (when indicated) if at all possible [IIa].

When should completion angiography be performed, and what action should be taken if a residual thrombus is found?

Always use completion angiography when done [I]. If a residual thrombus is found, consider using intraoperative local thrombolysis.

What should be done in case of graft occlusion?

For graft occlusion, always correct the mechanical cause of the graft occlusion if at all possible.

When open surgery is conducted, what should be considered for inflow and outflow corrections?

When open surgery is conducted, consider using endovascular options for inflow and outflow corrections.

When should preoperative or intraoperative thrombolysis be considered as an adjuvant?

Consider using preoperative or intraoperative thrombolysis as adjuvant if open surgery did not clear the thrombus burden well enough.

Should thrombolysis be consiodered for very mild ALI (Rutherford class I)?

Do NOT use thrombolysis if ALI is very mild (Rutherford class I).

When should percutaneous catheter-directed thrombolysis be considered as an alternative to surgery?

Always consider percutaneous catheter-directed thrombolysis as an alternative to surgery for Rutherford class IIa.

What else should be cosndered?

Consider using suction thrombectomy or aspiration as an adjuvant.

What agents are preferable to use in this condition?

Use tPA or Urokinase as preferable agents.

Should plasma fibrinogen levels be routinely monitored?

Do not routinely monitor plasma fibrinogen levels.

Should Heparin be continued during thrombolysis?

Do NOT continue using heparin during thrombolysis.

If bleeding occurred, what steps should be taken based on the severity of the bleeding?

If a bleeding occured, continue treatment if minor, and stop if major.

What should be done if ALI is caused by a thrombosed popliteal artery aneurysm and what method should not be used?

If ALI is caused by thrombosed popliteal artery aneurysm, repair the aneurysm, and use vein graft if at all possible. Do NOT use stent grafting.

When should four compartment fasciotomy be used?

Use four compartment fasciotomy if compartment syndrome is evident or suspected clinically, or if the ischaemia was profond or prolonged. Do not use fasciotomy routinely.

Under what conditions should emergency fasciotomy be performed?

Perform emergency fasciotomy within no more than 2 hours of diagnosing compartment syndrome.

Qs ON FOLLOW UP

What type of medication should patients be kept on if the cause of Acute Limb Ischaemia (ALI) was an embolism?

Keep patients on anticoagulation if the cause of ALI was an embolism.

What should be considered for patients with a thrombosed prosthetic graft?

Also consider anticoagulation for thrombosed prosthetic graft.

What medication should always be considered for long-term patients with ALI?

Always consider antiplatelet or anticoagulation + statin for long term patients.

CHAPTER 12
STEP-BY-STEP
CHARTS QUESTIONS &
ANSWERS

ILIAC ANGIOPLASTY - CHART QUESTIONS

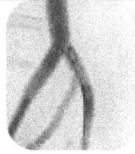

INSERT PIGTAIL & DO FINAL CHECK | **16**

What steps can be taken to ensure that no embolization requiring treatment has occurred?

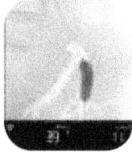

BALLOON THE STENT | **15**

What action should be taken if the stent is not fully molded?

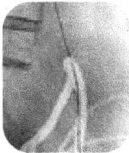

DEPLOY THE STENT | **14**

What action should be taken with the stent at this stage?

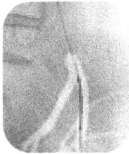

INSERT AND POSITION STENT | **13**

What actions should be taken to check at this stage ?

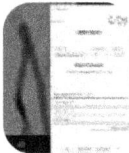

STAGE 4:
Perform Left
CIA Stenting

SELECT APPROPRIATE STENT | **12**

What kind of stent is appropriate to use?

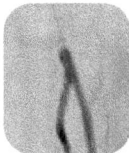

STAGE 3:
Perform Left
CIA Balloon
Angioplasty

DEFLATE THE BALLOON - CHECK | **11**

What should you do at this stage regarding the lesion's treatment and the potential need for repeat balloon angioplasty?

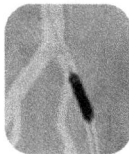

INFLATE THE BALLOON | **10**

How long is a balloon should be left inflated after being inflated to nominal pressure?

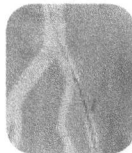

HEPARIN

INSERT APPROPRIATE BALLOON | **09**

What part of the lesion should the balloon cover?

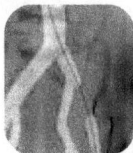

INSERT STIFF WIRE | **08**

What benefits are provided by using a stiff wire?

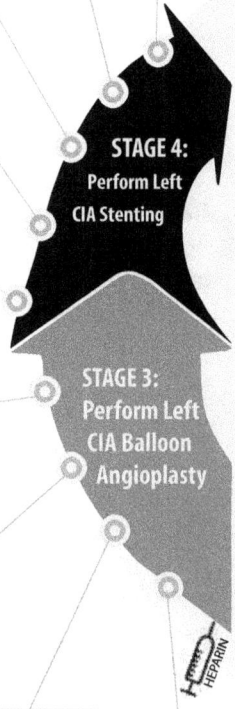

01 | START YOUR CASE

What preparations, including positioning and local anesthesia, are needed before starting a left iliac angioplasty?

02 | INSERT THE GUIDEWIRE

What guidewire is recommended for use, and how is its placement verified using fluoroscopy?

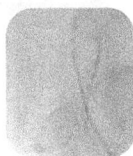

03 | INSERT SHEATH

What sheath size is needed at this stage?

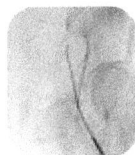

STAGE 1:
Secure access via right groin. Cross the iliac lesion.

HEPARIN

04 | CROSS THE ILIAC LESION

What steps would you take to exchange the J wire for a Glidewire, and what method would you use to cross the lesion?

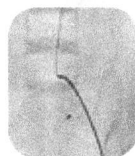

STAGE 2:
Perform angiogram

05 | EXCHANGE COBRA TO PIGTAIL

What is the correct positioning of the pigtail tip, and how should the contrast injector, frame rate, and C-Arm angles be set, specifically with regards to CC and RAO angles?

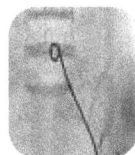

06 | Perform Digital Subtraction Angiography (DSA)

What's the benefit of DSA at this stage?

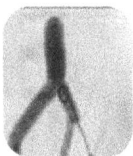

07 | ASSIGN DSA AS A ROADMAP

What advantages does the roadmap provide?

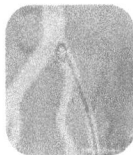

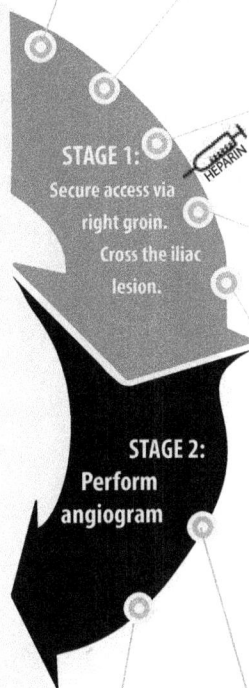

ILIAC ANGIOPLASTY - CHART ANSWERS

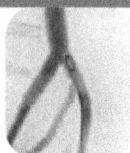

INSERT PIGTAIL & DO FINAL CHECK | **16**

Move further to femoro-popliteal and tibial arteries to ensure no embolisation needing treatment has occurred.

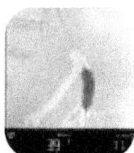

BALLOON THE STENT | **15**

Repeat ballooning if need be, and in more than one side.

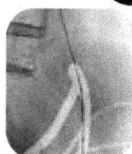

DEPLOY THE STENT | **14**

Self-expanding stents deploys using self-radial force. They are likely to require molding to the artery wall.

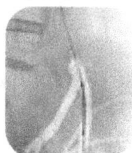

INSERT AND POSITION STENT | **13**

Be careful not to affect the internal iliac artery orifice. The best method to avoid this is by ensuring a correct C-Arm positon.

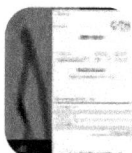

STAGE 4: Perform Left CIA Stenting

SELECT APPROPRIATE STENT | **12**

Select self-expanding stent, suitable in diameter, and length.

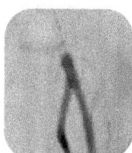

DEFLATE THE BALLOON - CHECK | **11**

Check the lesion is treated well and responded sufficiently. Repeat balloon angioplasty if need be.

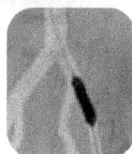

STAGE 3: Perform Left CIA Balloon Angioplasty

INFLATE THE BALLOON | **10**

Balloon is inflated to nominal pressure and is left inflated for 2min.

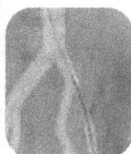

HEPARIN

INSERT APPROPRIATE BALLOON | **09**

Ensure the balloon covers the whole lesion but not the branches (Here the IIA) where possible.

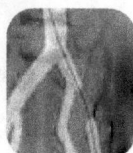

INSERT STIFF WIRE | **08**

This will secure the balloon positioning and then the stent deployment.

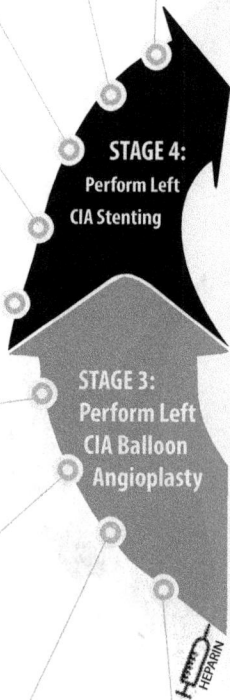

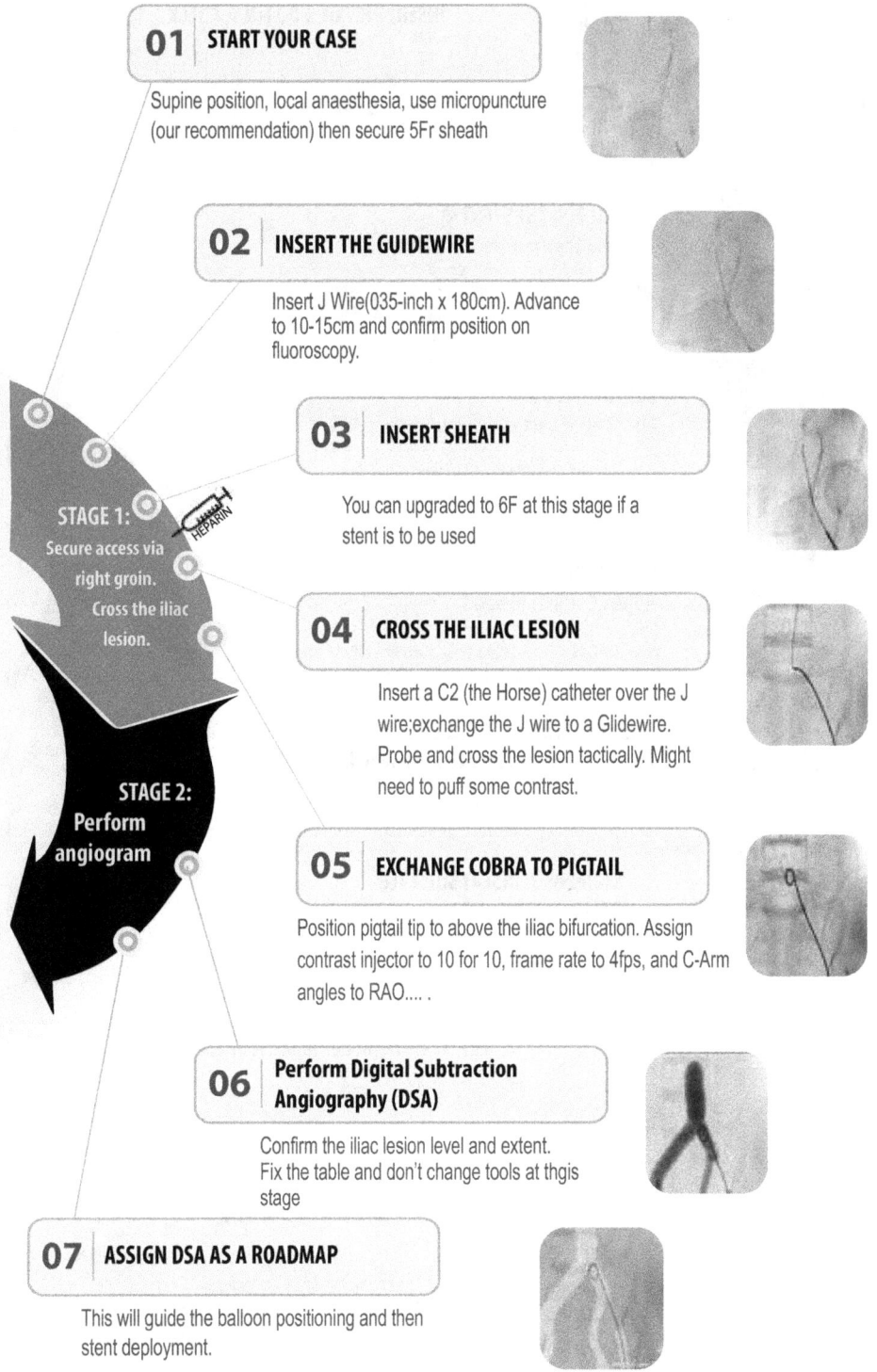

01 | **START YOUR CASE**

Supine position, local anaesthesia, use micropuncture (our recommendation) then secure 5Fr sheath

02 | **INSERT THE GUIDEWIRE**

Insert J Wire(035-inch x 180cm). Advance to 10-15cm and confirm position on fluoroscopy.

03 | **INSERT SHEATH**

You can upgraded to 6F at this stage if a stent is to be used

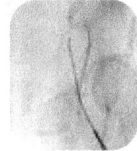

STAGE 1:
Secure access via right groin. Cross the iliac lesion.

HEPARIN

04 | **CROSS THE ILIAC LESION**

Insert a C2 (the Horse) catheter over the J wire;exchange the J wire to a Glidewire. Probe and cross the lesion tactically. Might need to puff some contrast.

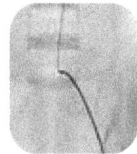

STAGE 2:
Perform angiogram

05 | **EXCHANGE COBRA TO PIGTAIL**

Position pigtail tip to above the iliac bifurcation. Assign contrast injector to 10 for 10, frame rate to 4fps, and C-Arm angles to RAO.... .

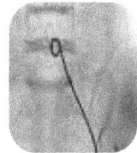

06 | **Perform Digital Subtraction Angiography (DSA)**

Confirm the iliac lesion level and extent. Fix the table and don't change tools at thgis stage

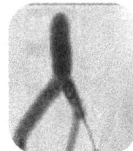

07 | **ASSIGN DSA AS A ROADMAP**

This will guide the balloon positioning and then stent deployment.

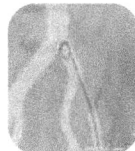

SFA ANGIOPLASTY - CHART QUESTIONS

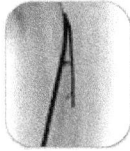

INSERT PIGTAIL & DO FINAL CHECK | **16**

How can you verify that no treatable embolization has taken place?

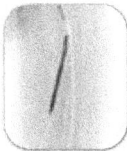

BALLOON THE STENT
Mold the stent to the wall | **15**

If the stent isn't fully molded, what steps should you take?

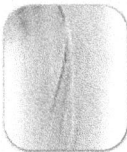

DEPLOY THE STENT
Check each part while deploying | **14**

What steps should be undertaken regarding the stent at this juncture?

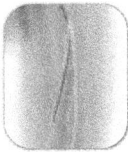

INSERT STENT if needed
Adjust C-Arm if needed | **13**

What kind of stent is appropriate to use? What actions should be taken to check at this stage ?

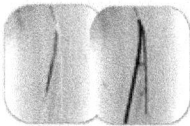

STENOSIS 2: DEFLATE & CHECK.
Check, +/- repeat inflation if needed. | **12**

Check the lesion is treated well and responded sufficiently. Repeat balloon angioplasty if need be.

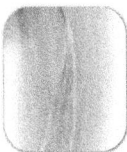

STENOSIS 2: INSERT SUITABLE
BALLOON & INFLATE | **11**

inflate balloon to nominal pressure and leave inflated for 2min.

STENOSIS 1: DEFLATE & CHECK.
Check, +/- repeat inflation if needed. | **10**

At this stage, how should you address the lesion's management and the possibility of requiring a subsequent balloon angioplasty?

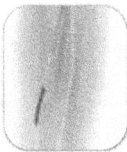

STENOSIS 1: INSERT SUITABLE
BALLOON & INFLATE | **09**

Which segment of the lesion should be encompassed by the balloon? Once inflated, for how long should the balloon remain inflated and at what pressure?

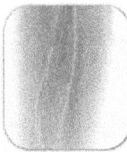

STAGE 4:
Perform Left
CIA Stenting

STAGE 3:
Perform Left
CIA Balloon
Angioplasty

HEPARIN

01 | **START YOUR CASE**

What considerations, including equipment selection and patient assessment, are necessary before performing a left SFA angioplasty?

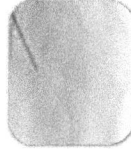

02 | **INSERT THE GUIDEWIRE**

Which guidewire is suitable for the procedure, and how is its position confirmed using fluoroscopy?

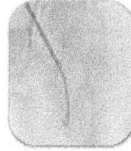

03 | **INSERT SHEATH**

At this phase, what size of sheath is required?

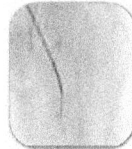

04 | **RUN A DSA**
Femoral and Popliteal arteries

How does DSA add value at the current phase?

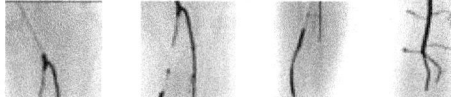

05 | **RUN A DSA**
Tibials, Peroneal and Foot Arteries

What's the benefit of DSA at this stage?

06 | **CROSS THE SFA LESION**

How would you go about replacing the J wire with a Glidewire, and which technique would you employ to traverse the lesion?

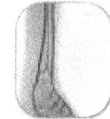

07 | **INSERT STIFF WIRE**
Use 0.018 wire. Take catheter out

What advantages does utilizing a stiff wire offer?

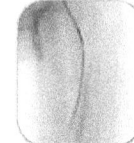

08 | **CENTRE TO LESION. DO DSA & ROADMAP**

What benefits does the roadmap offer?

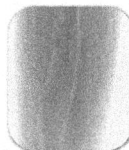

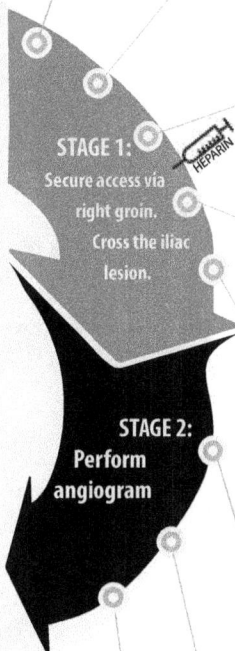

STAGE 1:
Secure access via right groin.
Cross the iliac lesion.

HEPARIN

STAGE 2:
Perform angiogram

SFA ANGIOPLASTY - CHART ANSWERS

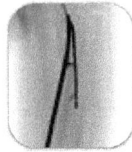

INSERT PIGTAIL & DO FINAL CHECK | **16**

Check femoro-popliteal and tibial arteries to ensure no embolisation needing treatment has occurred.

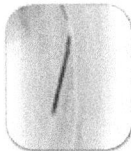

BALLOON THE STENT
Mold the stent to the wall | **15**

Repeat ballooning if need be, and in more than one side.

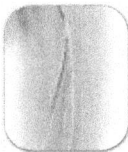

DEPLOY THE STENT
Check each part while deploying | **14**

Self-expanding stents deploys using self-radial force. They are likely to require molding to the artery wall.

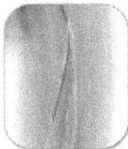

STAGE 4:
Perform Left
CIA Stenting

INSERT STENT if needed
Adjust C-Arm if needed | **13**

Be careful not to affect the profunda artery orifice. The best method to avoid this is by ensuring a correct C-Arm positon.

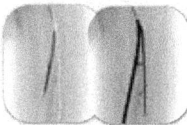

STENOSIS 2: DEFLATE & CHECK.
Check, +/- repeat inflation if needed. | **12**

Check the lesion is treated well and responded sufficiently. Repeat balloon angioplasty if need be.

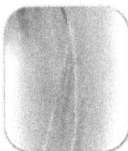

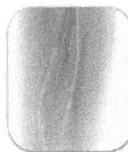

STAGE 3:
Perform Left
CIA Balloon
Angioplasty

STENOSIS 2: INSERT SUITABLE
BALLOON & INFLATE | **11**

inflate balloon to nominal pressure and leave inflated for 2min.

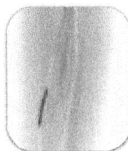

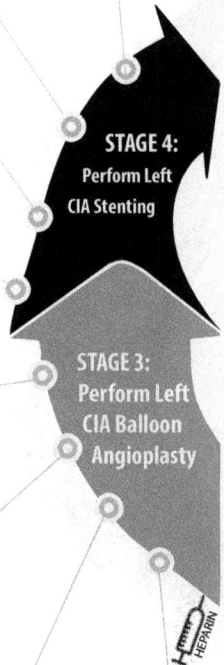

HEPARIN

STENOSIS 1: DEFLATE & CHECK.
Check, +/- repeat inflation if needed. | **10**

Check the lesion is treated well and responded sufficiently. Repeat balloon angioplasty if need be.

STENOSIS 1: INSERT SUITABLE
BALLOON & INFLATE | **09**

inflate balloon to nominal pressure and leave inflated for 2min.

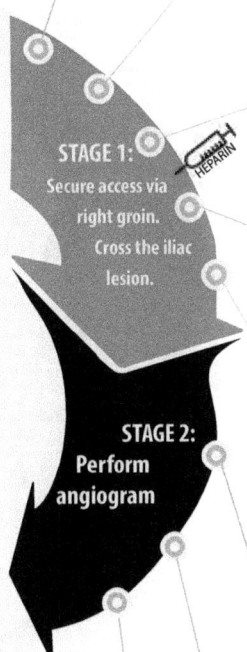

01 | **START YOUR CASE**

Antegrade SFA procedure starts here. Supine position, local anaesthesia, micro-puncture and sheath

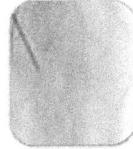

02 | **INSERT THE GUIDEWIRE**

Insert J Wire .035-inch x 180cm. Advance to proximal SFA and confirm position on fluoroscopy.

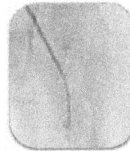

03 | **INSERT SHEATH**

Use 4 or 5Fr sheath. Use 4F sheath if this is for diagnostic angiogram only.

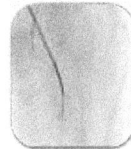

STAGE 1:
Secure access via right groin. Cross the iliac lesion.

HEPARIN

04 | **RUN A DSA**
Femoral and Popliteal arteries

Check and confirm anatomy

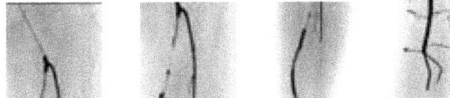

STAGE 2:
Perform angiogram

05 | **RUN A DSA**
Tibials, Peroneal and Foot Arteries

Check and confirm anatomy

06 | **CROSS THE SFA LESION**

Insert a CXI catheter and exchange the J wire to a Glidewire. Probe and cross the lesion tactically. Might need to puff some contrast. Might need to use 0.018 wire.

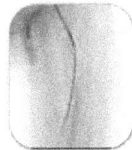

07 | **INSERT STIFF WIRE**
Use 0.018 wire. Take catheter out

Use 0.018 wire. Take catheter out. Check end of wire in lower popliteal artery.

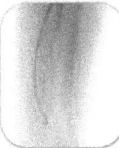

08 | **CENTRE TO LESION. DO DSA & ROADMAP**

Fix position on the lesion and ensure lesion marked. Fix the C-Arm position.

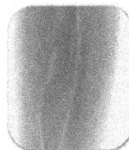

TIBIAL ANGIOPLASTY - CHART QUESTIONS

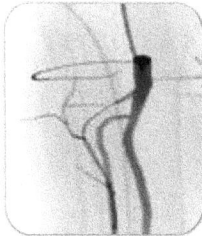

DO FINAL CHECK 11

What measures can be adopted to confirm that there hasn't been any embolization necessitating intervention?

STAGE 4:
Perform Left CIA Stenting

STAGE 3:
Perform Left CIA Balloon Angioplasty

HEPARIN

DEFLATE & CHECK.
Check, +/- repeat inflation if needed. 10

How should you proceed with the lesion's treatment at this stage, and how do you determine the need for another balloon angioplasty?

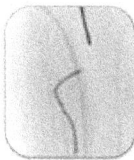

INSERT SUITABLE BALLOON & INFLATE 09

Over which portion of the lesion should the balloon be positioned? After inflation, how long should you maintain the balloon's inflation and at which pressure?

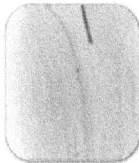

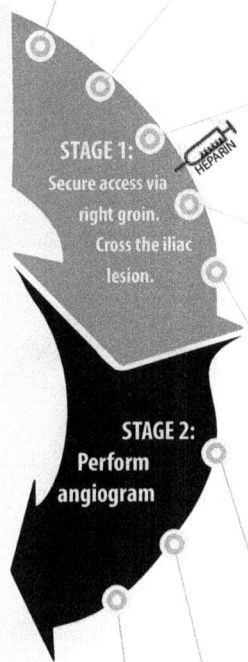

01 | **START YOUR CASE**

Before conducting a right AT angioplasty, which equipment choices and patient evaluations are essential?

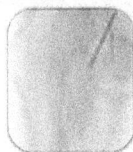

02 | **INSERT THE GUIDEWIRE**

How do you determine the appropriate guidewire for the procedure and verify its placement with fluoroscopy?

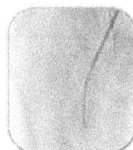

03 | **INSERT SHEATH**

During this stage, which sheath size is necessary?

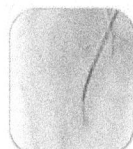

04 | **RUN A DSA**
Femoral and Popliteal arteries

How does DSA enhance the process during this phase?

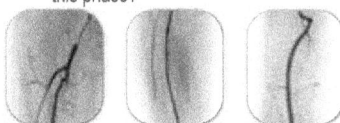

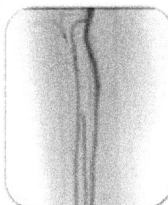

STAGE 1:
Secure access via right groin. Cross the iliac lesion.

HEPARIN

STAGE 2:
Perform angiogram

05 | **RUN A DSA**
Tibials, Peroneal and Foot Arteries

How does DSA enhance the process during this phase?

06 | **CROSS THE AT LESION**

What procedure would you follow to swap the J wire for a Glidewire, and what approach would you adopt to navigate through the lesion?

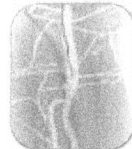

07 | **INSERT STIFF WIRE**
Use 0.018 wire. Take catheter out

What are the advantages of using a 0.018 stiff wire?

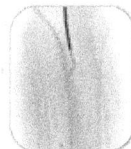

08 | **CENTRE TO LESION. DO DSA &**
ROADMAP

How does the roadmap enhance the procedure?

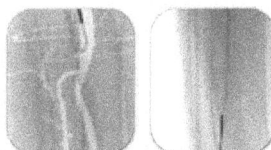

TIBIAL Angioplasty - CHART ANSWERS

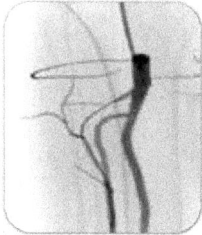

DO FINAL CHECK | **11**

Check femoro-popliteal and tibial arteries to
ensure no embolisation needing treatment has
occurred.

STAGE 4:
Perform Left
CIA Stenting

STAGE 3:
Perform Left
CIA Balloon
Angioplasty

HEPARIN

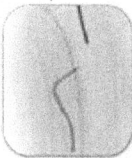

DEFLATE & CHECK.
Check, +/- repeat inflation if needed. | **10**

Check the lesion is treated well and responded
sufficiently. Repeat balloon angioplasty if need be.

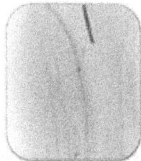

INSERT SUITABLE BALLOON & INFLATE | **09**

inflate balloon to nominal pressure and leave
inflated for 2min.

01 START YOUR CASE

Antegrade SFA procedure starts here. Supine position, local anaesthesia, micro-puncture and sheath

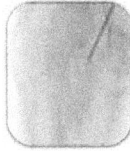

02 INSERT THE GUIDEWIRE

Insert J Wire .035-inch x 180cm. Advance to proximal SFA and confirm position on fluoroscopy.

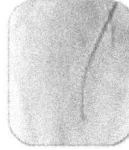

03 INSERT SHEATH

Use 4 or 5Fr sheath. Use 4F sheath if this is for diagnostic angiogram only.

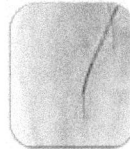

STAGE 1:
Secure access via right groin. Cross the iliac lesion.

HEPARIN

04 RUN A DSA
Femoral and Popliteal arteries

Check and confirm anatomy

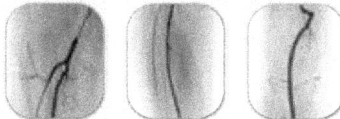

STAGE 2:
Perform angiogram

05 RUN A DSA
Tibials, Peroneal and Foot Arteries

Check and confirm anatomy

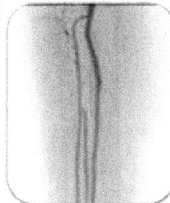

06 CROSS THE AT LESION

Insert a CXI catheter and exchange the J wire to a Glidewire, 0.018 or 0.014.
Probe and cross the lesion tactically. Might need to puff some contrast.

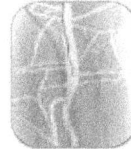

07 INSERT STIFF WIRE
Use 0.018 wire. Take catheter out

Use 0.018 wire. Take catheter out. Check end of wire in lower popliteal artery.

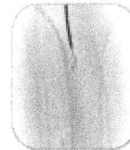

08 CENTRE TO LESION. DO DSA &
ROADMAP

Fix position on the lesion and ensure lesion marked. Fix the C-Arm position.

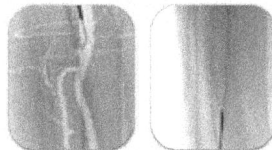

RENAL Angioplasty - CHART QUESTIONS

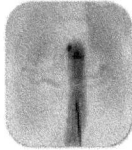

DO FINAL CHECK | 16

What to check?

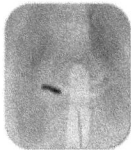

BALLOON THE STENT | 15

Can the ballooning be repeated?

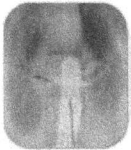

DEPLOY THE STENT | 14

How do self-expanding stents deploy in relation to
their self-radial force?
Why might self-expanding stents require molding
to the artery wall after deployment?

INSERT AND POSITION STENT | 13

What is the crucial element in securing accurate
stent placement and alignment?

SELECT APPROPRIATE STENT | 12

Which stent and what average diameter and
length to use?

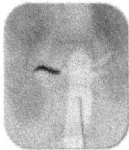

PERFORM BALLOON ANGIOPLASTY | 11

To what level of pressure should the balloon be inflated?
How long should the balloon be maintained in the inflated
state once it is inflated to the nominal pressure?

CROSS RENAL A. STENOSIS | 10

How should one progress with the wire while crossing
the lesion?
Where should the wire be positioned post lesion
crossing?

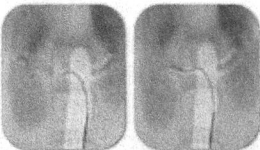

CANNULATE RENAL ARTERY | 09

Which catheter and Glidewire sizes are to be used
for insertion in this step? How is the catheter
formed and connected to the right renal artery?

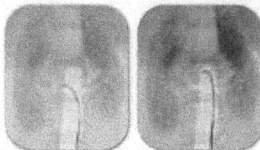

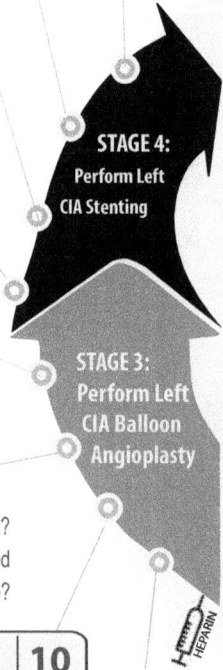

STAGE 4:
Perform Left
CIA Stenting

STAGE 3:
Perform Left
CIA Balloon
Angioplasty

HEPARIN

01 | **START YOUR CASE**

What factors, both in terms of equipment and patient evaluation, need to be considered prior to renal artery angioplasty?

02 | **INSERT THE GUIDEWIRE**

Which guidewire should be chosen for the procedure, and what method using fluoroscopy confirms its positioning?

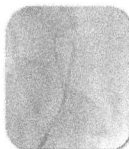

03 | **INSERT SHEATH**

What is the appropriate sheath size needed for this phase?

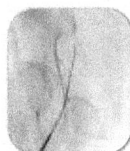

STAGE 1:
Secure access via right groin. Cross the iliac lesion.

04 | **PROCEED WITH THE GUIDEWIRE AND CATHETER**

Which guidewire and catheter should be utilized at this stage, and where are they intended to reach?

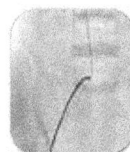

STAGE 2:
Perform angiogram

05 | **PREPARE TO PERFORM DSU**

Which catheter to use, what position, and what is the contrast injector parameters to use?

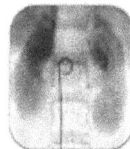

06 | **Attention to the sheath**

Which sheath to use now? is the 5Fr sheath usually enough?

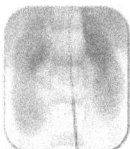

07 | **Perform Digital Subtraction Angiography (DSA)**

What about table position?

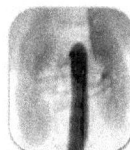

08 | **CREATE A ROADMAP**

How else can you inject the contrast?

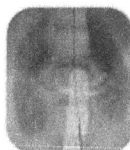

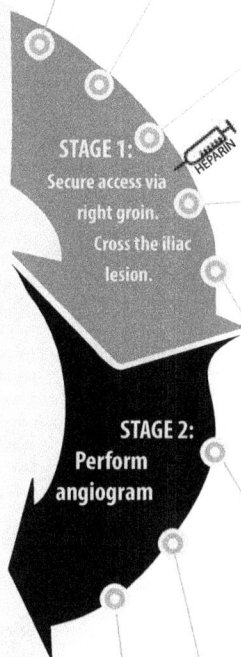

RENAL Angioplasty - CHART ANSWERS

DO FINAL CHECK
Use the sheath   **16**

Check for suitability, stent position and expansion,
and any complications

BALLOON THE STENT
Check each part while deploying   **15**

Repeat ballooning gently if need be

DEPLOY THE STENT
Check each part while deploying   **14**

Self-expanding stents deploys using self-radial
force. They might require molding to the artery
wall.

INSERT AND POSITION STENT
Adjust C-Arm if needed   **13**

Ensuring a correct C-Arm position.

STAGE 4:
Perform Left
CIA Stenting

SELECT APPROPRIATE STENT
Self-expanding stent in this case **12**

Select self-expanding stent, 2.5 mm in diameter,
and 15mm length.

STAGE 3:
Perform Left
CIA Balloon
Angioplasty

BALOON ANGIOPLASTY THE LESION **11**

Balloon is inflated to nominal pressure and is left
inflated for 2min.

HEPARIN

CROSS RENAL A. STENOSIS
'bury' the wire within the renal area **10**

Gently proceed with the wire, cross the lesion, and
bury the wire into the renal area.

CANNULATE RENAL ARTERY
Choose suitable length and diameter **09**

Insert Cobra catheter and 0.018 Glidewire. Form
the catheter in aorta and hook it to the right renal
artery

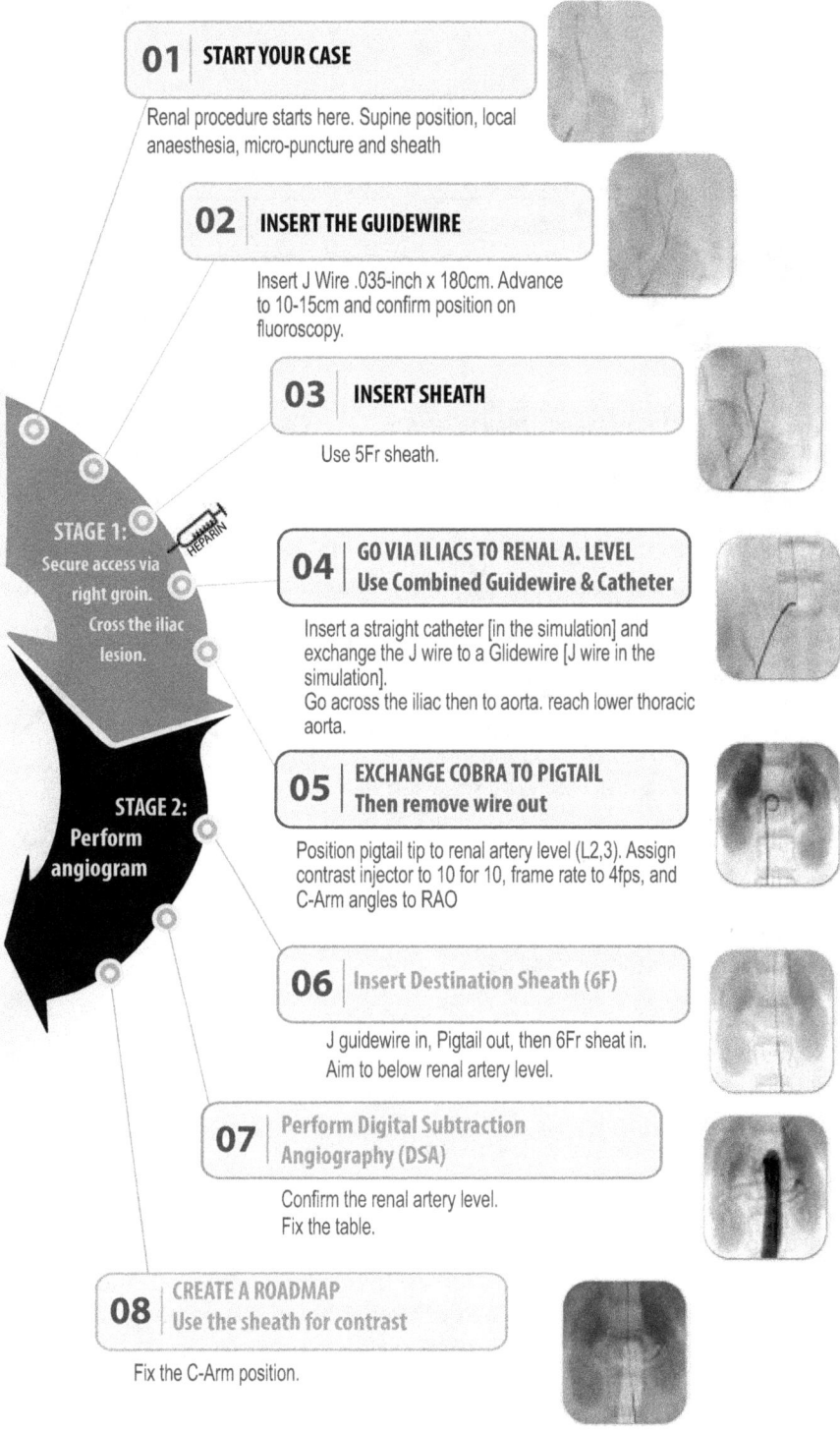

01 | START YOUR CASE

Renal procedure starts here. Supine position, local anaesthesia, micro-puncture and sheath

02 | INSERT THE GUIDEWIRE

Insert J Wire .035-inch x 180cm. Advance to 10-15cm and confirm position on fluoroscopy.

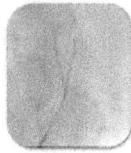

03 | INSERT SHEATH

Use 5Fr sheath.

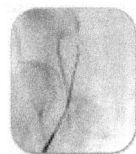

STAGE 1:
Secure access via right groin. Cross the iliac lesion.

HEPARIN

04 | GO VIA ILIACS TO RENAL A. LEVEL
Use Combined Guidewire & Catheter

Insert a straight catheter [in the simulation] and exchange the J wire to a Glidewire [J wire in the simulation].
Go across the iliac then to aorta. reach lower thoracic aorta.

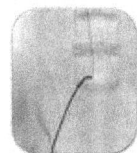

05 | EXCHANGE COBRA TO PIGTAIL
Then remove wire out

Position pigtail tip to renal artery level (L2,3). Assign contrast injector to 10 for 10, frame rate to 4fps, and C-Arm angles to RAO

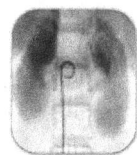

STAGE 2:
Perform angiogram

06 | Insert Destination Sheath (6F)

J guidewire in, Pigtail out, then 6Fr sheat in. Aim to below renal artery level.

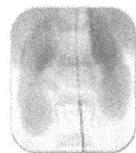

07 | Perform Digital Subtraction Angiography (DSA)

Confirm the renal artery level.
Fix the table.

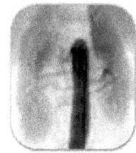

08 | CREATE A ROADMAP
Use the sheath for contrast

Fix the C-Arm position.

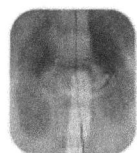

EVAR - CHART QUESTIONS

DO A FINAL CHECK | **17**

How do you confirm that the sealing is effective before finishing the procedure?

USE LARGE BALLOON TO MOULD | **16**

What could be the implications if the stent is not properly molded to the sealing zones?

CHOSE EVAR LIMB, INSERT & DEPLOY | **15**

How should the C/L limb stent be positioned in relation to the main body to ensure sealing at the modular stent? Why is the overlapping of the C/L limb stent with the main body crucial for the modular stent's sealing?

LT/ CONFIRM INITERNAL ILIAC A. | **14**

How do you guarantee the C-Arm is in the correct position, specifically in the Right Anterior Oblique (RAO) view, to vividly display the landing zone?

CHECK POSITION WITHIN STENT | **13**

How can you ensure the proper positioning of the pigtail within the stent?
What is crucial about the pigtail's movement within the stent body?

LT/ PROCEED TO GATE CANNULATION | **12**

After straightening the pigtail, to which location should it be withdrawn with the wire? What does cannulating the gate entail in this procedure?

STAGE 4: Balloon Molding of stents and completion angiogram

STAGE 3: Complete limbs cannulation & Deployment

HEPARIN

01 | START YOUR CASE

What are the first steps conducted in EVAR?

02 | RT - INSERT GUIDEWIRE

How do you correctly insert the Rosen wire, and what are its specifications?
To what length should the Rosen wire be advanced, and how is its position confirmed?
What is the purpose of setting up Proglide in this procedure?What size sheath should
be inserted following the Proglide setup for percutaneous access?

03 | SETUP THE LT SIDE

After the micro-puncture, what size and type of sheath should be inserted?

04 | LT/ INSERT GUIDEWIRE

How do you correctly insert the Rosen wire, and what are its
specifications? To what length should the Rosen wire be advanced,
and how is its position confirmed?

STAGE 1:
Secure access
via both groins.
Setup stiff wire
(right) &
pigtail
catheter
(left)

HEPARIN

05 | RT/ CANNULATE THE AORTA

How should the aorta be cannulated, and which components
are involved in reaching the descending aorta?

06 | RT/ EXCHANGE TO STIFF WIRE

Which guidewire to use, and once the exchange has been
made, what should be done with the catheter?

STAGE 2:
Insert EVAR Main
Body. Check
position.
Deploy the
EVAR Body

HEPARIN

07 | LT/ CANNULATE THE AORTA

What steps need to be followed to cannulate the aorta
with both the Glidewire and the catheter?

08 | RT/ SELECT EVAR BODY
Select appropriate size and length

How do you determine the appropriate size and length when
selecting an EVAR body? What factors need to be
considered to ensure the correct selection of an EVAR body?

RT/DEPLOY MAIN BODY | **11**

What is the process for deploying the
main body top, and what checks are
performed to ensure proper
placement?

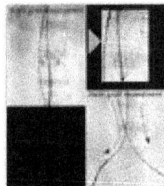

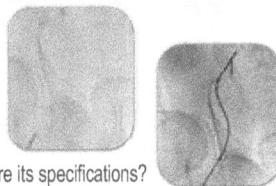

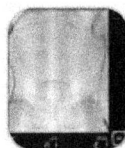

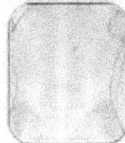

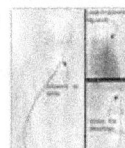

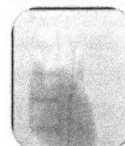

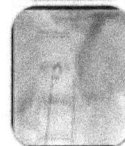

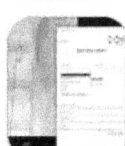

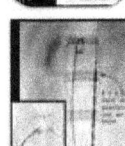

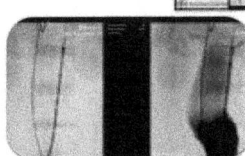

09 | RT/ INSERT & ORIENT EVAR BODY

How do you properly orient the EVAR stent during the
procedure? What adjustments need to be made to the
EVAR stent after the C-Arm position is altered?

10 | POSITION C-ARM. RUN DSA

How should the fluoroscope be
angled in relation to the center line of
the infrarenal aorta?

EVAR - CHART ANSWERS

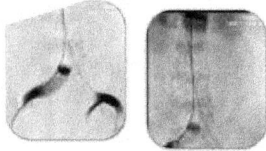

DO A FINAL CHECK
Ensure good sealing, no kinking or leaks | **17**

Once sealing is confirmed, withdraw the
catheters and wires and finish the procedure.

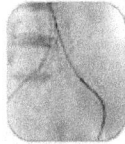

USE LARGE BALLOON TO MOULD
Apply Balloon on sealing zones | **16**

Balloon should be used to mould the stent onto the
sealing zones and to ensure a smooth opposiiton.

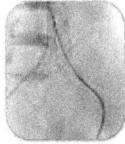

STAGE 4:
Balloon Moldi
stents and com
giogram

CHOSE EVAR LIMB, INSERT & DEPLOY
Ensure good overlap | **15**

The C/L limb stent should overalp with the main body
to ensurer sealing at the modular stent. The stent
should also not extend over the IIA.

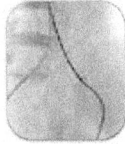

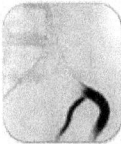

STAGE 3:
Complete
limbs
cannulation &
deployment

LT/ CONFIRM INITERNAL ILIAC A.
Using a contrast via the sheath | **14**

Ensure approporiate C-Arm position (RAO) to clearly
show the landing zone.

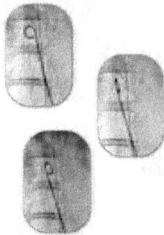

CHECK POSITION WITHIN STENT | **13**

Remove BERN catheter out and replace it with a
PIGTAIL. Take wire out and position the pigtail within the
stent. Ensure pigtail can turn freely within the stent body.
Can also use COda balloon for this purpose.

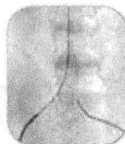

HEPARIN

LT/ PROCEED TO GATE CANNULATION | **12**
Adjust C-Arm if needed

Insert Glidewire in pigtail to straighten it. Withdraw pigtail
to mid aorta with the wire. Remove pigtail and insert
BERN catheter. Cannualte the gate.

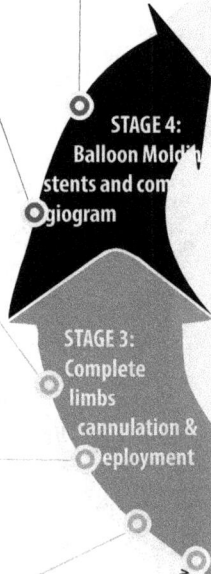

01 START YOUR CASE

EVAR starts here. Supine position, general anaeasthesia, micro-puncture and sheath

02 RT - INSERT J WIRE

Insert Rosen wire .035-inch x 180cm. Advance to 10-15cm and confirm position on fluoroscopy. Setup proglide (for percutaneous access), Insert 6F sheath.

03 MOVE TO LT SIDE
LT/ Micro-sheath in.

Micro-puncture and sheath are all assumed done for you.

04 LT/ INSERT J WIRE

Insert Rosen wire .035-inch x 180cm. Advance to 10-15cm and confirm position on fluoroscopy. Setup proglide (for percutaneous access), Insert 6F sheath.

STAGE 1:
Secure access
via both groins.
Setup stiff wire
(right) &
pigtail
catheter
(left)

HEPARIN

05 RT/ CANNULATE THE AORTA

Insert C2 catheter and exchange the J wire to a Glidewire. Cannulate the aorta to descending aorta (both guidewire and catheter).

06 RT/ EXCHANGE TO LINDQUEST
Then remove catheter out

Take the J Wire out and exhange it to a Lindquest. Take the Catheter out.

STAGE 2:
Insert EVAR Main
Body. Check
position.
Deploy the
EVAR Body

HEPARIN

07 LT/ CANNULATE THE AORTA &
EXCHANGE TO PIGTAIL

Exchange the J wire to Glidewire --> cannulate the aorta to the diagram level (both glidewire and catheter). Exchange C2 catheter to Pigtail. Position the tip at renal arteries level.

08 RT/ SELECT EVAR BODY
Select appropriate size and length

RT/DEPLOY MAIN BODY **11**

09 RT/ INSERT & ORIENT EVAR BODY
Land at renal a. level

Deploy main body top --> check all good --> deploy to bifurcation --> check all good.

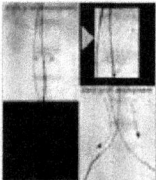

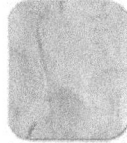

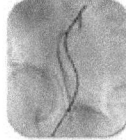

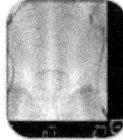

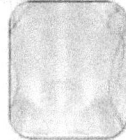

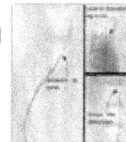

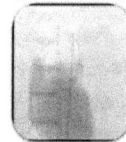

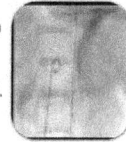

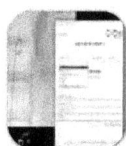

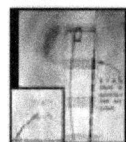

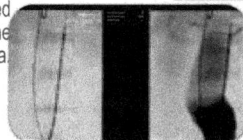

Orient the EVAR stent. Adjust after changing C-Arm position

POSITION C-ARM. RUN DSA
Confirm the renal arteries level **10**

The fluoroscope should be angled perpendicular to the center line of the infrarenal aorta.

CHAPTER 13
ENDOVASCULAR
MIND MAPPING
QUESTIONS &
ANSWERS

ENDOVASCULAR MIND MAPPING QUESTIONS

Provide a detailed mind map illustrating the steps and considerations involved in setting up and securing <u>vascular access</u>? Your mind map should encompass the following aspects:

1. The general approach to vascular access.
2. The principles of planning ahead when considering vascular access.
3. Best practices and methods for securing the vascular access once established.
4. Address the unique challenges and techniques associated with:
   - a. Accessing a bypass.
   - b. Utilizing proximal and brachial access.
   - c. Approaching a pulseless femoral artery.
5. Strategies and measures to handle vascular access complications.

Present a mind map on setting up and managing a <u>vascular sheath</u>, focusing on the following:
- Basic setup
- Sizing
- Sheath management practices
- Strategies for addressing potential failures.

Create a mind map detailing the use and management of <u>vascular guidewires</u>, emphasizing on the following:
- Guidewire properties
- Handling techniques
- Lesion interaction
- Common types of guidewires.

Illustrate a mind map on the utilization and management of <u>vascular catheters</u>, focusing on the following:
- Catheter properties.
- Catheter tip features.
- Techniques for handling catheters.
- Common types of catheters

Create a mind map detailing the process of <u>passing guidewires and catheters</u> through lesions, emphasizing the following scenarios:
- Instances when guidewires bounce away.
- Techniques for navigating through diseased arteries.
- Challenges faced when wires do not pass through the lesion.

Present a mind map focused on endovascular imaging, highlighting:
- The process of performing DSA (Digital Subtraction Angiography).
- Techniques to enhance imaging quality.
- Considerations for flow rate.
- Importance and adjustment of image rate

Create a mind map centered on selective catheterization, covering:
- The general methodology of how to perform it.
- Techniques specific to brachiocephalic catheterization.
- Approaches for visceral catheterization.
- Guidelines for infrainguinal catheterization?"

VASCULAR ACCESS MIND MAP

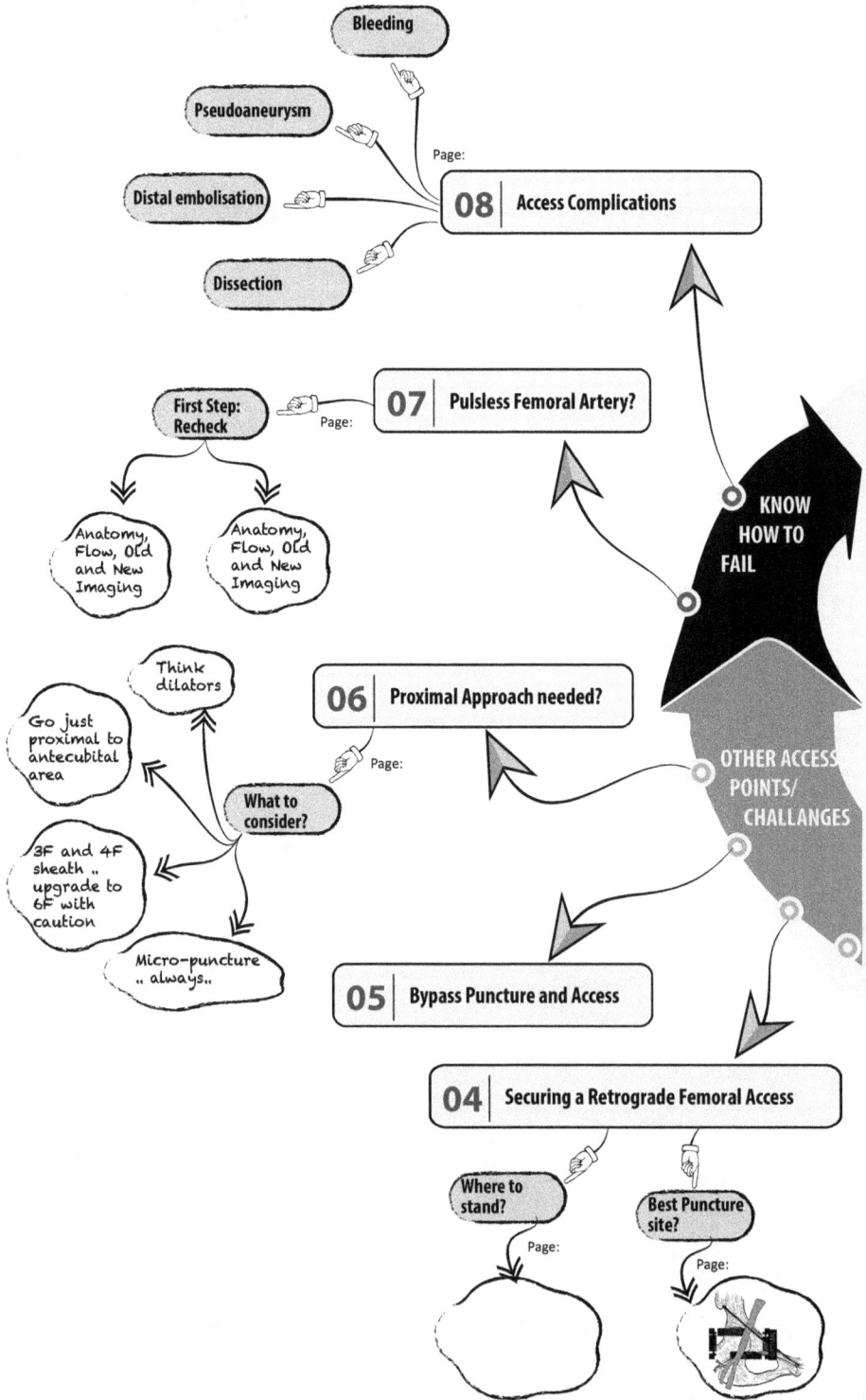

Bleeding

Pseudoaneurysm

Distal embolisation

Dissection

Page:

08 | **Access Complications**

07 | **Pulsless Femoral Artery?**

Page:

First Step: Recheck

Anatomy, Flow, Old and New Imaging

Anatomy, Flow, Old and New Imaging

Think dilators

Go just proximal to antecubital area

3F and 4F sheath .. upgrade to 6F with caution

What to consider?

Micro-puncture .. always..

06 | **Proximal Approach needed?**

Page:

KNOW HOW TO FAIL

OTHER ACCESS POINTS/ CHALLANGES

05 | **Bypass Puncture and Access**

04 | **Securing a Retrograde Femoral Access**

Where to stand?

Page:

Best Puncture site?

Page:

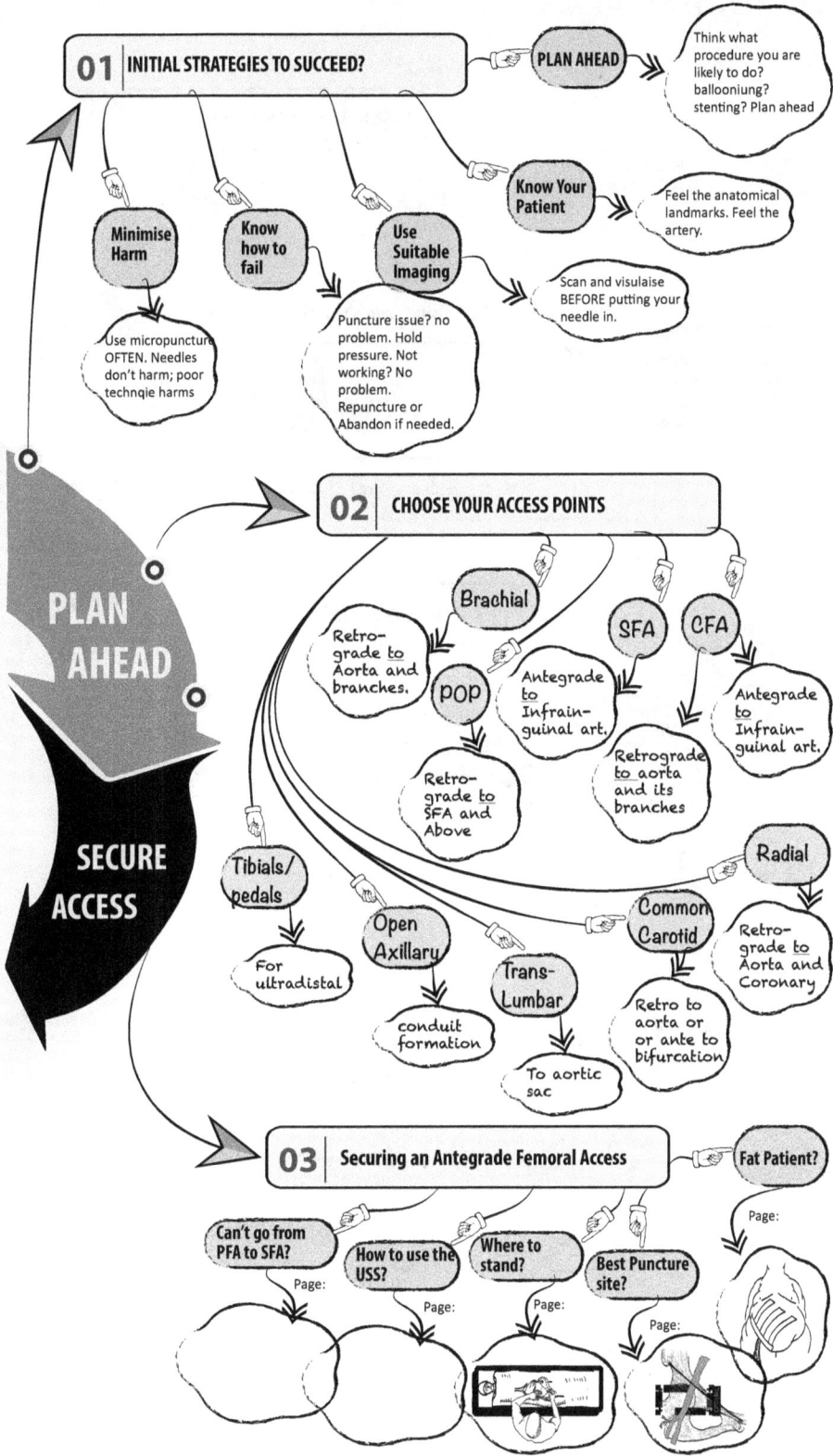

01 | INITIAL STRATEGIES TO SUCCEED?

PLAN AHEAD

Think what procedure you are likely to do? ballooniung? stenting? Plan ahead

Know Your Patient

Feel the anatomical landmarks. Feel the artery.

Minimise Harm

Know how to fail

Use Suitable Imaging

Scan and visualise BEFORE putting your needle in.

Use micropuncture OFTEN. Needles don't harm; poor technqie harms

Puncture issue? no problem. Hold pressure. Not working? No problem. Repuncture or Abandon if needed.

PLAN AHEAD

SECURE ACCESS

02 | CHOOSE YOUR ACCESS POINTS

Brachial

Retro-grade to Aorta and branches.

SFA

CFA

POP

Antegrade to Infrain-guinal art.

Antegrade to Infrain-guinal art.

Retrograde to aorta and its branches

Retro-grade to SFA and Above

Tibials/ pedals

For ultradistal

Open Axillary

conduit formation

Trans-Lumbar

To aortic sac

Common Carotid

Retro to aorta or or ante to bifurcation

Radial

Retro-grade to Aorta and Coronary

03 | Securing an Antegrade Femoral Access

Fat Patient?

Page:

Can't go from PFA to SFA?

Page:

How to use the USS?

Page:

Where to stand?

Page:

Best Puncture site?

Page:

VASCULAR SHEATH MIND MAP

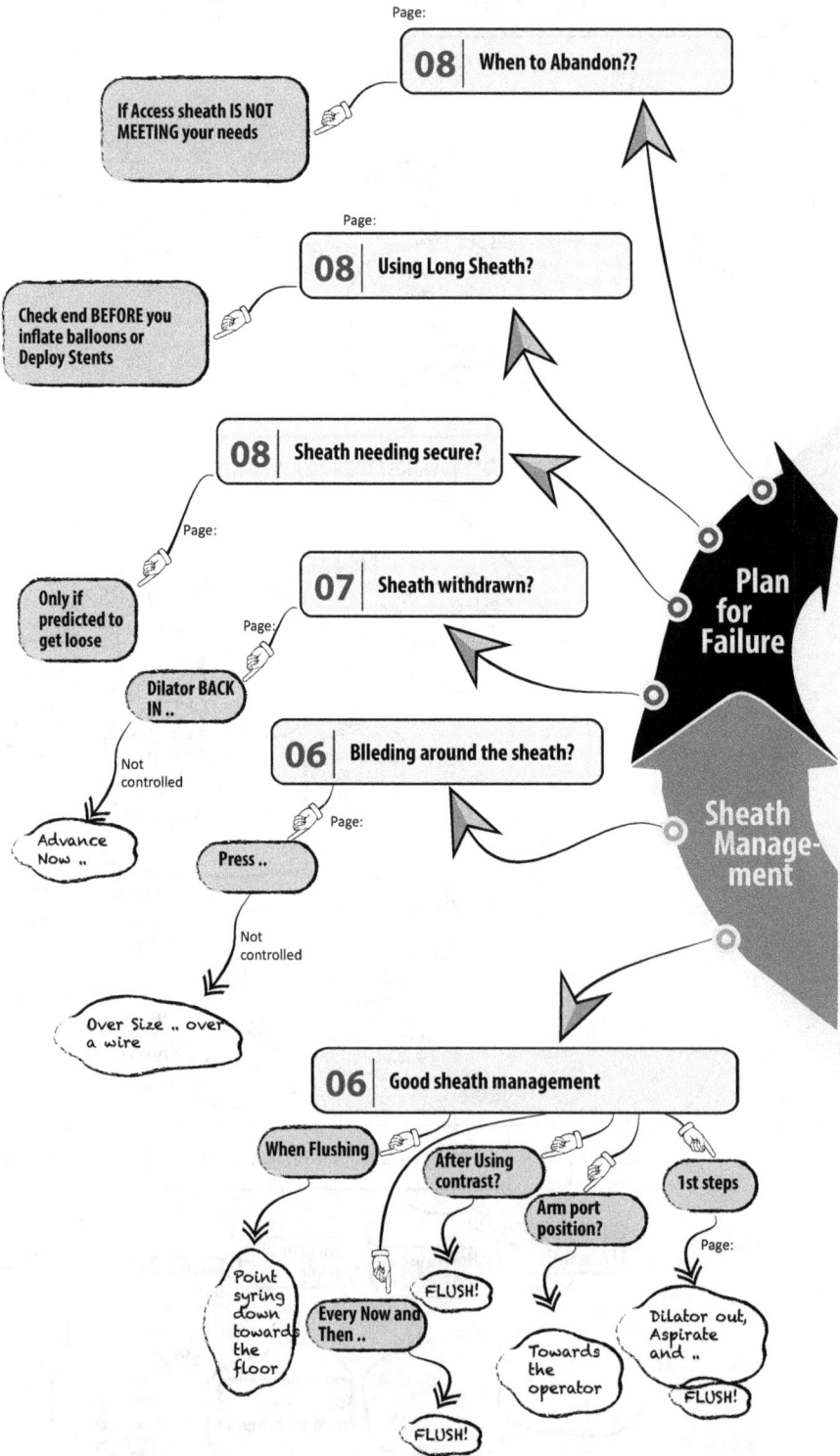

Page:

08 | **When to Abandon??**

If Access sheath IS NOT MEETING your needs

Page:

08 | **Using Long Sheath?**

Check end BEFORE you inflate balloons or Deploy Stents

08 | **Sheath needing secure?**

Page:

Only if predicted to get loose

07 | **Sheath withdrawn?**

Page:

Dilator BACK IN ..

Not controlled

Advance Now ..

06 | **Blleding around the sheath?**

Page:

Press ..

Not controlled

Over Size .. over a wire

Plan for Failure

Sheath Manage-ment

06 | **Good sheath management**

When Flushing

After Using contrast?

Arm port position?

1st steps

Page:

Point syring down towards the floor

Every Now and Then ..

FLUSH!

Towards the operator

Dilator out, Aspirate and ..

FLUSH!

FLUSH!

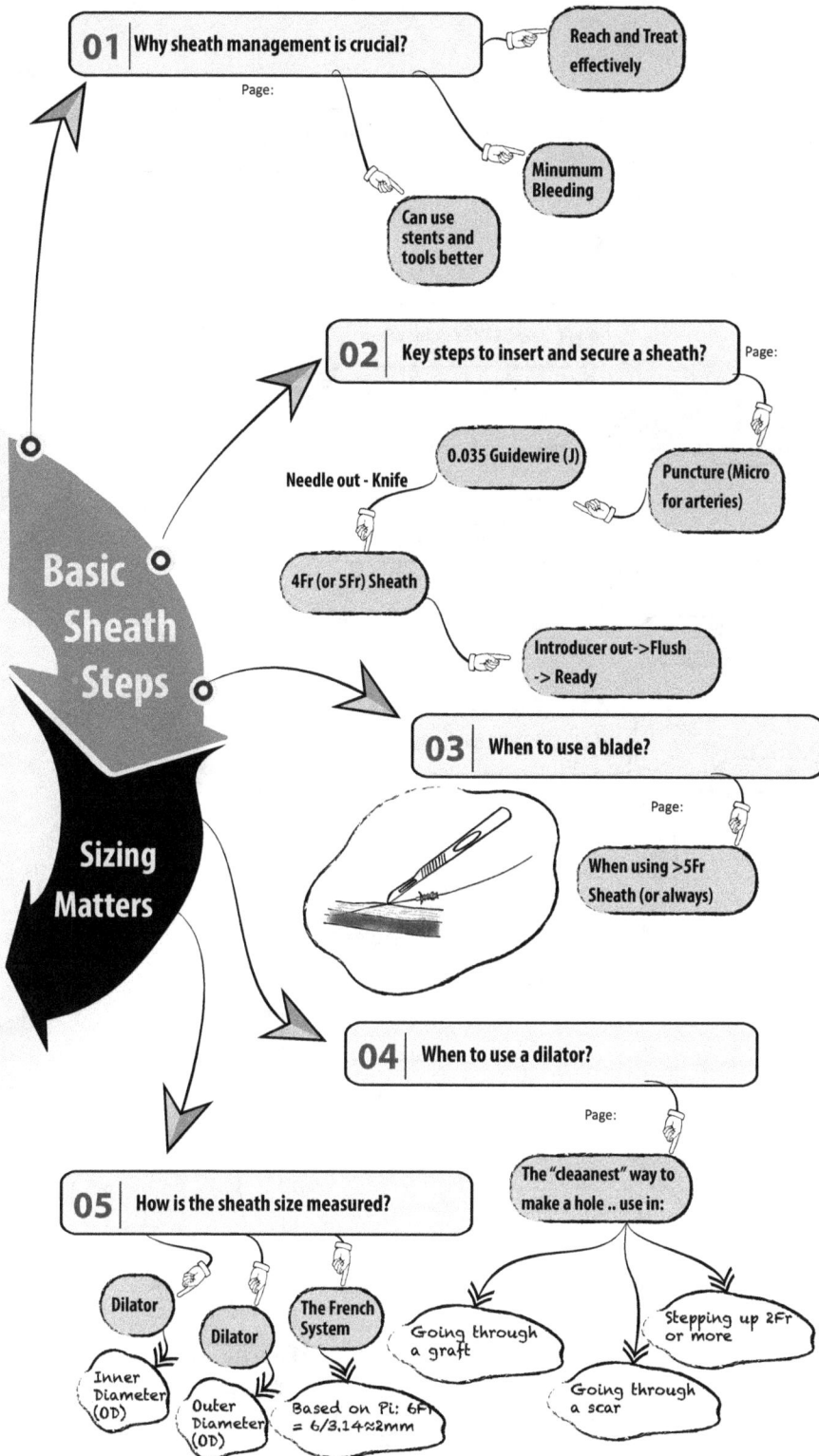

01 | Why sheath management is crucial?

Page:

Reach and Treat effectively

Minumum Bleeding

Can use stents and tools better

02 | Key steps to insert and secure a sheath?

Page:

0.035 Guidewire (J)

Puncture (Micro for arteries)

Needle out - Knife

4Fr (or 5Fr) Sheath

Introducer out->Flush -> Ready

Basic Sheath Steps

Sizing Matters

03 | When to use a blade?

Page:

When using >5Fr Sheath (or always)

04 | When to use a dilator?

Page:

The "cleaanest" way to make a hole .. use in:

05 | How is the sheath size measured?

Going through a graft

Stepping up 2Fr or more

Going through a scar

Dilator

Dilator

The French System

Inner Diameter (OD)

Outer Diameter (OD)

Based on Pi: 6Fr = 6/3.14≈2mm

VASCULAR GUIDEWIRES MIND MAP

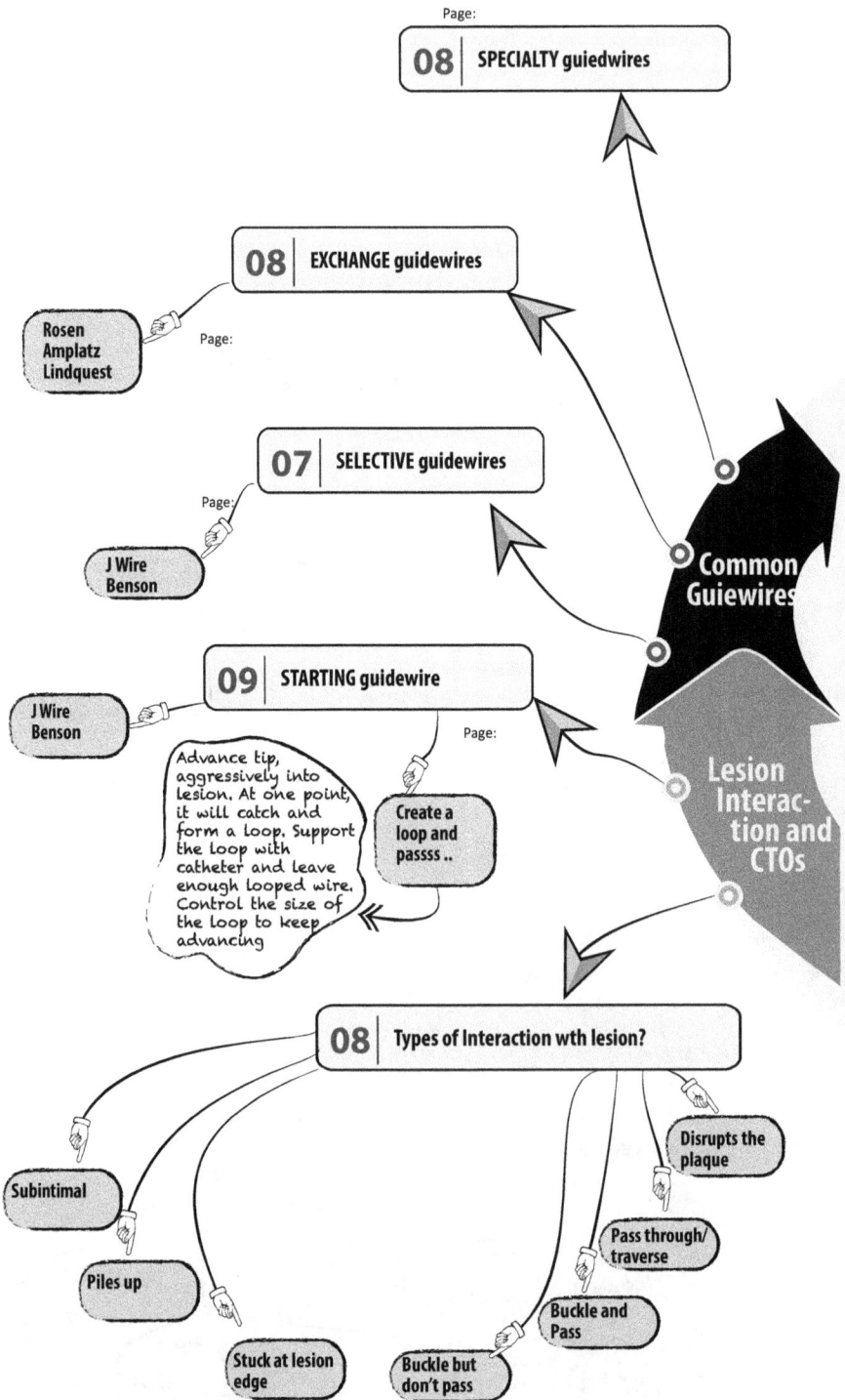

Page:

08 | SPECIALTY guiedwires

08 | EXCHANGE guidewires

Rosen
Amplatz
Lindquest

Page:

07 | SELECTIVE guidewires

Page:

J Wire
Benson

09 | STARTING guidewire

J Wire
Benson

Page:

Advance tip, aggressively into lesion. At one point, it will catch and form a loop. Support the loop with catheter and leave enough looped wire. Control the size of the loop to keep advancing

Create a loop and passss ..

Common Guiewires

Lesion Interac-tion and CTOs

08 | Types of Interaction wth lesion?

Disrupts the plaque

Pass through/traverse

Subintimal

Buckle and Pass

Piles up

Buckle but don't pass

Stuck at lesion edge

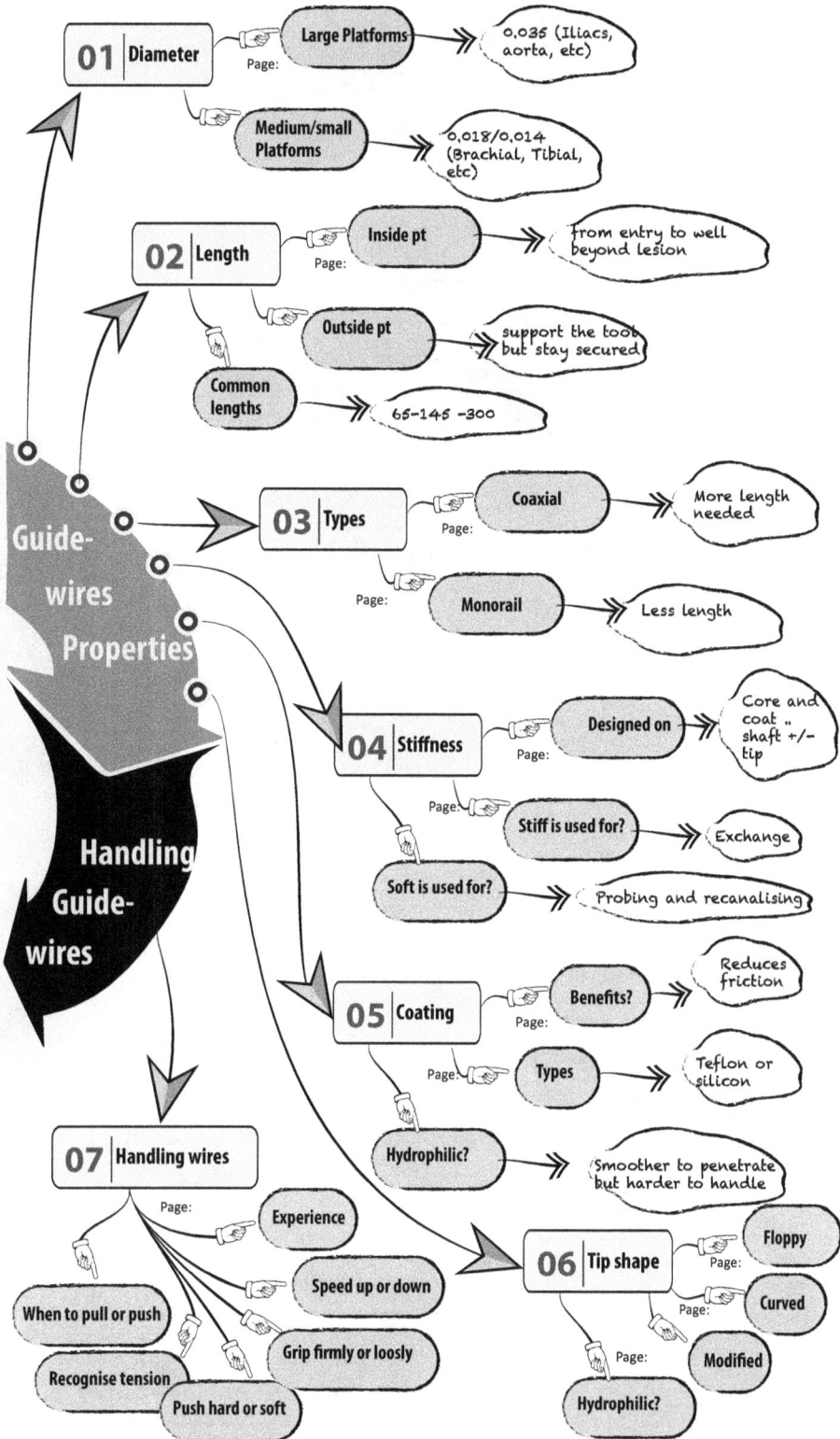

01 | Diameter — Page:
- ☞ **Large Platforms** → 0,035 (Iliacs, aorta, etc)
- ☞ **Medium/small Platforms** → 0,018/0,014 (Brachial, Tibial, etc)

02 | Length — Page:
- ☞ **Inside pt** → from entry to well beyond lesion
- ☞ **Outside pt** → support the tool but stay secured
- ☞ **Common lengths** → 65-145 -300

03 | Types — Page:
- ☞ **Coaxial** → More length needed
- ☞ **Monorail** → Less length — Page:

04 | Stiffness — Page:
- ☞ **Designed on** → Core and coat " shaft +/- tip
- ☞ **Stiff is used for?** → Exchange — Page:
- ☞ **Soft is used for?** → Probing and recanalising

05 | Coating — Page:
- ☞ **Benefits?** → Reduces friction
- ☞ **Types** → Teflon or silicon — Page:
- **Hydrophilic?** → Smoother to penetrate but harder to handle

06 | Tip shape
- ☞ **Floppy** — Page:
- ☞ **Curved** — Page:
- **Modified**
- **Hydrophilic?** — Page:

07 | Handling wires — Page:
- ☞ **Experience**
- ☞ **Speed up or down**
- ☞ **Grip firmly or loosly**
- ☞ **Push hard or soft**
- **When to pull or push**
- **Recognise tension**

Guide-wires Properties

Handling Guide-wires

VASCULAR CATHETERS MIND MAP

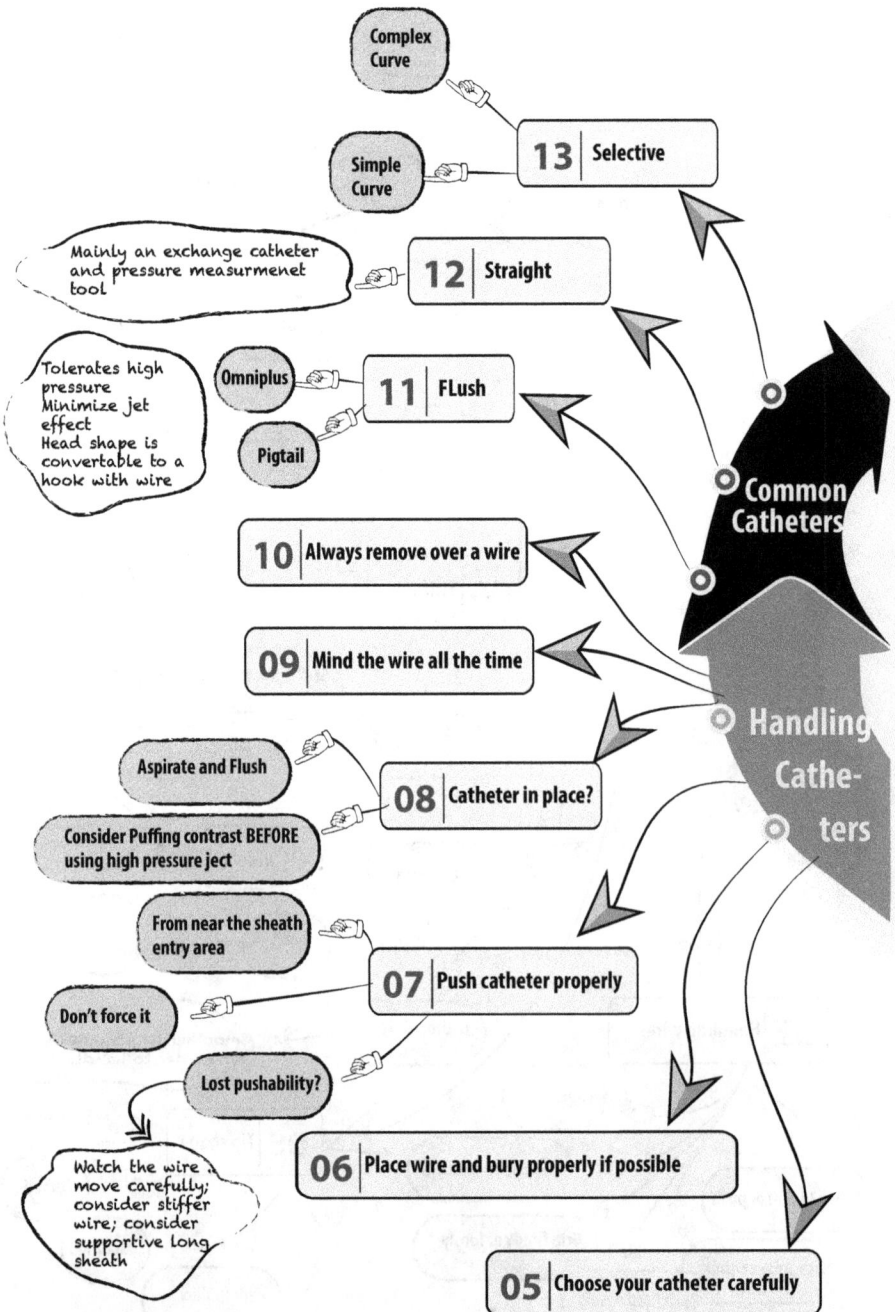

Complex Curve

Simple Curve

13 | Selective

Mainly an exchange catheter and pressure measurmenet tool

12 | Straight

Tolerates high pressure
Minimize jet effect
Head shape is convertable to a hook with wire

Omniplus

Pigtail

11 | FLush

10 | Always remove over a wire

09 | Mind the wire all the time

Aspirate and Flush

Consider Puffing contrast BEFORE using high pressure ject

08 | Catheter in place?

From near the sheath entry area

07 | Push catheter properly

Don't force it

Lost pushability?

Watch the wire move carefully; consider stiffer wire; consider supportive long sheath

06 | Place wire and bury properly if possible

05 | Choose your catheter carefully

Common Catheters

Handling Cathe-ters

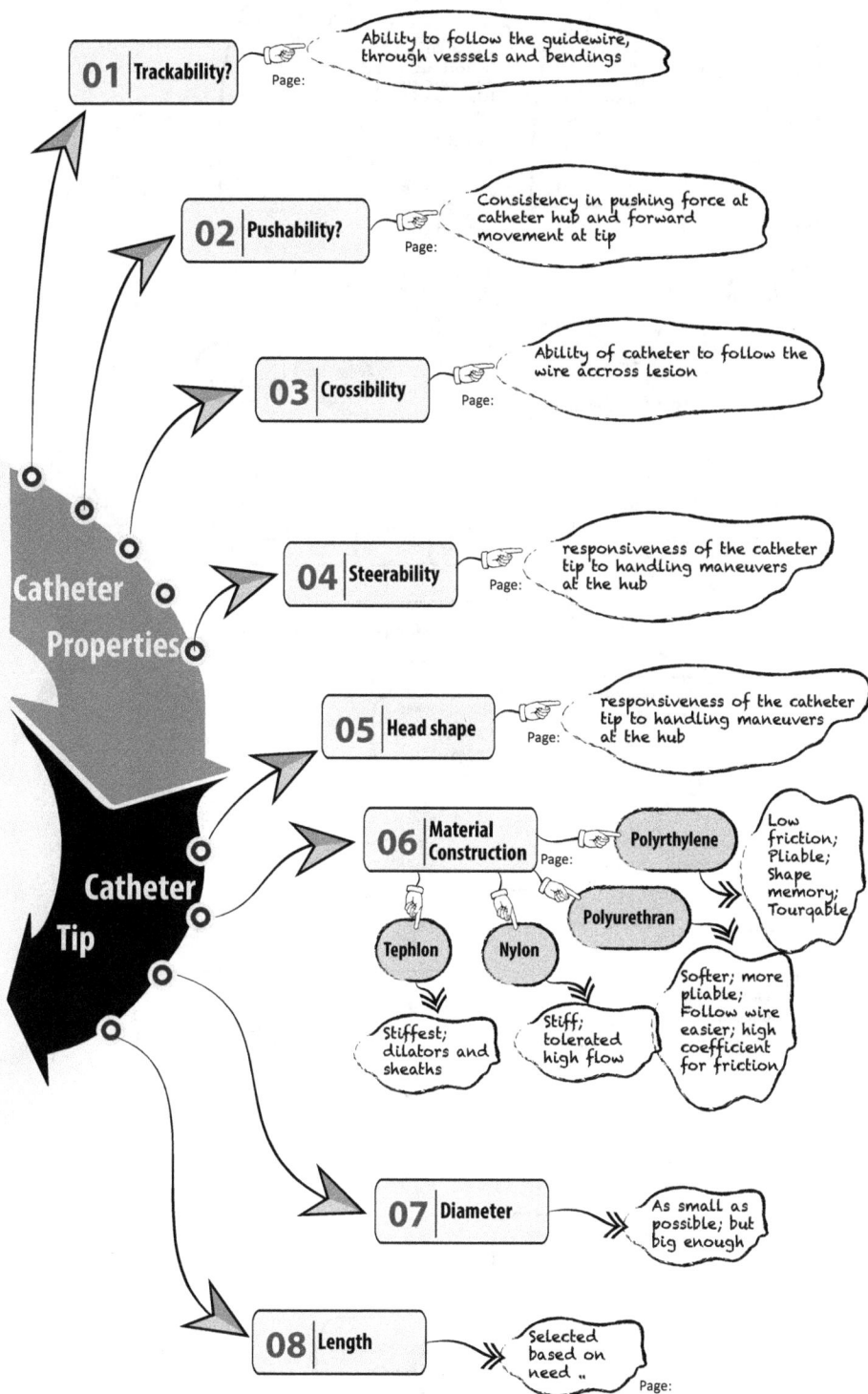

01 | Trackability? — Ability to follow the guidewire, through vesssels and bendings
Page:

02 | Pushability? — Consistency in pushing force at catheter hub and forward movement at tip
Page:

03 | Crossibility — Ability of catheter to follow the wire accross lesion
Page:

04 | Steerability — responsiveness of the catheter tip to handling maneuvers at the hub
Page:

Catheter Properties

05 | Head shape — responsiveness of the catheter tip to handling maneuvers at the hub
Page:

06 | Material Construction
Page:

Polyrthylene — Low friction; Pliable; Shape memory; Tourqable

Polyurethran — Softer; more pliable; Follow wire easier; high coefficient for friction

Tephlon — Stiffest; dilators and sheaths

Nylon — Stiff; tolerated high flow

Catheter Tip

07 | Diameter — As small as possible; but big enough

08 | Length — Selected based on need ..
Page:

PASSING WIRES AND CATHETERS MIND MAP

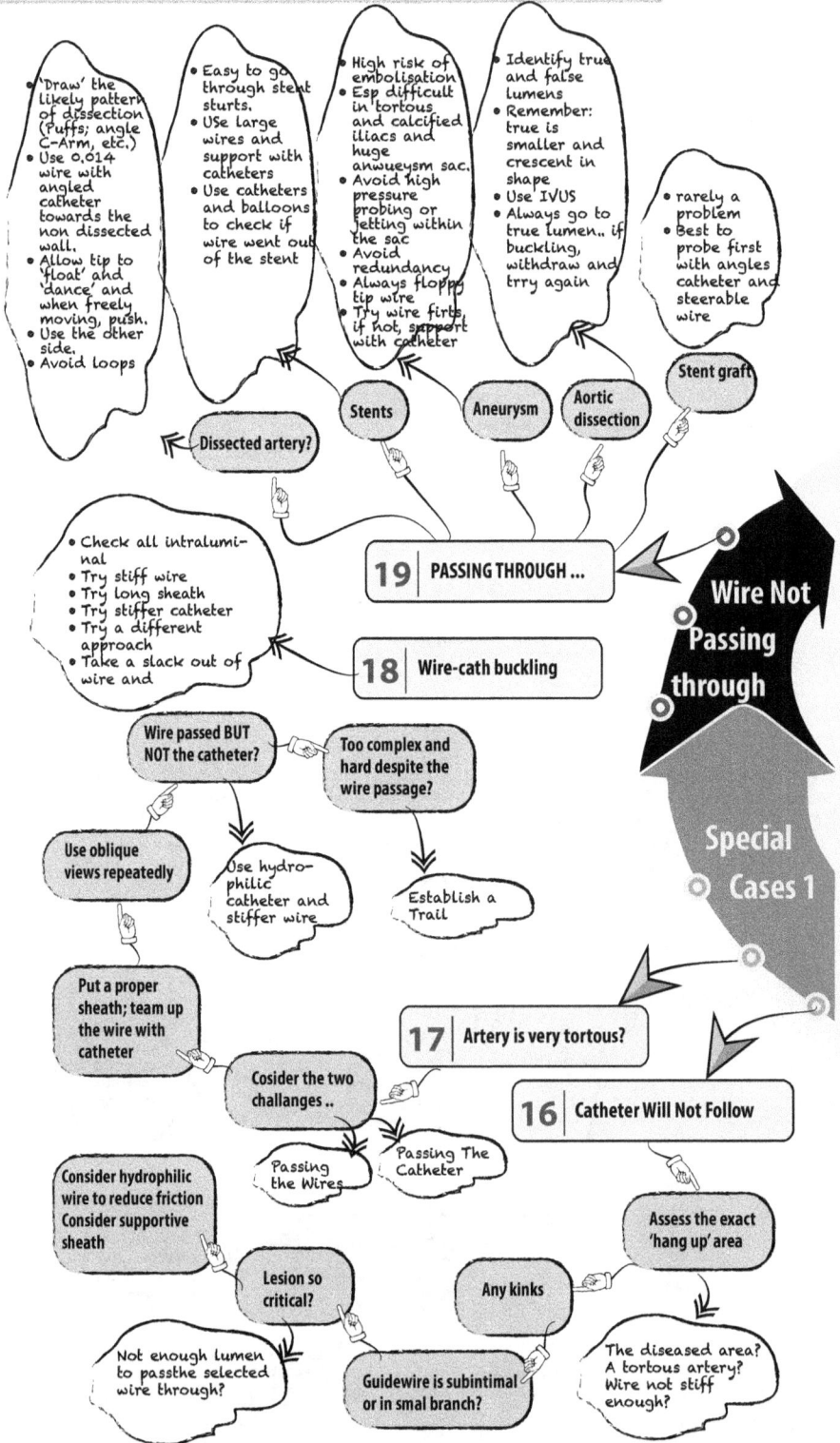

- 'Draw' the likely pattern of dissection (Puffs; angle C-Arm, etc.)
- Use 0.014 wire with angled catheter towards the non dissected wall.
- Allow tip to 'float' and 'dance' and when freely moving, push.
- Use the other side.
- Avoid loops

- Easy to go through stent sturts.
- Use large wires and support with catheters
- Use catheters and balloons to check if wire went out of the stent

- High risk of embolisation
- Esp difficult in tortous and calcified iliacs and huge anwueysm sac.
- Avoid high pressure probing or jetting within the sac
- Avoid redundancy
- Always floppy tip wire
- Try wire firts, if hot, support with catheter

- Identify true and false lumens
- Remember: true is smaller and crescent in shape
- Use IVUS
- Always go to true lumen.. if buckling, withdraw and trry again

- rarely a problem
- Best to probe first with angles catheter and steerable wire

Stent graft

Dissected artery?   **Stents**   **Aneurysm**   **Aortic dissection**

Wire Not Passing through

19 | PASSING THROUGH ...

- Check all intraluminal
- Try stiff wire
- Try long sheath
- Try stiffer catheter
- Try a different approach
- Take a slack out of wire and

18 | Wire-cath buckling

Special Cases 1

Wire passed BUT NOT the catheter?   **Too complex and hard despite the wire passage?**

Use hydrophilic catheter and stiffer wire

Use oblique views repeatedly

Establish a Trail

Put a proper sheath; team up the wire with catheter

17 | Artery is very tortous?

Cosider the two challanges ..

16 | Catheter Will Not Follow

Passing the Wires   Passing The Catheter

Consider hydrophilic wire to reduce friction Consider supportive sheath

Assess the exact 'hang up' area

Lesion so critical?   **Any kinks**

Not enough lumen to passthe selected wire through?   **Guidewire is subintimal or in smal branch?**   The diseased area? A tortous artery? Wire not stiff enough?

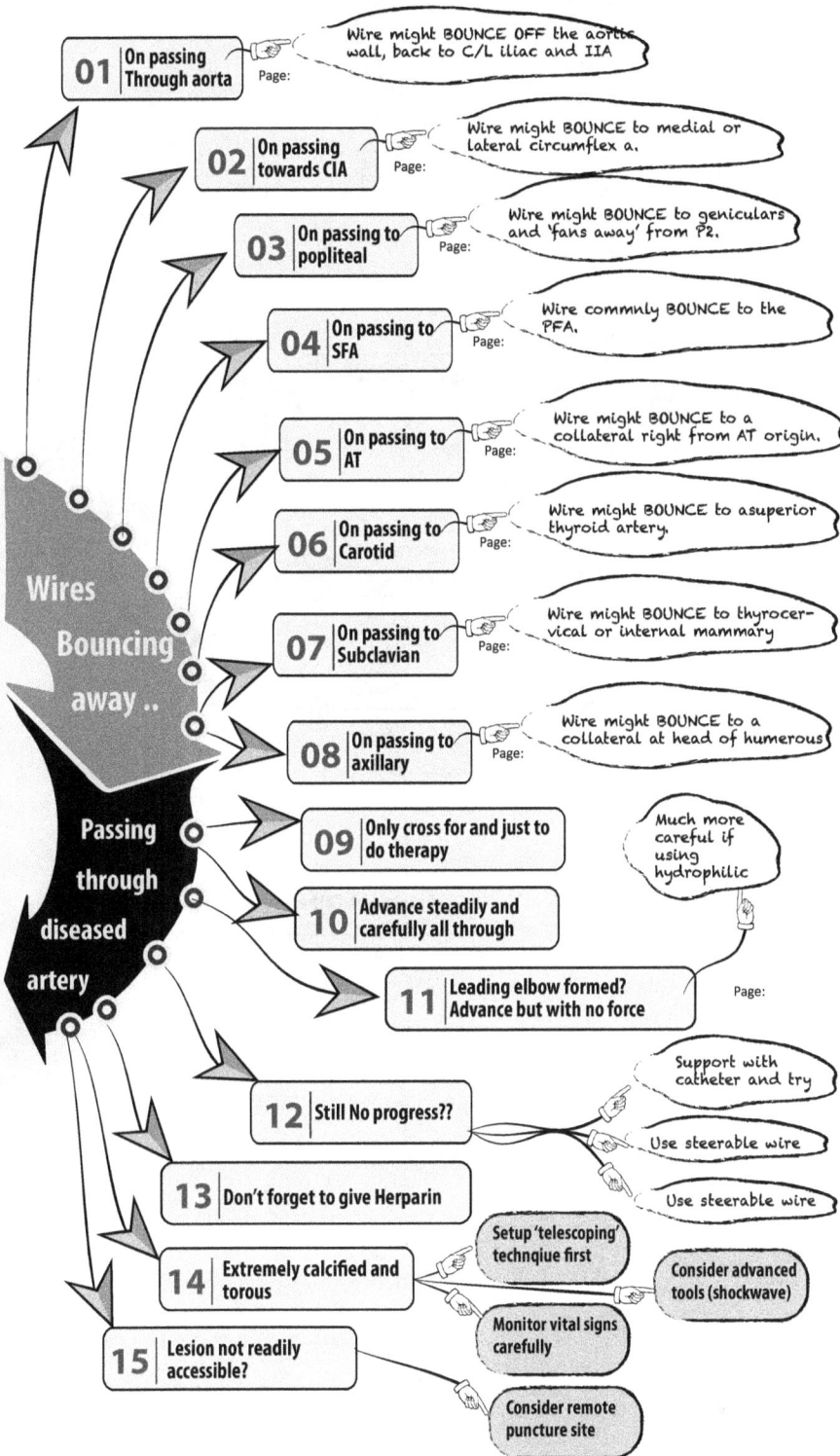

01 | On passing Through aorta — Page:
Wire might BOUNCE OFF the aortic wall, back to C/L iliac and IIA

02 | On passing towards CIA — Page:
Wire might BOUNCE to medial or lateral circumflex a.

03 | On passing to popliteal — Page:
Wire might BOUNCE to geniculars and 'fans away' from P2.

04 | On passing to SFA — Page:
Wire commnly BOUNCE to the PFA.

05 | On passing to AT — Page:
Wire might BOUNCE to a collateral right from AT origin.

06 | On passing to Carotid — Page:
Wire might BOUNCE to asuperior thyroid artery.

07 | On passing to Subclavian — Page:
Wire might BOUNCE to thyrocer-vical or internal mammary

08 | On passing to axillary — Page:
Wire might BOUNCE to a collateral at head of humerous

Wires Bouncing away ..

Passing through diseased artery

09 | Only cross for and just to do therapy

10 | Advance steadily and carefully all through
Much more careful if using hydrophilic

11 | Leading elbow formed? Advance but with no force — Page:

12 | Still No progress??
Support with catheter and try
Use steerable wire
Use steerable wire

13 | Don't forget to give Herparin

14 | Extremely calcified and torous
Setup 'telescoping' technqiue first
Consider advanced tools (shockwave)
Monitor vital signs carefully

15 | Lesion not readily accessible?
Consider remote puncture site

ENDOVASCULAR IMAGING MIND MAP

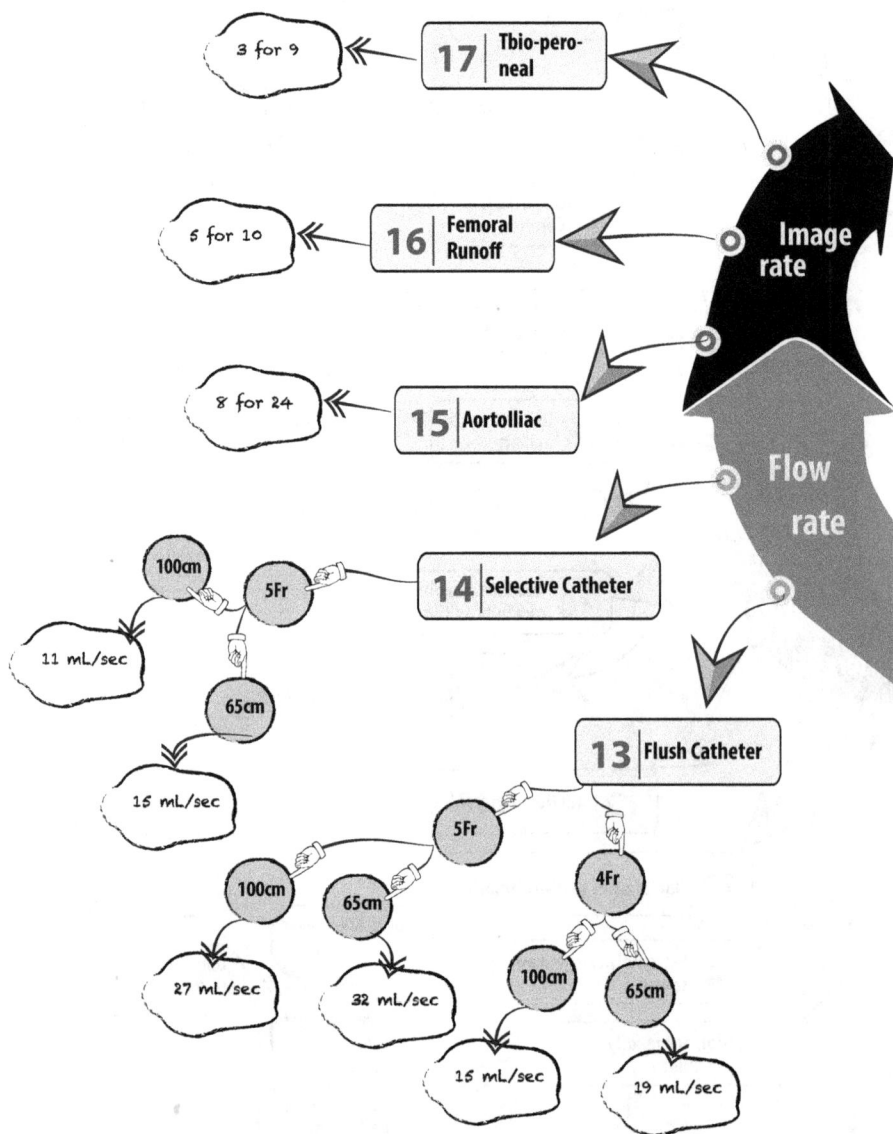

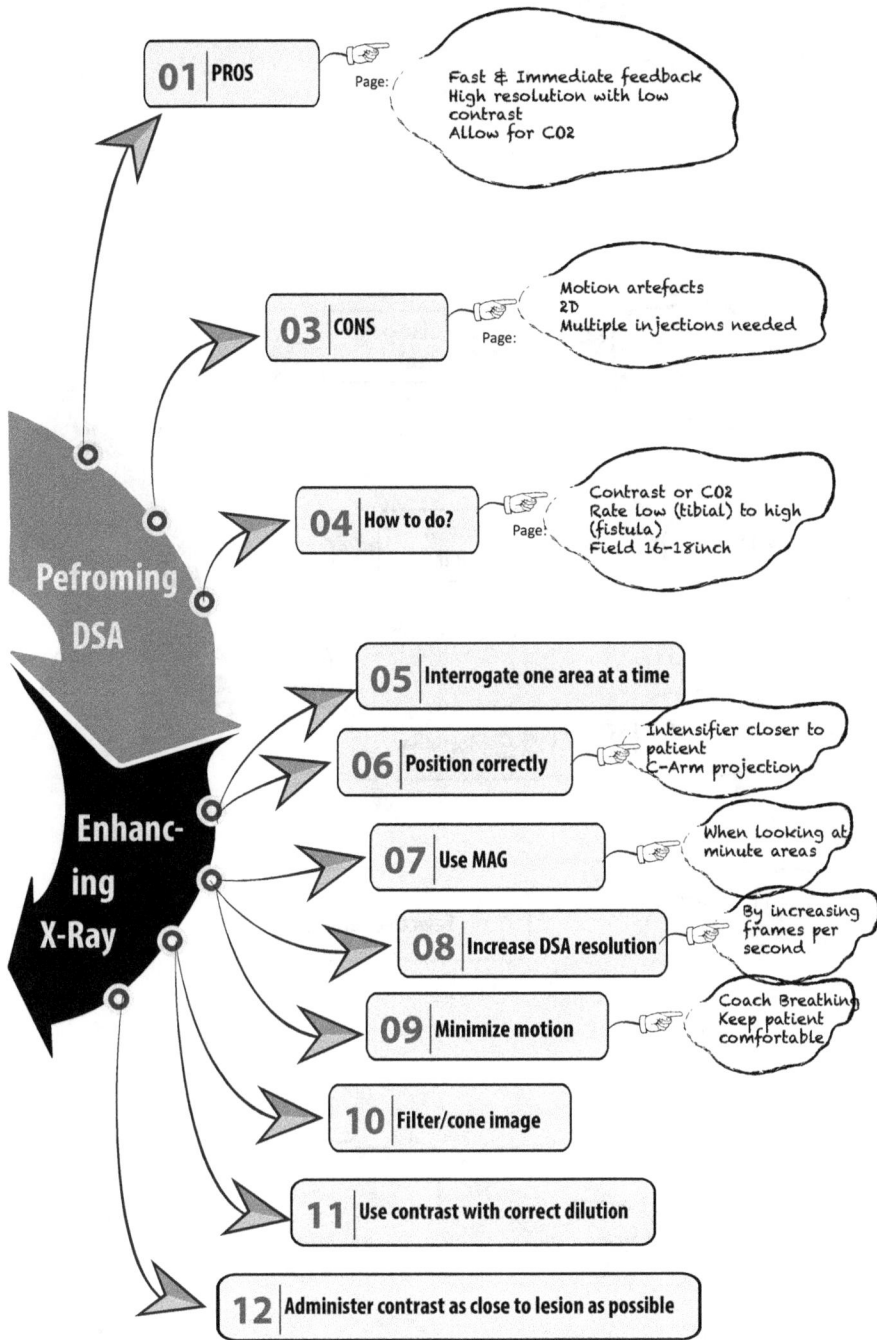

Peforming DSA

01 | PROS
Page:
Fast & Immediate feedback
High resolution with low contrast
Allow for CO2

03 | CONS
Page:
Motion artefacts
2D
Multiple injections needed

04 | How to do?
Page:
Contrast or CO2
Rate low (tibial) to high (fistula)
Field 16-18inch

Enhancing X-Ray

05 | Interrogate one area at a time

06 | Position correctly
Intensifier closer to patient
C-Arm projection

07 | Use MAG
When looking at minute areas

08 | Increase DSA resolution
By increasing frames per second

09 | Minimize motion
Coach Breathing
Keep patient comfortable

10 | Filter/cone image

11 | Use contrast with correct dilution

12 | Administer contrast as close to lesion as possible

SELECTIVE CATHETERISATION MIND MAP

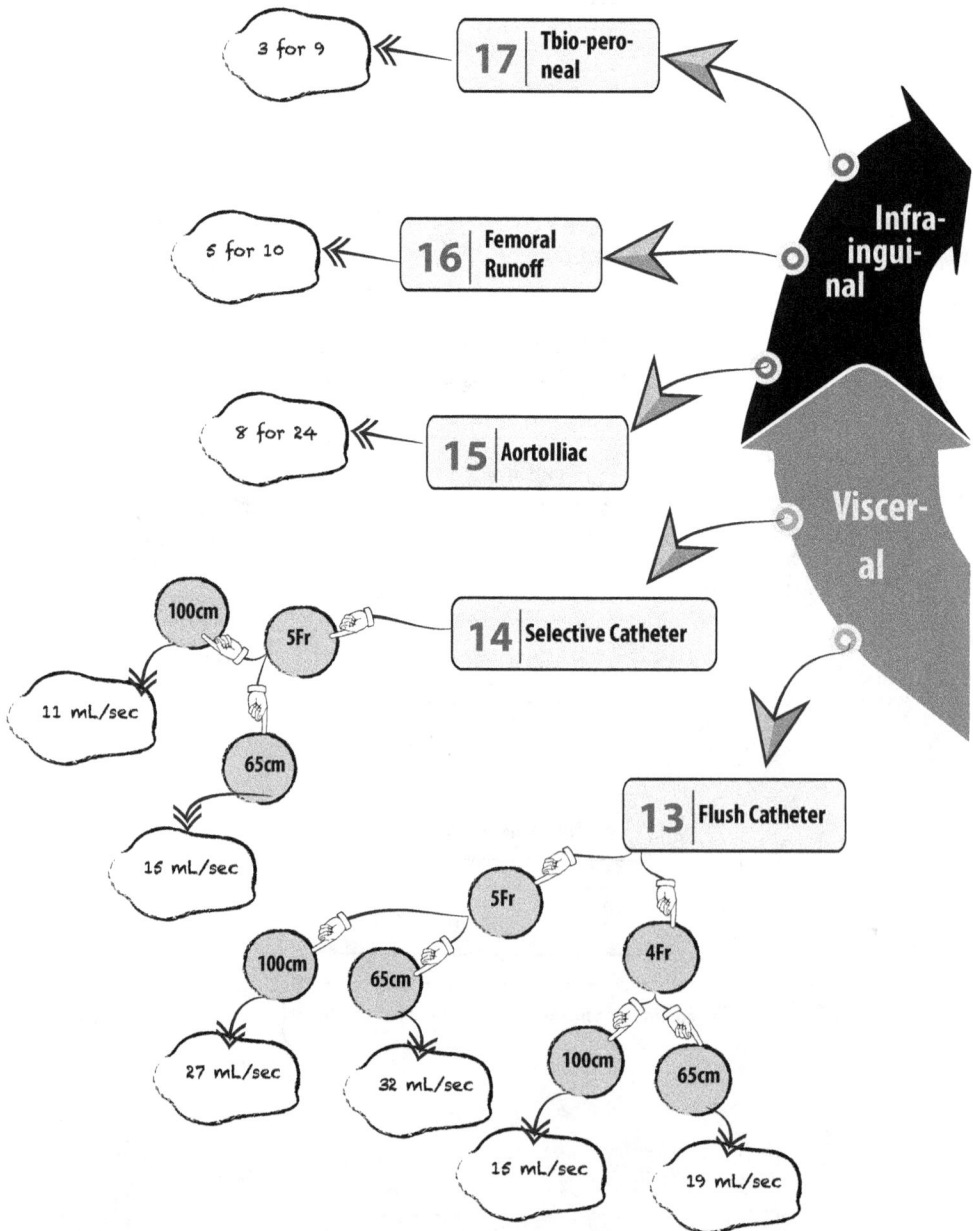

3 for 9 ← **17** Tbio-pero-neal

5 for 10 ← **16** Femoral Runoff

8 for 24 ← **15** Aortolliac

Infra-ingui-nal

Viscer-al

14 Selective Catheter
100cm
5Fr
11 mL/sec
65cm
15 mL/sec

13 Flush Catheter
5Fr
4Fr
100cm
27 mL/sec
65cm
32 mL/sec
100cm
15 mL/sec
65cm
19 mL/sec

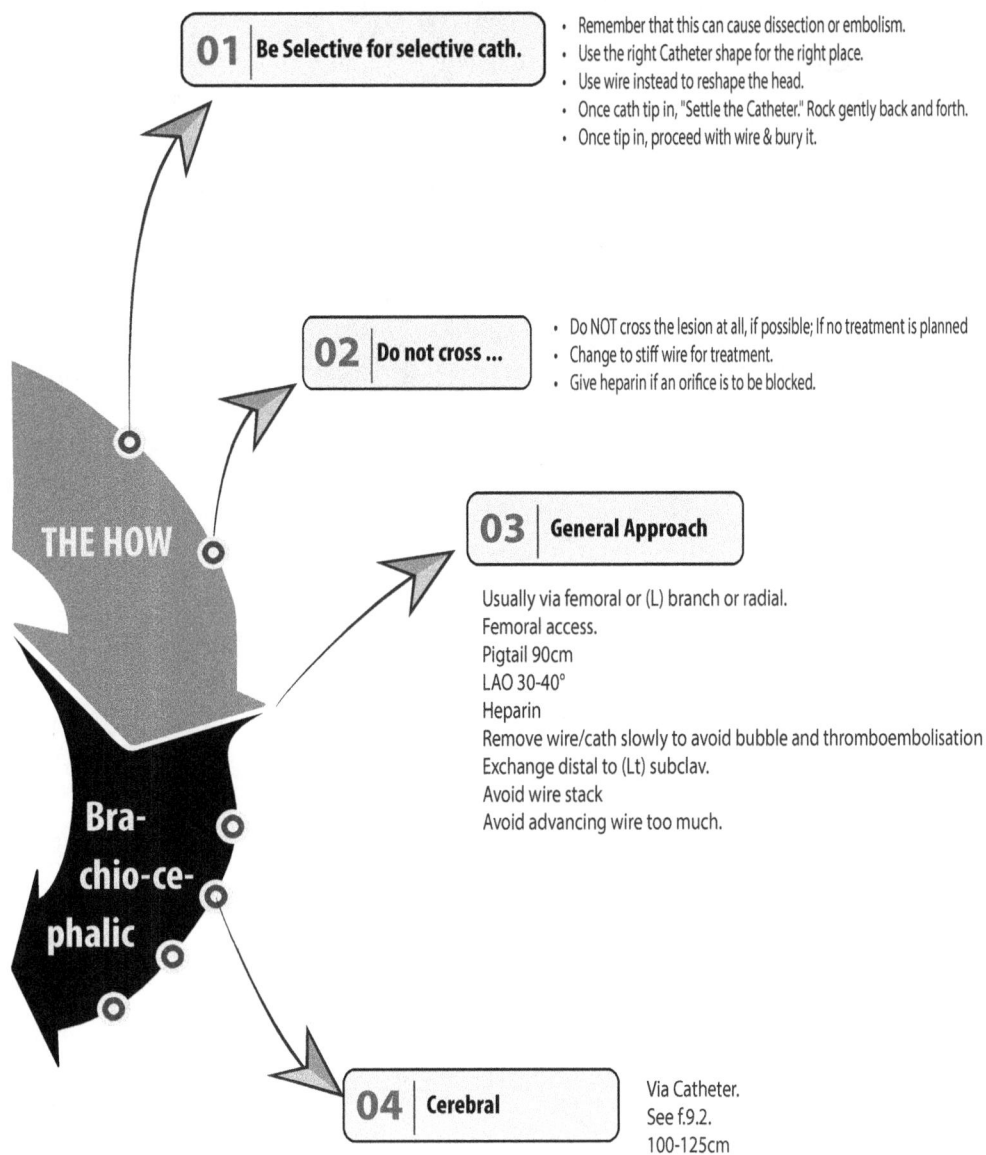

01 | **Be Selective for selective cath.**

- Remember that this can cause dissection or embolism.
- Use the right Catheter shape for the right place.
- Use wire instead to reshape the head.
- Once cath tip in, "Settle the Catheter." Rock gently back and forth.
- Once tip in, proceed with wire & bury it.

02 | **Do not cross ...**

- Do NOT cross the lesion at all, if possible; If no treatment is planned
- Change to stiff wire for treatment.
- Give heparin if an orifice is to be blocked.

03 | **General Approach**

Usually via femoral or (L) branch or radial.
Femoral access.
Pigtail 90cm
LAO 30-40°
Heparin
Remove wire/cath slowly to avoid bubble and thromboembolisation
Exchange distal to (Lt) subclav.
Avoid wire stack
Avoid advancing wire too much.

THE HOW

Bra-chio-ce-phalic

04 | **Cerebral**

Via Catheter.
See f.9.2.
100-125cm

CHAPTER 14
ENDOVASCULAR TOOLS AND DEVICES

GUIDEWIRES

What is the tip length and weight for each of the following:

Asahi Gladiu

ASAHI GLADIU
3cm soft tip
1g to cause 2mm bend in the distal 10mm of the wire

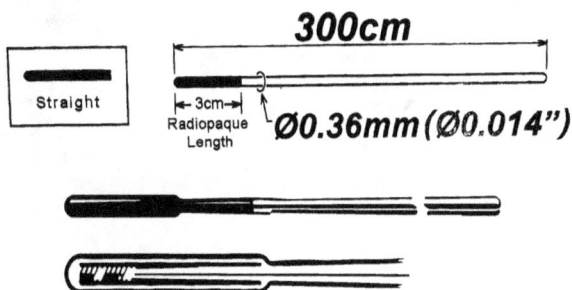

Command 18ST

COMMAND 18ST
3cm soft tip
4g to cause 2mm bend in the distal 10mm of the wire

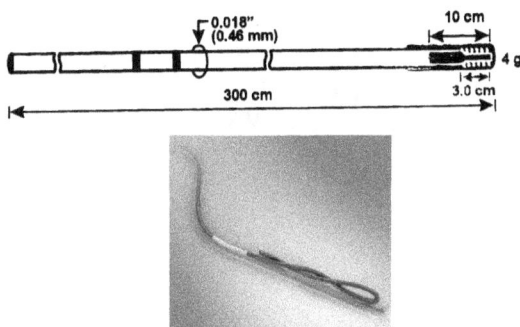

V18 Guidewire

8 cm soft tip

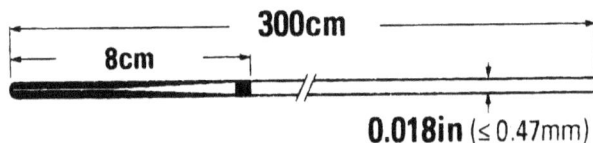

Radiofocus Glidewire Advantage

GLIDEWIRE ADVANTAGE
1cm soft tip
0.018

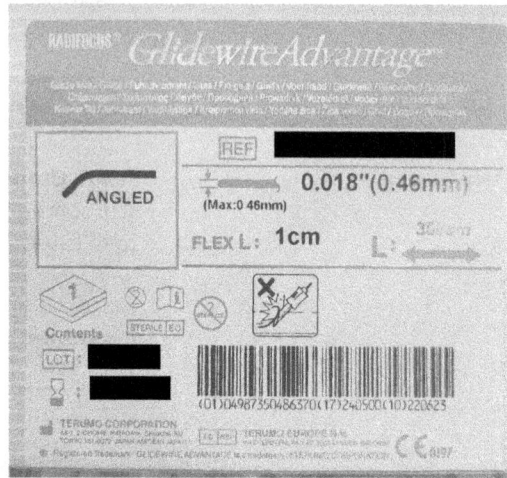

Barewire

BAREWIRE
3cm soft tip
0.014

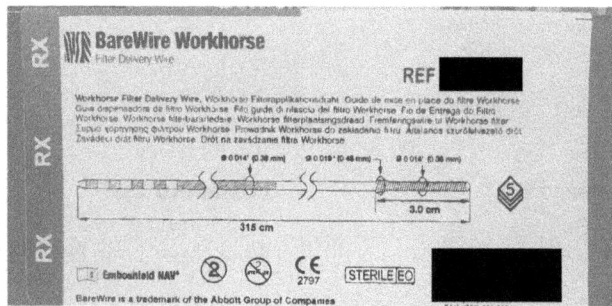

Platinum plus

PLATIMUN PLUS
3cm soft tip
0.018

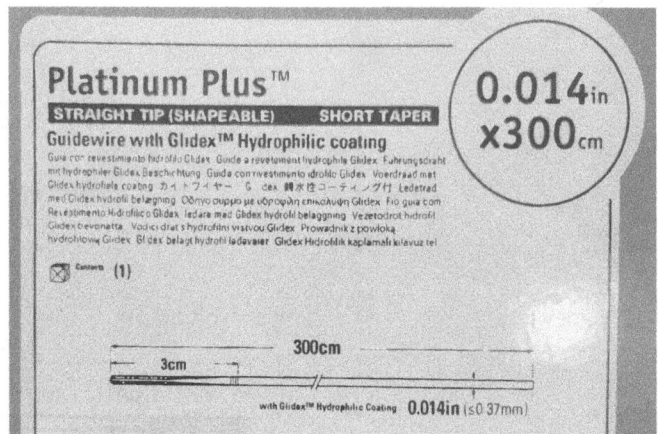

Asahi Sion

ASAHI SION
1cm soft tip angles
0.036

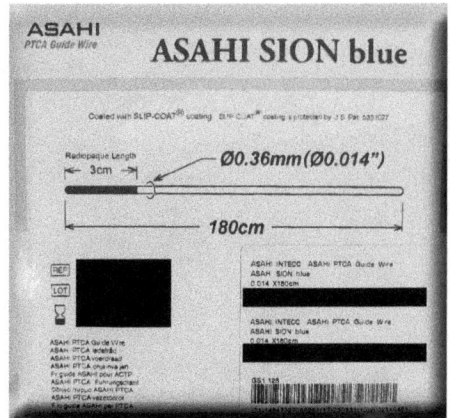

Terumo Radiofocus

TERUMO RADIOFOCUS
3cm soft tip straight
0.036

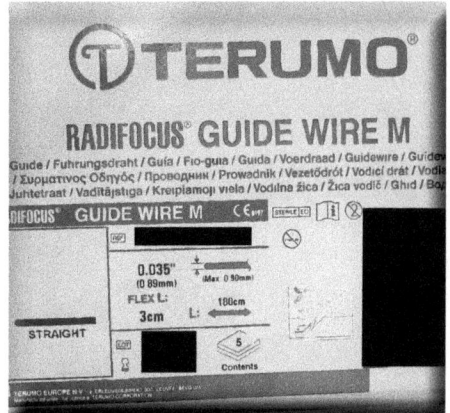

CTO 18

TCTO 18
3cm soft tip straight
0.036

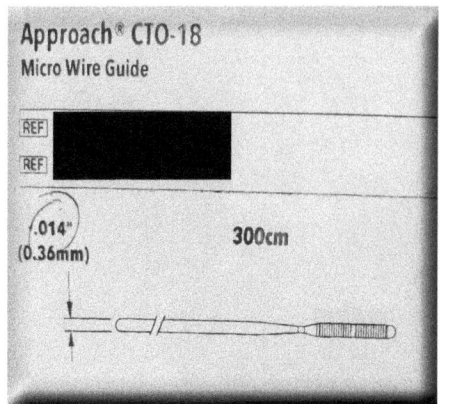

SPECIALIST CATHETERS

What are the key features of the following catheters:

CXI Support Catheter

CXI SUPPORT CATHETER
Most Suitable For distal angioplasy Due to:
*a braided kink-resistant catheter.
*stainless-steel braised (better torque and pushability)
*hydrophilic distal 40cm (pushability and trackability)
* angled tip (selective catheterization)
* markers at tip, 5,10,15cm for better visibility
* Length marker (showing progressing through the sheath)

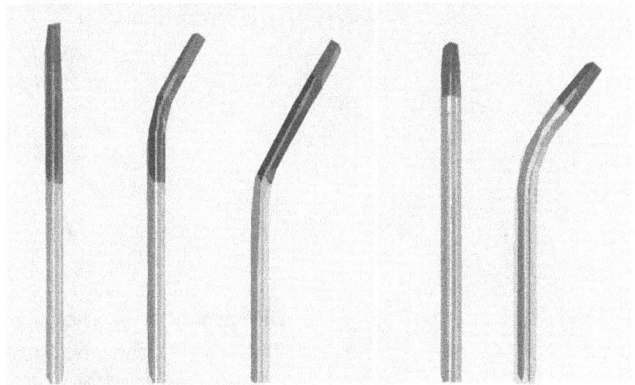

NaviCross Support Catheter

NAVICROSS SUPPORT CATHETER
Double-braided stainless steel.
12mm Tapered Tip.
Straight and 30° Angled Tips.
Telescope Technique.
Hydrophilic Mcoat™.
Three Radiopaque Markers.
These features make it a versatile and effective tool

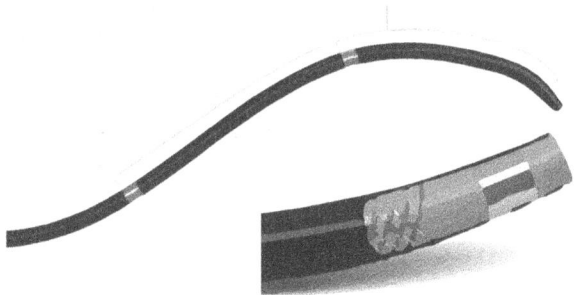

Thrombosuction catheters

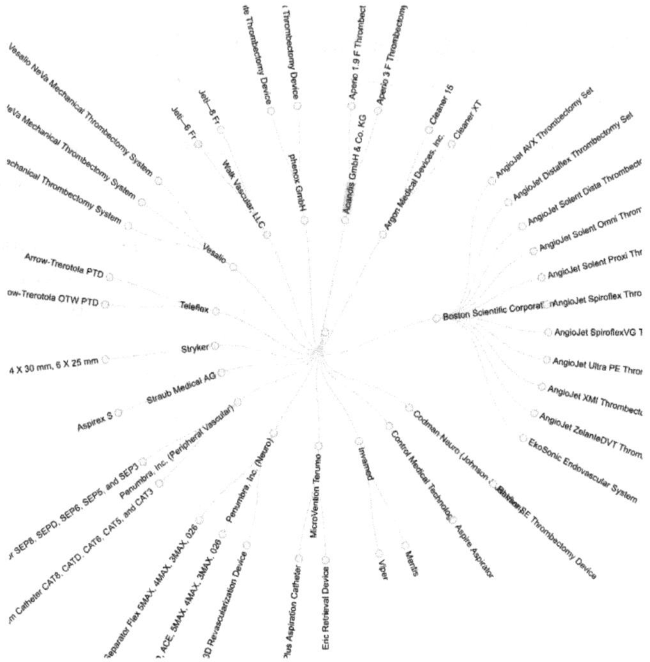

Directional Atherectomy
Devices

Directional or excisional atherectomy
Plaque is removed by cutting in one direction; captured in the nose cone or part of the catheter, then removed

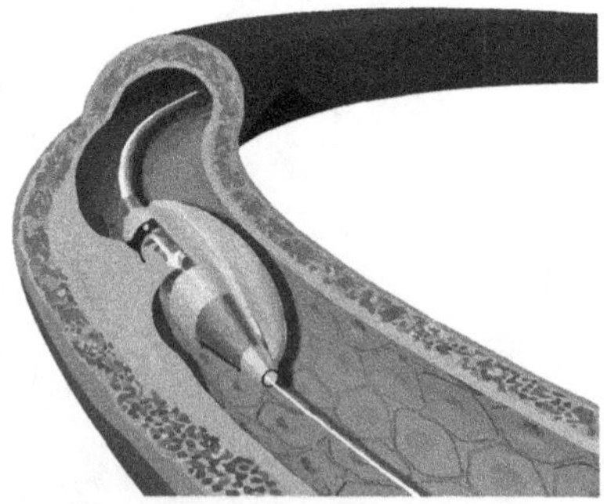

Examples: Turbo-Hawk and SilverHawk peripheral plaque excision systems (Medtronic)

Benefits:
Avoids barotrauma, potentially decreasing the risk of neointimal hyperplasia and dissection
Removes plaque without leaving a foreign body

Limitations:
Requires large sheath size
May cause distal embolization or perforation
Limited by tortuosity, calcification, and lesion length

Risks:
Death: 0.9%
Myocardial infarction: 1.3%
Target lesion revascularization: 11.8%
Major amputation: 1.4%

Rotational atherectomy

Rotational Atherectomy:

High-speed rotating burr with diamond-coated tips ablates plaque into small particles; cleared by blood flow

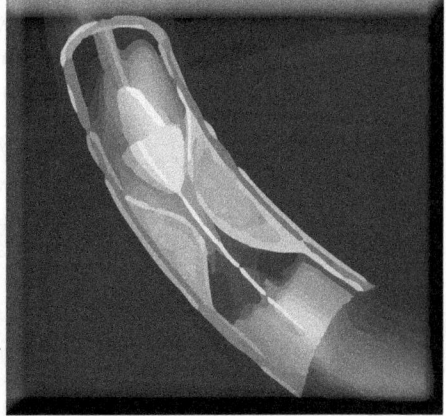

Examples: Rotablator rotational atherectomy system (Boston Scientific)
Effectiveness: Heavily calcified lesions; reduces plaque without significant vessel wall injury or dissection
Potential Issues: Slow flow phenomenon, no reflow phenomenon, distal embolization, perforation, spasm, or dissection
Risks: Death (1%), myocardial infarction (1.2-1.3%), emergency CABG (1-2.5%)

Chocolate Balloon

Structure:
Braided shaft
Atraumatic tapered tip
Distal end with semi-compliant balloon
Nitinol constraining structure (CS) for fast deflation and uniform re-wrap

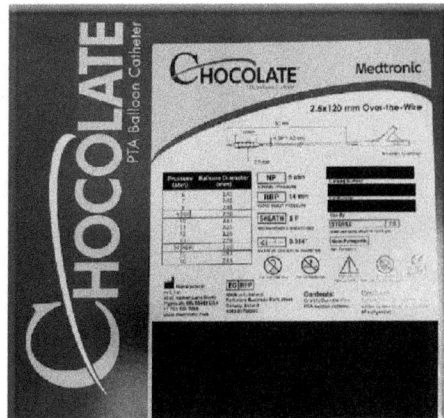

Compatibility:
0.014" and 0.018" systems
Compatible with 0.014" and 0.018" guidewires, respectively
Length: Overall catheter lengths range from 120-150 cm
Balloon Features:
Expands to known diameters at specific pressures
Available in multiple sizes
Contains two radiopaque markers for positioning

Shockwave Balloon

Shockwave balloon angioplasty catheter
Uses sonic pressure waves to break up calcium deposits in narrowed or blocked arteries
Advantages:
Minimally invasive
Less pain, shorter recovery time
Effective for calcified lesions
Low risk of complications
Disadvantages:
Newer procedure, less long-term safety data
More expensive
Not suitable for all patients
Overall: Safe and effective for calcified lesions, with the benefits of minimal invasiveness and low complications, but with considerations regarding cost and suitability for all patients.

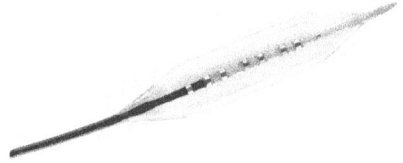

STENTS

What are the key features of the following catheters:

Zilver Flex Stents

Zilver Flex Stent:
Made of nitinol, known for flexibility and durability
Type: Self-expanding, doesn't require an external balloon for expansion
Benefits:
Less traumatic to the vessel
Allows for more precise deployment
Usability: Relatively easy to insert
and deploy
Effectiveness:
The 5-year primary patency rate
for Zilver Flex stents in the iliac ar-
tery was 74%. The 5-year primary
patency rate for Zilver Flex stents
in the femoropopliteal artery
was 86%. The 5-year freedom
from major adverse limb events (MALE) for Zilver Flex stents was 81%.
The rate of stent thrombosis at 5 years for Zilver Flex stents was 2.4%.
Stents that were placed in the iliac artery had a higher rate of stent
thrombosis than stents that were placed in the femoropopliteal artery.

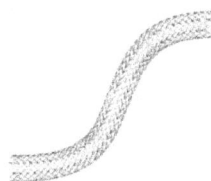

Viabhan Stent

Viabhan Stent

Lengths: Up to 25 cm, suitable for long or complex lesions
Design: Low profile, minimizing discomfort or pain post-procedure
Visibility: Radiopaque markers for easy imaging
Technology: Proven CBAS Heparin Surface technology to prevent blood
clots and restenosis
Material: Synthetic expand-
ed polytetrafluoroethylene
(ePTFE)
Coating: Heparin-coated
fabric to prevent blood clots
Variety: Available in differ-
ent sizes and lengths
Risk: Low, but potential
complications include:
Bleeding
Infection
Thrombosis
Restenosis
Effectiveness:
Primary patency rates are typically in the range of 60-70% at 5 years.
Secondary patency rates are typically in the range of 80-90% at 5 years.
Restenosis rates are typically in the range of 20-30% at 5 years.

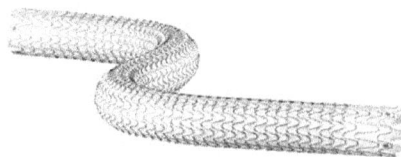

Supera stent

3 key features:
High compression resistance. Once deployed, takes shape (round open lumen) even if calcium.
Low chronic outward force.
Hence deployed 1:1
High flexibility and fracture resistance.

Effectiveness: Primary patency rate at 3 years: 94%. Freedom from target lesion revascularization (TLR) at 3 years: 92%. Restenosis rate at 3 years: 6%.

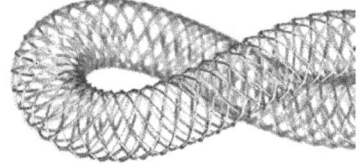

Advanta V12 stents

Features:
PTFE film covering technology.
316L stainless steel struts.
Low profile design.
Multiple FDA approved indications for use.
Radiopaque markers.

Effectiveness:
Primary patency rate at five years: 96.4%.
Freedom from target lesion revascularization (TLR) at five years: 93.5%. Restenosis rate at five years: 7.2%.

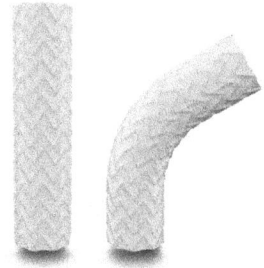

Zilver PTX

Paclitaxel-coated stent.
The Zilver PTX stent is coated with paclitaxel
Nitinol stent.
Self-expanding stent.
Long lengths and diameters.
Radiopaque markers.

Effectiveness:
Primary patency rate at 5 years: 75.2%. Freedom from target lesion revascularization (TLR) at 5 years: 64.8%. Restenosis rate at 5 years: 24.8%.

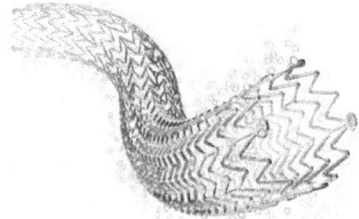

Index

REFERENCES AND FURTHER READING

Vascular and Endovascular Surgery: A Companion to Specialist Surgical Practice 2023
Editors: Ian Loftus MD FRCS, Robert J. Hinchliffe MD FRCS
Publisher: Elsevier
ISBN-10: 070208462X
This text serves as an essential companion to specialists seeking an in-depth understanding of vascular and endovascular surgery. With its comprehensive and up-to-date approach, this 7th edition provides invaluable insights into the field.

Endovascular Skills: Guidewire and Catheter Skills for Endovascular Surgery, Fourth Edition 2019
Editors: Peter A. Schneider
Publisher: CRC Press
ISBN-10: 1482217376
A definitive guide that delves deep into the techniques and skills essential for endovascular surgery. It stands as an invaluable resource for both budding and seasoned surgeons aiming to hone their craft and expand their toolkit.

Vascular and Endovascular Surgery at a Glance 2014
Authors: Morgan McMonagle, Matthew Stephenson
Publisher: Wiley-Blackwell
Edition: 1st
ISBN-10: 1118496035
Dimensions: 21.72 x 0.81 x 28.07 cm
A concise yet comprehensive overview of vascular and endovascular surgery presented in an illustrative format. It's designed to provide quick insights, making it an essential read for those wanting a rapid yet thorough understanding of the domain.

Rutherford's Vascular Surgery and Endovascular Therapy, 9th Edition 2018
Authors: Anton N Sidawy, Bruce A Perler
Publisher: Elsevier
ASIN: B07BYT4S6C
Rutherford's Vascular Surgery and Endovascular Therapy stands as a seminal text in the field of vascular surgery. This 9th edition, authored by leading experts Anton N Sidawy and Bruce A Perler, continues to uphold the esteemed legacy of the series. With its comprehensive coverage of both traditional and endovascular techniques, the book serves as a fundamental guide for vascular surgeons, interventionalists, and trainees.